DISC

CHILDREN with TRAUMATIC BRAIN INJURY

CHILDREN with TRAUMATIC BRAIN INJURY

A Parents' Guide

Edited by Lisa Schoenbrodt, Ed.D., CCC-SLP

Woodbine House ■ 2001

© 2001 Woodbine House

All rights reserved. Published in the United States of America by Woodbine
House, 6510 Bells Mill Road, Bethesda, MD 20817-1636. 800-843-7323.
http://www.woodbinehouse.com

Cover Illustration: Charlotte Fremaux

Figure 1 in Chapter 1 reprinted from *Know Your Brain,* NIH Publication No.
92-3440-a (National Institute of Neurological Disorders and Stroke, 1992).

Library of Congress Cataloging-in-Publication Data

Children with traumatic brain injury: a parents' guide / edited by Lisa Schoenbrodt
    p. cm.
    Includes bibliographical references and index.
    ISBN 0-933149-99-9 (pbk.)
        1.Brain-damaged children—Rehabilitation. 2. Brain—Wounds and injuries—
Patients—Rehabilitation. 3. Brain damage—Complications. I. Schoenbrodt, Lisa,
1961-

RJ496.B7 C49 2001
618.92'8043—dc21

                                                                    2001017732

Manufactured in the United States of America

10   9   8   7   6   5   4   3   2   1

TABLE

OF

CONTENTS

ACKNOWLEDGEMENTS

There were many people who were involved throughout the development and completion of this book. First, each chapter author is an expert in his or her discipline. Each of them took a great deal of time to pack as much information as possible into their chapters. I am grateful for their time, effort, attention to detail, and speedy responses to my constant deluge of e-mails and phone calls. One author I particularly want to acknowledge is Joan Carney, who helped tremendously with facilitating the transfer of information to and from chapter authors, and who provided a constant source of support—thank you.

I also wish to acknowledge Susan Stokes at Woodbine House for her constant support of the project and for always being so flexible and available in the editing process. In addition, I would like to thank Nancy Gray, who compiled the Glossary and Resource Guide. I would also like to acknowledge several of my colleagues who helped with proofing and revising throughout this project: Lura Vogelman, Gerry Simon, Bernandine Kremer, Jacqueline Gesell, Libby Kumin, Romayne Smith, and anyone else I forgot. Finally, I would like to thank my parents, Margaret and Fred Schoenbrodt, my husband, Scott, and my children, David Karl, Matthew Scott, and Amy Elizabeth Myers, who were, as always, forever patient and always supportive during this project.

One more important thank you is to all the families who provided parent statements and photographs for the book. Your firsthand knowledge is what lends credence to this book. It is to them and to all children and families whose lives have been altered by traumatic brain injury that this book is dedicated.

INTRODUCTION

Lisa Schoenbrodt, Ed.D., CCC-SLP

The very words that make up the term "traumatic brain injury" indicate that something deeply upsetting has occurred. Webster's Dictionary defines trauma as "a severe wound caused by a sudden physical injury; an emotional shock causing lasting and substantial damage to a person's psychological development." In fact, a traumatic brain injury (TBI) can mean all that and more, not only to the individual who had the injury, but to the family as well.

In my experience, families of children with traumatic brain injury are in a category all their own. For the most part, their children were "normal," healthy children who were on the path of life and all it has to offer. Suddenly, the trauma hit, and life as it once was is no longer. Not only are you spending every minute, day and night, in the hospital with your child, but you are also flooded with unfamiliar medical jargon. Once you have mastered the medical language and your child is ready to return to school, a new flood of terminology is quickly released—from the educational system.

Your child will be as unique in his pattern of recovery as he is as an individual. You may talk to other parents whose child shows none of the same symptoms as your child and had a completely different recovery pattern. For instance, your child may have accompanying physical deficits, along with problems thinking and remembering, whereas another family's child may have some problems remembering words and learning new information, and have a lot of emotional stress as a result. This variability is very typical of traumatic brain injury and sometimes very frustrating for parents.

Some of this variability has to do with your child's age when he was injured, as well as the nature of the injury itself. In this book, we wanted to include information on children with TBI of *all* ages—from birth through high school age—so, some of the information may be more or less relevant to your child, depending on his age. And, although we focus primarily on closed head injuries (as opposed to injuries in which something such as a bullet penetrates the skull), there are many different areas of the brain that can be injured, to different degrees, and with different effects.

It is my hope that this book will help you to gain a better understanding of most, but maybe not all, of the issues you will face on the journey with your child through recovery. The information you learn will be increasingly important as your child ventures back out into the community.

You will find that many people who interact with your child—friends, teachers, specialists, administrators, and others—aren't as familiar with TBI as you soon will be. Often you may find yourself in the position of educating others about TBI and how it has affected your child.

In order to introduce you to the major issues you will face, I have included chapters by professionals who are experts in their various disciplines. These chapters address the major problem areas you may face, including evaluation, treatment, advocacy, and legal issues. This is not to say that all children will exhibit the same level of complications that are described in each chapter. (Your child may also have some deficits that are not described in this book, simply because the variability of issues is so large.) The chapter authors describe the range of issues that most commonly occur, and try to include as many examples as possible to help make terminology less foreign. Most chapters include a portion of a case study about "Johnny," who represents a composite of many different children with TBI and was created to highlight what each of us thought to be more "typical" issues facing children with TBI. I hope that this example will help you to understand the content in each chapter and to relate it to what you and your child may be experiencing.

Also included throughout the book are passages and statements made by real-life parents of children who have and may continue to have the same experiences you are having. Their comments are provided to give you some perspective on what is presented in each chapter. They also may help substantiate what you may be feeling.

In addition, you will notice that there is a glossary of terminology and resource lists of reading materials and organizations you may wish to contact for more information and for support services. I strongly urge you to contact your local, state, and national organizations for support groups and updates to legislation regarding traumatic brain injury. Many parents I have spoken with were grateful to be able to contact groups who understood about their needs and could link them with support groups or other families who shared their experiences.

You will also note that throughout the book, the personal pronouns "he" and "she" are used alternately by chapter to refer to children with traumatic brain injury. In addition, the terminology "traumatic brain injury" or "TBI" is used consistently throughout the book. You may see this same condition referred to elsewhere as "acquired brain injury," "head injury," or "brain injury." I chose to use the term "traumatic brain injury" because it is the one that is most often used by medical and special education professionals. In addition, it is the terminology that is used in the federal Individuals with Disabilities Education Act (IDEA) in listing specific disabilities that can qualify a student for special educational assistance.

When you have finished this book, I hope you will find that you have enough information to get you and your child started down the road to rehabilitation. This is a road that will no doubt be filled with bumps and turns, but one that you and your family do not have to travel alone. This book should help you discover ways to navigate the medical and educational systems and to find additional information and support for you and your child. Everyone involved with the compilation of this book wishes you patience and hope for the future.

1
WHAT IS TRAUMATIC BRAIN INJURY?

James R. Christensen, M.D.

Your child has had a traumatic brain injury (TBI). What does this mean? Perhaps you have previously known someone who had a TBI, or have seen an actor on television or video portraying someone who has had a brain injury. You are probably asking yourself, "Will my child turn out like that?"

Although certain types of problems are common in children with TBI, each injury is unique, and consequently, each child's outcome is also unique. It is important to first understand head injury in general, and then your child's head injury in particular.

■ What Is Traumatic Brain Injury?

When you are first told that your child has had a traumatic brain injury, you may have trouble understanding what this means. After all, the brain is not visible like other body parts, and the function of the brain is mysterious to most of us. This often makes it difficult to understand and appreciate what has happened.

To determine whether someone has had a TBI, we rely on clinical evidence (observations) that the brain is not functioning properly.

For example, there may be a period of loss of consciousness, weakness in one part of the body, or difficulty in thinking or speaking. When this type of evidence occurs in association with an injury to the head, we call this a Traumatic Brain Injury (TBI)—meaning that the brain has been injured by *traumatic* or physical forces. A TBI is not progressive. That is, the damage to the brain does not get worse over time. How the damage manifests itself, however, can change.

◾◾ Who Gets TBIs?

Unfortunately, as you know, no one is immune from the risk of having a TBI. In fact, you may be asking yourself, "Why should I bother

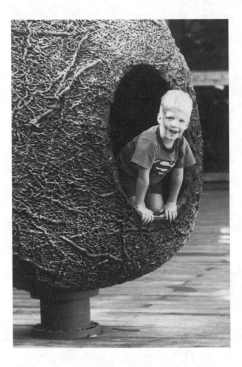

reading this section, since my child has already had an injury?" The short answer is that you need to understand who gets head injuries and why so that you can prevent future head injuries for you and your child. It is important to think of head injuries as events that can be modified or prevented, instead of thinking of them as unavoidable accidents. While some head injuries *may* be unavoidable, we can only prevent things over which we take some control.

One of the highest risk factors for sustaining a TBI is having had one before. As you will read in future chapters, people with TBIs often have problems in thinking abilities and impulse control, which can result in unsafe behavior. This places them at higher risk for being in harm's way yet again. It is vital to be aware of this risk and to take steps to prevent yet another TBI.

We know a great deal about who gets TBIs, when and why. There are two peaks in incidence related to age—the first in the late teen and early adult years, and the second in the elderly. Boys are twice as likely as girls to sustain a TBI. A shocking statistic is that, by age 16, boys in the U.S. have a 4 percent chance, and girls a 2.5 percent chance, of sustaining a TBI (ranging in severity from mild to very severe). In other words, about 4 out of every 100 boys and 2.5 out of every 100 girls have a traumatic brain injury by age 16.

Children from families with lower socioeconomic status are more likely to have TBIs. This is largely related to:

1. decreased access to preventative measures (for example, bicycle helmets), and
2. lack of safe play areas.

Certain behaviors also increase the risk for TBI. In particular, using alcohol or drugs are high risk behaviors for TBI. Children with problems such as attention-deficit/hyperactivity disorder (AD/HD) are also at much higher risk for injury. This is because they are more likely to engage in risky physical behavior, act impulsively, or overlook possible danger due to inattentiveness.

As you can imagine, common causes of TBIs vary with the age of the child. Also, different causes of injury can result in different injuries and severity of injury. Infants and toddlers most often sustain injuries related to falls, and, unfortunately, child abuse. As children become more independent and begin to play outside, run, and ride bicycles, injuries occur in these settings. The majority of head injuries at this age (roughly from age 5-12) are from falls, but these tend to be milder head injuries. Most *severe* brain injuries in this age group occur when motorized vehicles hit children who are walking or riding bicycles. In adolescence, too, automobile crashes are responsible for the majority of severe brain injuries. But in this age group, the child is most likely either to be driving or to be a passenger in the car.

▪▪ A Simple Review of the Brain

To understand how traumatic brain injury affects the brain, it is essential to first understand some basics about the structure and function of the brain.

The Central Nervous System (CNS) is made up of the brain and the spinal cord. While the spinal cord is also susceptible to trauma, the implications of a spinal cord injury are very different from those of a brain injury, and consequently will not be addressed here.

The brain controls or *mediates* the function of the entire body. It is responsible for all of the things we think and do. Just as importantly, it is also responsible for keeping us from doing the things we shouldn't do. It is responsible for our ability to sense things around us; to think, plan, and organize; to communicate through speech and gestures; to move the body and all of its parts, doing things for ourselves, and moving ourselves from one place to another. It controls basic bodily functions, such as our breathing, blood pressure, heart rate, and bowel and bladder function. And it is responsible for our personality, our emotions, and the ability to control them and our behavior. It makes us who we are.

The brain is the consistency of gelatin and is housed within the skull. Between the skull and the surface of the brain are three membranes collectively called the *meninges:*
1. the dura mater (attached to the inner surface of the skull),
2. the arachnoid (the middle layer), and,
3. the pia mater (attached to the surface of the brain).

In the subarachnoid space (between the arachnoid and the pia) is a layer of watery fluid called cerebrospinal fluid (CSF), which acts as a cushion for the brain during movement. Inside the brain are spaces called ventricles. It is here that the CSF is made. The CSF then flows out through the ventricular system into the subarachnoid space, where it is eventually absorbed into the blood stream.

Parts of the Brain

You will hear people talking about the different parts of the brain and what these parts "do." The brain may be divided into three major parts: the forebrain, midbrain, and hindbrain. The forebrain is the portion of the brain that has become so highly developed and specialized in humans. It is made up of the cerebrum (cerebral hemispheres and the basal ganglia) and the diencephalon (thalamus and hypothalamus).

The Forebrain

The Cerebrum. There are two cerebral hemispheres—right and left—divided down the center by a deep fissure. The surface of the hemispheres is deeply fissured and grooved. The grooves are called sulci, and the ridges between the grooves are called gyri. The hemispheres are the seat of the highest skills of the brain, allowing us to think, communicate, and perform highly skilled, finely coordinated tasks.

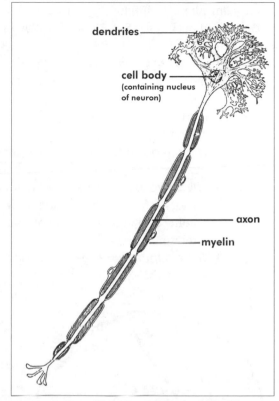

The outer "gray matter" portion of the cerebral hemispheres is called the cortex, and is where the cell bodies of the nerve cells (neurons) are located. Underneath the gray matter is the white matter. This area contains the axons, which are projections from the neurons. Through these axons, impulses travel to other parts of the brain and body to communicate with

Figure 1: *From "Know Your Brain," published by NIH, National Institute of Neurological Disorders and Strokes.*

other nerve cells or muscles. The axons are coated with an insulating substance called myelin (which is why they appear white). Myelin allows the nerves' messages to travel faster.

There is a dominant and a nondominant hemisphere. As a general rule, the dominant hemisphere controls verbal functions: speech and language, including reading and writing, and calculations. It usually also controls the dominant hand. The nondominant hemisphere is more involved with visual functions: copying, drawing, understanding things we see, visual memory, and rhythm. Since the left side of the brain controls the movement and interprets the sensation for the right side of the body (and vice versa), the left hemisphere is the dominant hemisphere for most people. (Even in left-handed people, the left hemisphere is still more likely to control speech and language function, even though the motor control of the left hand will be in the right hemisphere.)

Each hemisphere is subdivided into four lobes: frontal, temporal, parietal, and occipital. (See Figure 2.) Each lobe is involved in different functions:

- **The frontal lobes** assist in coordinated fine movement, the motor aspect of speech, executive function (thinking abilities that allow us to have goal-directed behavior), motivation, social skills, and certain parts of what we call personality.
- **The temporal lobes** are important for memory, receptive language, and musical awareness.
- **The parietal lobes** are important in the interpretation of sensory information (including high level skills such as reading and understanding of spatial relationships) and attention.
- **The occipital lobes** perceive and interpret visual stimuli seen by the eyes.

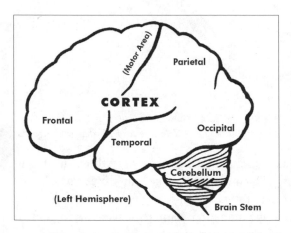

Figure 2: *This is a view of the brain from the side. It shows the four lobes of the cerebrum (frontal, temporal, parietal, and occipital), as well as the cerebellum and the brainstem. (Reprinted with the author's permission from Frances Bateson,* **The Brain Injury Guidebook***, The Brain Injury Association of Maryland.)*

The basal ganglia are areas located at the base of the cerebral hemispheres. They communicate back and forth with the hemispheres, helping with habitual movements and posture, and with certain cognitive abilities.

The Diencephalon. The last part of the forebrain is the diencephalon, made up of the thalamus and the hypothalamus. The thalamus is the "relay station" and distribution center for sensation from the body to the cortex. The hypothalamus is responsible for certain basic bodily functions such as the autonomic (involuntary) control over heart rate, body temperature, and fluid balance. It also has a role in emotional control.

The Midbrain and Hindbrain (Brainstem)

The cerebellum, part of the hindbrain, is located under the occipital lobes and connects to the rest of the brain by tracts, or bundles of nerve fibers, which enter the brainstem. The cerebellum is responsible for equilibrium and the coordination of voluntary muscle activity. It also plays a role in the modulation of muscle tone—the amount of tension, or resistance to movement, in a muscle.

The midbrain and the hindbrain (pons and medulla oblongata minus the cerebellum) are sometimes referred to collectively as the "brainstem." The brainstem connects to the diencephalon at the top end, and the spinal cord at the "tail end." The brainstem is responsible for basic bodily functions such as breathing and heart rate. Through the brainstem pass all of the pathways that run between the spinal cord and the brain. These pathways carry messages to the brain concerning sensation, and from the brain to the rest of the body to control movement and posture. Ten out of twelve of the cranial nerves also originate in and emerge from the brainstem. These nerves supply sensation and movement to the head and neck structures. Additionally, pathways that awaken and alert the entire brain originate in the brainstem. Abnormal function of these pathways can cause coma.

Of course, the above is a simplistic view of brain function. Many functions are less compartmentalized than the above scheme would suggest. That is, most areas of the brain rely heavily on the function of other parts of the brain in carrying out their "work."

A good example of how functions of different parts of the brain are related involves the frontal lobes' role in "executive function"—that is, in putting together what other parts of the brain are doing, and organizing this function into goal-directed behavior. The frontal lobes cannot do what they do without other parts of the brain doing their part. Additionally, the frontal lobes are not the exclusive location of this executive function. Another example of the distribution of function is the cerebellum. Studies are finding that besides having a role in the functions described above, the cerebellum also plays a role in behavior and cognition. These are some of the reasons it is difficult to predict how a particular brain injury will affect a particular child. Your child's physician will be able to tell you how the function of the injured area of the brain may be affected in general, but will be unable to predict specific effects with absolute certainty.

■■ What Happens to the Brain When It's Injured?

When the head is hit by something, or the head is abruptly stopped or sped up, physical forces and energy are transferred to the head and brain, and can result in injury.

You may hear several different terms to describe this injury. Although they sound different, they are used interchangeably by some professionals. This can lead to some confusion. It is not uncommon for families to say, "He didn't have a brain injury. I was told he had a head injury." Let's go over some definitions:

Head Injury refers to a traumatic injury to the head, and could result in a fracture to a bone in the skull or face, or bruises or cuts to the head and face. A head injury may or may not include an injury to the brain.

A *Closed Head Injury (CHI)* is one in which there is no penetration or opening from the outside through the dura (the tough membrane inside the skull that covers the brain). This is the most common kind of head injury, and is the type of head injury that we will be talking about in this book, unless otherwise specified.

In contrast, an *Open Head Injury* is one in which there is an opening or penetration from the outside through the skull and dura (as with a gunshot wound).

The term *Traumatic Brain Injury (TBI)* means that there is evidence of brain involvement associated with the head injury. This brain involvement is demonstrated by:

1. altered level of consciousness (for example, drowsiness, lethargy, confusion, coma); or
2. neurologic signs, such as localized weakness, that indicate that part of the brain has been injured.

The term traumatic brain injury (TBI) is obviously the more specific one to use when the brain is involved. However, specifying whether there was a closed versus open head injury is also important. This is because it clarifies the type of TBI that is likely to be associated with the head injury. The TBI associated with a closed head injury is more likely

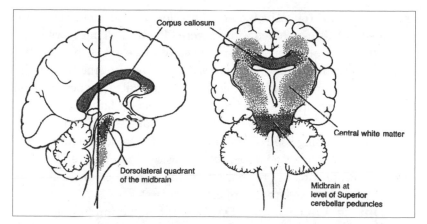

Figure 3: *Brain regions particularly involved by diffuse axonal injury (DAI). Reprinted from S.H. Auerbach, "Neuroanatomical Correlates of Attention and Memory Disorders in Traumatic Brain Injury: An Application of Neurobehavioral Subtypes,"* Journal of Head Trauma Rehabilitation, *1(3), 4; reprinted by permission of Aspen Publishers, Inc. ©1986.)*

to be diffuse—meaning it affects multiple areas throughout the brain. The TBI associated with an open head injury is more likely to be focal—meaning it affects a localized area of the brain. To be perfectly clear when describing your child's injury, it is often best to say "Closed (or Open) Head Injury with (or without) Traumatic Brain Injury."

Immediate Injuries

The injuries that are caused by trauma are divided into "immediate" and "delayed" injuries. Immediate injuries are those that occur immediately at the time of the injury, and are due to the physical forces injuring or disrupting parts of the brain. There are two main types of immediate injuries: contusions and diffuse axonal injury (DAI).

Contusions. Contusions are bruises. When an area of the brain is bruised, some of the cells in that area of the brain can be totally disrupted or broken apart, and consequently die. Other cells can be partially injured or stunned, and therefore unable to function for a period of time (seconds to weeks).

Where contusions are located depends on the circumstances of the injury. If a stationary head is hit with an object (for example, struck with a hammer), the contusion will be in the cortex at the point of contact, and there will possibly be another bruise on the opposite side of the brain (180 degrees from the other bruise). These are often called "coup" (hit) and "contrecoup" (opposite the hit) contusions. This is *not* how contusions are typically distributed with a severe Closed Head Injury with TBI.

With a severe injury, there is usually more speed and energy involved in the injury, and the head is often moving at the time of the accident. The contusions with this type of injury usually occur as the head is suddenly stopped, and then a split second later, the brain is suddenly stopped by hitting against the inside of the skull. This results in the brain crushing itself on prominent rough parts of the inner table (surface) of the skull. Consequently, contusions with severe TBIs tend to occur in areas of the frontal lobes, the temporal lobes, and the brainstem. (Refer back to Figure 2.)

Diffuse Axonal Injury (DAI). As the name implies, a diffuse axonal injury is an injury to the axons (the extensions of the neurons or nerve cells), which occurs diffusely throughout the brain (not in one small localized area). This injury is also referred to as a *shearing injury*. Because axons often extend long distances in the brain, they are particularly vulnerable to twisting movements of the brain at the time of the injury. As the head and brain are accelerated and spun violently and then brought to a quick stop, the brain is twisting on itself. This can stretch the axons so far that they are physically pulled apart. This results in immediate loss of function of that neuron, and in its death. As with contusions, certain parts of the brain are more vulnerable to DAI, as shown in Figure 3.

Delayed Injuries

Unfortunately, once the accident has taken place, the immediate injuries have already occurred and cannot be modified. Fortunately, the secondary or "delayed" injuries are yet to occur. This makes it vital to try to prevent or minimize secondary injuries, as well as to optimize your child's health, when he is first hospitalized. There are several types of secondary or delayed injuries that can occur, including bleeding (hemorrhages), herniation syndromes, edema, and damage from the neurotoxic cascade. Let's look at what these type of injuries are.

Bleeding. Bleeding can occur anywhere inside the head as a result of blood vessels being torn or disrupted. This bleeding can occur:

- within the brain itself (intraparenchymal or intracerebral hemorrhage),
- into the ventricles (intraventricular hemorrhage), or
- into the spaces surrounding the brain:

- between the skull and the dura
  (epidural hematoma),
- under the dura (subdural hematoma), or
- under the arachnoid layer of the meninges,
  into the cerebrospinal fluid (subarachnoid
  hemorrhage).

The consequences of this bleeding depend on the amount of blood, how fast it accumulates, and the location. Wherever the blood is located, it will take up space. This can be a problem, since the brain is within a closed, rigid space (except in infants with open sutures, or if a large part of the skull is missing). Because this space is usually filled with the brain, the cerebrospinal fluid, and the blood within the blood vessels, any additional blood that occupies space will mean one of two things: something else has to give, or there will be increased pressure within that space.

If a hemorrhage or other space-occupying lesion occurs very slowly, the brain will have time to adjust. It can squeeze some fluid out of the brain or the cerebrospinal fluid space, or decrease the amount of blood in the blood vessels, and thus make room for the extra blood. However, if a hemorrhage occurs very rapidly and occupies a significant amount of space, it will place the brain under increased pressure. If there is increased pressure within the space inside the head (intracranial pressure, ICP), the circulation will have to adjust itself to ensure that there is still enough blood flow to the brain to keep it nourished. If the blood flow is not sufficient, this can result in a further injury to the brain due to lack of oxygenation and blood flow *(hypoxic ischemic injury)*.

Herniation Syndrome. If there is a localized mass or area of swelling that pushes on and deforms the brain, it may result in a herniation syndrome. This occurs when the brain tries to squeeze itself into another space within the intracranial space, resulting in high pressure on focal areas of the brain and its blood vessels. This can lead to further localized brain injury and stroke.

Edema. Edema or swelling of the brain can also occur after head trauma, and can result in increased intracranial pressure (ICP). The swelling can be localized in an area of contusion, or it can be diffuse. It is more common in children than in adults. It can cause the same type of complications as bleeding.

For most severe injuries, an intracranial pressure monitor will be placed temporarily. This is a device that is surgically implanted

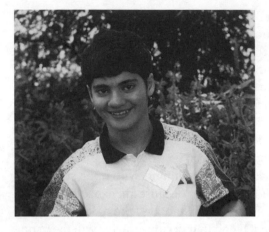

inside the head and sends information about internal pressures to a monitor. This technology has revolutionized the care of patients with TBI. It allows the medical and surgical staff to recognize problems early, to use appropriate medications and interventions to control ICP, and to recognize when there may be a problem that might be improved with surgery. This helps a great deal in preventing secondary injuries.

Damage from Neurotoxic Cascade. In recent years, we have also begun to study the role of the neurotoxic cascade in TBI. This neurotoxic cascade is a chain of events in the metabolism of the neurons that is set in motion by an insult (in this case, by trauma), and results in the further injury and possible death of the neuron. There is currently much investigation underway, searching for ways to modify or prevent the secondary injuries occurring as a result of this process.

Determining How and Where Your Child's Brain Is Injured

The ability to take pictures of the brain has revolutionized the care of children with TBI. Two types of "pictures" are generally taken in determining the type and location of your child's brain injury: 1) CT (computerized tomography) scans, and 2) MRIs (magnetic resonance imaging). Both of these techniques show cross sections of the brain.

Initially, when your child is acutely ill, CT scans will be done. This is because they can be done very quickly. They also show, with very high accuracy, injuries that will respond to medical and surgical interventions. They show most of the types of injuries discussed above, although DAI may not show up well.

MRIs show much greater detail of the brain, but take much longer to do. Consequently, they are usually done later, to document the permanent injuries in more detail. They are much more sensitive to DAI than CT scans.

Neither of these tests causes any pain. Your child's head must remain still during image-taking, however, so sedation is sometimes needed. (This is more likely during an MRI.) CT has the disadvantage of exposure to X-rays, but the amount of radiation used today is very small. MRIs do not entail any radiation exposure, but use harmless magnetic fields instead.

It is important to remember that the above techniques give a picture of the structure of the brain, but do not show function. Also, they do not have the resolution to show injury at the microscopic or cellular level. Consequently, they will give a general picture of the areas of the brain that are seriously injured, but have limitations. How your child is actually functioning often tells more about the brain injury than the pictures can.

▪▪ How Is the Severity of Injury Classified?

Parents are understandably anxious to learn what their child's chances are for a good recovery. And in fact, there are a variety of methods of predicting outcome based on different indicators of severity of injury. While none of these predict with 100 percent certainty, they do provide a framework for identifying who is at high or low risk for long-term complications related to their injury. This can help in planning your child's care and in deciding how to use your family's resources.

The severity of a brain injury is usually expressed as Mild, Moderate, or Severe. The three major methods of assessing severity are:
1. using the Glasgow Coma Scale,
2. observing the length of coma, and
3. observing the length of posttraumatic amnesia.
These three major predictors of severity reflect the depth and duration of neurologic dysfunction. That is, they offer an indication of how long, and to what degree, function is and will be abnormal.

The Glasgow Coma Scale

The Glasgow Coma Scale (GCS) is a scale developed by neurosurgeons. It is used in the intensive care setting, to follow patients in an objective way, to detect improvement or deterioration. It consists of three subtests: best eye, verbal, and motor response. The total possible score ranges from 3 (no response) to 15 (alert and oriented). To predict long-term outcome, either the initial or the first GCS after resuscitation is the one most commonly used.

Severity is rated according to the following scores:
- Mild—GCS 13-15;
- Moderate—GCS 9-12;
- Severe—GCS 3-8.

To give you an idea of what these scores correlate with, most people begin to open their eyes spontaneously at a GCS of 8-9.

:: GLASGOW COMA SCALE

ACTIVITY	BEST RESPONSE
Eye Opening	
Spontaneous	4
To speech	3
To pain	2
None	1
Verbal	
Oriented	5
Confused	4
Inappropriate words	3
Nonspecific sounds	2
None	1
Motor	
Follows commands	6
Localizes pain	5
Withdraws to pain	4
Abnormal flexion [bending]	3
Abnormal extension [straightening]	2
None	1

Teasdale, G. & B. Jennet. "Assessment of Coma and Impaired Consciousness: A Practical Scale." Lancet 2:81-84, 1974.

Length of Coma

Whether or not your child is in coma, and how long he remains in coma, is one of the parameters that reflects the severity of brain injury. Unfortunately, there are multiple definitions of coma. Although everyone agrees that coma is a period of unresponsiveness or unconsciousness, not everyone agrees on the degree of responsiveness that indicates the end of coma.

In a neurosurgical setting, spontaneous eye opening is sometimes used as a marker for the end of coma. The problem in using this definition for children with very severe injuries is that everyone with a TBI will eventually begin to spontaneously open their eyes. However, a very small minority will not regain any further ability to interact with their environment. Because of this, in a rehabilitation setting, coma is most commonly considered to be over when the child begins to follow simple commands. This proves to the observer that some meaningful interaction with the environment has taken place—the child has understood a spoken or gestured command, and proven his understanding by responding as requested. Some experts disagree with using this as the end point of coma. However, when the duration of coma is defined this way, it has been shown to correlate to long-term outcome.

Research has found that six hours or more of coma indicates a severe TBI. However, the International Classification of Diseases classifies severity of TBI as follows:

- Mild TBI—less than one hour of coma (usually momentary loss of consciousness or none at all);
- Moderate TBI—1-24 hours of coma;
- Severe TBI—24 or more hours of coma.

Posttraumatic Amnesia

The third major predictor of severity is the length of Posttraumatic Amnesia (PTA). As the name implies, PTA is a period of amnesia or memory disturbance during the period after (*post*) the trauma. It is, however, much more than just a period of memory disturbance. It is a period of confusion, disorientation, and sometimes agitation. During this period, your child will remember many old memories that were adequately stored in the brain prior to the accident. However, his ability to remember new information will be impaired. This leads to disorientation and the inability to remember things that are happening on a daily basis.

PTA provides a very good indication of how memory and cognition will be affected over the long term. It is often a more useful indicator of severity than is the duration of coma. This is especially true when there is no coma or short coma or when your child wakes up immediately after sedation is withdrawn in the intensive care unit, so the actual length of coma is not really known. Severity based on length of PTA is usually described in the following way:

PTA	Severity
<1 hour	Mild
1-24 hours	Moderate
1-7 days	Severe
>7 days	Very severe

Although you may be saying, no one "measured" PTA in your child, you can take comfort in the fact that retrospective analysis of PTA is rather accurate. When parents answer the question, "When did your child come back to himself?" their response is usually fairly close to the answer obtained by objectively measuring when PTA ends. Consequently, your child's physician can use this historical information concerning the approximate length of PTA, and it will be useful in classification of severity.

Which Indicators Are Most Important?

Sometimes children with TBI don't fit neatly into the above classification systems. This is because there are some variables that can change the classified severity from one category to another. For example, if a CT scan shows a focal injury, that injury, by definition, cannot be a mild injury, and the severity is either moderate or severe. Also, if the length of PTA reflects a higher degree of severity, it takes precedent over the other indicators. For example, a child who has a GCS of 14 when admitted to the hospital and momentary loss of consciousness at the scene of the accident would, on the basis of those parameters, have had a mild TBI. However, if that same child then has a period of PTA lasting seven days, he has had a very severe TBI, not a mild one. (The great weight or significance given to PTA can be appreciated by remembering that a severe injury can be defined as more than twenty-four hours of either coma *or* PTA.)

❚❚ What Do the Different Degrees of Severity Mean?

Once you know the degree of severity of your child's TBI, it will help steer him, your family, and his care providers in the right direction. Everyone involved in his care will have a good idea of what problems to look for and how closely to look for them, as well as what types of assistance and treatment will probably be needed. This is because we know the relative risk for certain problems for each of the different levels of severity of injury.

The general rules (and remember that all rules have exceptions) are that children and adolescents with mild TBI usually do very well, without long-term complications. Children with moderate TBI are at high risk for at least temporary (if not permanent) cognitive and behavioral problems. And children with severe TBI are at very high risk for permanent cognitive and behavioral problems, and motor (movement) problems as well.

Later chapters will discuss the cognitive, behavioral, and motor problems, so we will not go into them here in any great depth. To give you an idea, however, the cognitive deficits are usually not a general reduction of the child's abilities (as occurs in mental retardation, for example). Rather, there are specific symptoms that interfere with the child's ability to think and perform. Examples of these symptoms include difficulty remembering new things, maintaining attention, and organizing thoughts and actions, as well as a need for increased time to process and respond to information. The behavior problems are often a direct extension of these thinking problems. Other behavioral symptoms might include disinhibition—speaking or acting without thinking, resulting in socially unacceptable behavior; inability to initiate ideas, thoughts, or actions; and difficulty in controlling emotions. The motor problems can range from a slight slowing of reaction time to major difficulties moving and coordinating movement.

The Severe TBI Spectrum

You will note that there is a very wide range of injury classified as "severe." Given this wide range, it is useful to understand the differences between the "milder" and the "more severe" ends of the "severe TBI" spectrum. At the severe end of the spectrum (where the outcome is worse) are children who have an initial GCS of 3 or 4. Some studies have shown that virtually all children in this category have at least moderate disabilities that persist over time. In contrast, those with GSC 5-8 have a lesser degree of disability. In one study, 65 percent of people with this degree of severity had at least moderate disabilities. At the milder end of the spectrum, with short length of coma, PTA is often a more reliable predictor of outcome than is the duration of coma. At this end of the spectrum, with hours of coma and days or weeks of PTA, the long-term problems will be in the areas of cognition and behavior, as described above. When coma lasts for weeks, however, the cognitive deficits will be more severe (with some reduction of overall cognitive abilities), and the possibility of significant and lasting motor problems is more likely.

Unfortunately, there are rare children with extremely severe TBIs who do not make a significant recovery and remain in what is called a persistent vegetative state (PVS). In this state, the child opens his eyes and has normal wake-sleep cycles, but does not have any meaningful interactions with the environment. Fortunately, PVS is rare, thanks to today's acute trauma systems and rapid response and treatment.

■ What Other Factors Are Useful in Predicting Severity?

The Age Factor

What about age? Does it make a difference in how TBI affects a child? The answer is a qualified yes, but maybe not in the ways that you expect.

Compared to adults, children and adolescents are less likely to die from a brain injury. It also seems that children with mild TBI have fewer symptoms after their injuries than adults do. While there is a suggestion that they may also do better with moderate and severe TBIs, some studies argue that this is not the case.

We do know that adolescents seem to have the best outcome, and the younger the child at the time of the injury, the worse the outcome. For example, children who sustain their TBI under the age of nine years have a much higher incidence of reading disability. In a group of very severely injured children and adolescents (average length of coma=seven weeks), the correlation between length of coma and cognition differed according to the age when injured. For the same length of coma, those under ten years of age had a greater reduction in intelligence, compared with those over ten years of age.

This information may seem puzzling if you have heard the general rule of brain injury recovery: that the younger one is at the time of the injury, the better one does after the injury. Why does TBI *not* follow this rule? This general rule is based on the fact that the younger brain is more "plastic." It is not yet as "hardwired" as an older brain. Consequently, uninjured portions of the brain are able to take over function that normally would have occurred in another part (which has been injured, and therefore is unable to perform this function). If this is true in general of younger, more plastic brains, why isn't it true after TBI?

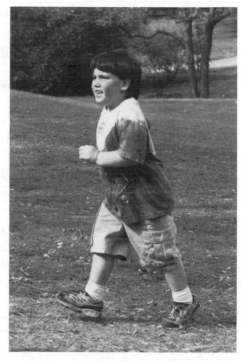

There are many possible explanations. Plasticity works best when a discrete area of the brain has been injured, and the rest of the brain is uninjured and can consequently function well enough to assume new functions and abilities. Since traumatic injury is so diffuse and widespread throughout the brain, the brain may be at a disadvantage in assuming these new functions. The younger brain may be more susceptible to the effects of trauma, due to its different physical and chemical properties. Also, remember that younger children often sustain different types of trauma than older children, which may result in differences in the primary injury. However, the following reason may be one of the most important. The types of specific neuropsychological deficits that result from TBI—memory, attention, and organizational difficulties—are extremely important in learning *new* things. If someone has already learned a great deal (like an older adolescent) before sustaining a TBI, he will look and function much better than a younger person with the same injury who still has many things to learn in life and school.

The Role of Secondary or Delayed Injury

Besides age, the presence or absence of secondary or delayed injury plays a major role in determining long-term outcome. For example, the outcome will be worse if there is a stroke or a hypoxic-ischemic injury (due to lack of oxygen and blood flow) in addition to the traumatic injury. Instead of recovering from one injury, the child has to recover from two separate injuries, both of which have their own long-term problems. See Chapter 2 for information about complications of, and recovery from, secondary injuries.

■■ Case Study

Now that we've reviewed some of the basics of traumatic brain injury, let's look at how a typical TBI might occur and the initial effects it might have on a child. The case study about Johnny, below, is written in the type of language you may see in medical reports written about your own child and uses terminology introduced in this chapter.

Johnny is a thirteen-year-old boy, who was in good health when he was injured five years ago. He was a B student, with some mild learning problems and mild attention deficits. He lived with his mother, father, older sister, and younger brother.

At age eight years, he sustained a Closed Head Injury with Severe Traumatic Brain Injury (TBI), when he was struck by a car while riding his bicycle. He was unconscious at the scene of the accident, and was taken by helicopter to the area trauma center. On arrival in the emergency department, he had a Glasgow Coma Scale (GCS) score of 5/15. He was intubated and placed on a ventilator. His initial CT scan showed contusions in both frontal lobes, and small punctate [pinpoint] hemorrhages in the deep white matter (left more than right), compatible with diffuse axonal injury (DAI), sometimes called shearing injury. His intracranial pressure (ICP) was normal. He had no significant associated injuries.

Johnny's initial course [hospital stay] was complicated by pneumonia, which responded to antibiotics. He did not have any deterioration of his neurologic status, and his follow-up CT scans remained stable. He was off the ventilator by day 5 of hospitalization. He began opening his eyes and was transferred from the intensive care unit (ICU) to the rehabilitation unit on day 6.

In the next chapter, we will use Johnny's story to introduce some of the medical issues that can be associated with TBI, as well as to talk about the rehabilitation of children with TBI. In later chapters, Johnny's story will be elaborated upon to help in clarifying and personalizing the many complex issues that arise when a child has a TBI.

▪▪ Conclusion

The early days after your child has sustained a TBI can be quite confusing and frightening for you and your family. It may seem as if an army of professionals is bustling around your child, trying to keep him alive and prevent possible complications. There might be so many tubes and wires coming out of your child's body that you wonder if he'll ever be able to do anything on his own again.

As you begin to grasp the severity of your child's injury, you may feel hopeful because his injury is considered less severe, or saddened because his injury is more severe. Regardless of the severity of a TBI, however, most children are able to recover quite a bit of their abilities during the months and years after the injury. However, nobody can say with any certainty how well your child will recover until he begins to awaken and make progress.

As a parent, the best thing you can do for your child right now is to hope for the best and to do today what needs to be done today. Help your child to stay as healthy and to function as well as he can, and most importantly, give him all the support and love you can.

▪▪ Parent Statements

At first my husband and I were just so glad that our daughter survived her car accident. We had no idea of the long-term implications of her brain injury. We are just starting to realize that she has changed forever and that our lives will never be the same.

🙐🙐

Our daughter has given us awareness of how precious life is.

🙐🙐

I prayed to have him live. I didn't know what I was asking. I think I would have done it again.

🙐🙐

When I got to the emergency room and this man with a badge that said "Hospital Chaplain" came out to meet me, I feared the worst.

❧

I don't think I'll ever use the words "I was in shock" lightly again. It was the weirdest feeling to just kind of step outside of myself and watch how I was thinking and reacting to what was happening to Bruce without really feeling any emotional connection to what was happening. I didn't realize that I was in shock at the time, though, and just kind of wondered what was wrong with me, that I could be so cool about the whole thing. My husband's reaction was totally different. He cried right off the bat.

❧

I never really thought about how the human brain worked before. It's just something you kind of take for granted. There are so many different parts that need to work together for your brain to function "normally," and so many ways that function can be disrupted.

❧

For the longest time, I was stuck on the thought that this was something I could have prevented somehow. If only I'd left work five minutes earlier that day, or taken a different route, or stopped at 7-11 for a snack…. But you can't keep beating yourself over the head with the "if only's." None of us would ever have chosen to do (or not do) what we did if we could have predicted the results.

❧

You can only take in so much information when you're feeling shocked and overwhelmed. I just wanted to hear that Justin would be OK, not a bunch of technical jargon.

❧

You reach a point where you want to understand what happened and why, and to understand your child's prognosis. I think we all reach that point at different times, and nobody should try to rush you.

REHABILITATION
AND MEDICAL
CONCERNS

James R. Christensen, M.D.

■ Rehabilitation

What Is Rehabilitation?

What *is* rehabilitation? When does it start? How long does it last? What does it do? Will it really help? These are some of the questions that are usually going through parents' minds, both early and late after the injury.

Technically, "rehabilitation" is the process of restoring abilities that someone used to have, but lost, due to injury or illness. This is in contrast to "habilitation," which aims to help someone acquire abilities they never had.

Rehabilitation is a goal-directed process. Its goals are to optimize your child's health and functional abilities. FUNCTION, FUNCTION, FUNCTION! That's what rehabilitation should be about. It should help your child function better, doing things for herself, at home, in school, and in social settings with peers.

Because every traumatic brain injury is unique, your child's rehabilitation plan will be individualized to meet her unique needs. It

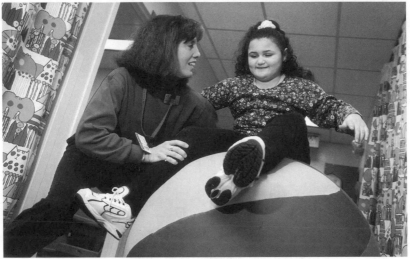

(Photo by Keith Weller.)

will, however, be similar to the plans for children with similar impairments and disabilities following TBI. That makes it possible to describe what the rehabilitation process will be like in general terms.

When Does Rehabilitation Begin?

It is generally accepted that the rehabilitation process should begin as soon as possible after the injury. In the past, rehabilitation did not begin until the patient was very medically stable and the acute medical stay was completed. Today rehabilitation begins in the intensive care unit (ICU), and continues as long as needed.

Obviously, the goals for a child in coma in an ICU are very different from the goals for a child with a mild TBI associated with some irritability and minor memory problems. And in fact, there are different stages of the rehabilitation process, with different objectives and goals.

For someone in coma who cannot participate in her own rehabilitation, there are two goals of rehabilitation in the early stages. First, doctors, nurses, and therapists will try to prevent complications that will prevent or retard recovery. For example, they will guard against muscle contracture that can limit movement or range of motion of joints. Second, the medical team will make certain that your child is in optimal health. For instance, they will treat infections, prevent excess weight loss through appropriate nutrition, and prevent bed sores.

As your child becomes more responsive and interactive, she will be able to actively cooperate and work toward rehabilitation goals.

How Does Rehabilitation Work?

During the recovery period, your child's brain is healing itself. Parts of the brain may have been so injured that they were not able to function properly for a period of time, but may eventually recover in days or weeks. Other parts of the brain, as discussed in Chapter 1, may have been permanently injured and the brain cells may have died. When this happens, the brain can accommodate for some of the changes due to a certain amount of "plasticity." It can learn to do some things that were previously done in the injured part of the brain. It may, however, never do them in the same manner or as efficiently as before. And there are some things that the brain may not be able to relearn.

If, during the recovery phase, part of the brain that has not been "working" properly starts to resume its previous function, recovery will occur rapidly. If, on the other hand, the brain needs to relearn certain functions, progress will proceed more slowly.

Given that the brain will be able to relearn some things and not others, it makes sense to take a two-pronged approach to the rehabilitation process. First, efforts should be made to help your child **relearn** to do things she can no longer do, as well as she can relearn those skills or functions. Second, your child should simultaneously be working on taking advantage of her abilities, and learning to use these abilities to **compensate** for her inabilities. That is, she should be learning to solve problems or do things in a different way if old methods no longer work. For example, she might learn to use a "day planner" to compensate for memory problems.

Who Is on the Rehabilitation Team?

The center of the team, of course, is you and your child. In addition, a variety of rehabilitation professionals will work with your child to optimize her health and assist in her recovery. The exact make-up of the professionals on the team will be tailored to meet her needs. Early in the course of recovery, after a very severe TBI, some or all of the following professionals who specialize in the rehabilitation of children with TBI might be involved:

- Physicians
- Nurses

- Nutritionist or dietitian
- Psychologist (to evaluate thinking abilities, looking for strengths and weaknesses in abilities such as attention, memory, and organizational abilities, and also to look at emotional well-being, motivation, and adjustment)
- Speech-language pathologist (to work on optimizing communication, as discussed in Chapter 5)
- Educator (to find learning strategies that will optimize learning in the classroom and assist with school re-integration)
- Swallowing therapist (who might be a speech-language pathologist or occupational therapist)
- Occupational therapist (to help relearn how to use the hands and arms for feeding skills, grooming skills, and other activities of daily living)
- Physical therapist (to help regain mobility skills)
- Social worker (to help you and your child adjust and cope, and to help your family explore available resources such as insurance and other funding resources)
- Recreational therapist or child life specialist (to help with adjustment to hospitalization and to help learn new leisure skills, if necessary)

As your child continues to recover and her abilities and disabilities change, the team will change too. Generally, the team shrinks when the time comes to work on long-term issues.

How Are Goals for Rehabilitation Set?

To come up with the goals and strategies needed to help your child regain skills, the team above will evaluate your child's abilities and disabilities. This period of evaluation is often frustrating to families, because they want treatment, not evaluations. But, the professionals who are going to assist in this process need to know:

1. what works and what doesn't work (impairments),
2. what your child can do (abilities), and
3. what she cannot do (disabilities).

Although it is painful to have your child's impairments and disabilities pointed out, it is part of the rehabilitation process. But the process should not dwell on the disabilities. Instead, it should capitalize on your child's abilities. It is through these abilities that your child will learn to function as well as possible. For example, if your child can move one side of her body well and has good head and trunk control, we know that she should be able to use these abilities to learn to walk again, even if the other side of her body is weak.

After evaluations are completed, the team will jointly set major goals for your child's rehabilitation. In the beginning, if your child requires acute intense rehabiliation, she will receive many hours of therapy, probably at least three hours a day. Usually, there is an emphasis on speech and language, physical, and occupational therapy, but your child's treatment will be tailored to her specific needs.

While team members are working with your child on actively learning and relearning skills, they will also be recommending other ways to help her function as well as possible. For example, they will recommend **environmental modifications**—or adaptations to her surroundings. These modifications can be either physical or behavioral. For example, the physical environment might be modified so your child can be more independent while using a wheelchair. Items might be placed within reach instead of on a high shelf, or a new sink might be installed so that she can roll up to it and wash and groom herself. The environment could also be modified to promote improved behavior. For instance, if she is agitated and easily over-excited, stimulating sights and sounds in the environment would be reduced, while still allowing her to be as oriented as possible.

Team members will also prescribe **assistive devices** or **adaptive equipment,** to help your child function as well as possible. Adaptive equipment will be used for specific reasons and during specific parts of the recovery to:

1. assist in and promote the recovery process,
2. optimize your child's physical and psychological independence, energy efficiency, and safety, and
3. to prevent secondary problems (such as deformities of the arms and legs).

A good example of adaptive equipment is a memory journal to substitute for or augment memory and to improve orientation (knowledge of where she is, what time it is, etc.). Braces, wheelchairs, or other equipment to help with motor skills are other common examples.

How Long Does the Recovery Process Take?

The recovery process will occur over a long period of time. The fastest recovery occurs at the beginning, and then gradually slows down. As a general rule, most of the natural recovery will occur in the first year after the injury. However, subtle (but sometimes significant) changes can continue to occur for two to five years after the injury. Depending on your child's age, she will also continue to develop at the same time. Unfortunately, her development will be affected by any impairments caused by the TBI.

During the rapid stages of recovery, your child's treatment and therapeutic goals need to change rapidly, sometimes on a daily basis. This is one reason that the intensity of rehab services will be highest at the beginning of the recovery. There are also other reasons. To use an old adage, "an ounce of prevention is worth a pound of cure." Most importantly, rehab services can sometimes prevent secondary problems, meaning your child's treatment will require fewer resources and energy down the road. For instance, one study showed that patients who were referred to rehab earlier had shorter stays and did at least as well as patients with similar injuries who were referred later. Those referred late spent time correcting secondary problems that were interfering with their progress.

As your child's recovery slows down, the intensity of therapy will also decrease. However, as long as your child continues to make progress toward her goals, continuing rehab (at an appropriate intensity) can be justified.

Where Should My Child Go for Rehab?

As you may have noticed, up until now, I have avoided saying that your child should go to this setting or that setting, for this or that part of her rehabilitation. Since all children with TBI and their problems are unique, plans need to be tailored to fit each child's needs. Some will need intense coordinated multidisciplinary rehabilitation, and others will need evaluations, counseling, and/or monitoring, all depending on the child's specific needs. Also, there is great variation throughout the country as far as rehabilitation services available.

In some areas, obtaining rehabilitation services may mean first going to a far-away city, and then trying to find local outpatient services at home, after the intense portion of the rehabilitation is complete. In other areas, rehabilitation services cover the whole spectrum, making it possible to receive intense coordinated multidisciplinary rehabilitation within the rehabilitation hospital, the home and community, and/or within a comprehensive day program (an outpatient program where comprehensive rehab is available). In these systems, appropriate outpatient and home health services (such as speech and language, occupational, or physical therapy) are also available when the intensive coordinated portion of rehabilitation is complete. (This comprehensive type of rehabilitation system is referred to as a "coordinated rehabilitation continuum.")

I do not want to give the impression that the quality of rehabilitation services in areas without these coordinated systems is substandard. There are highly qualified rehabilitation professionals in all areas of the country. However, in areas with fewer resources, you are going to need to be more resourceful and proactive in your child's care.

The major advantage of a coordinated rehabilitation continuum is that it allows your child to receive rehab services in the most functional and "normal" setting that is medically and behaviorally appropriate. Your child doesn't really need to learn to function in a hospital, but certainly does need to learn to function at home and school. Consequently, it is much more relevant for your child and family to work on goals at home and in a school-like setting (either in school or in a day hospital structured as a school setting).

If your child has been very severely injured, she will most likely be in an inpatient rehabilitation hospital, once she is discharged from the acute care hospital. How long she stays in this setting will depend on resources within your area. If there are no sources of acute intense rehab outside of the hospital, then your child may stay in the rehabilitation hospital as long as intense coordinated services are needed. If, however, you have access to a continuum of care, your child may be discharged from the rehab hospital and begin to receive outpatient services as soon as you can meet her medical and behavioral needs safely within your home. There is, of course, no perfect plan that works for everyone. Not only do rehab plans have to meet your child's needs, but they also have to take into consideration factors such as your family's work schedules and resources.

Obviously, you are going to be making a lot of decisions, and working with a lot of different people. You will be part of a rehabilitation team, whose members will change over time, depending on your family's and your child's needs. Early on, especially if your child has been severely injured, the team will be large. The key is that all team members should work together with you and your child, in a coordinated fashion, toward goals that you all agree upon. They should not only provide the appropriate evaluations and therapy, but should also teach you how to help your child during the recovery period, and how to eventually become an advocate and "care manager" for your child.

Initially, someone on your rehab team will take on the role as your case manager, to help you understand and participate with the rehab process so that you and your child get the most out of it. He or she will also help you understand long-term issues, so that you can utilize your resources such as insurance wisely. As time passes, your child's rehab team will shrink, but may still contain multiple professionals who can help you through the different transitions your child will face as she grows, develops, and matures.

What about Long-Term Rehabilitation?

We have been talking mostly about early acute rehabilitation services, but what about the long term? Earlier we said that rehab continues as long as there are goals and progress toward those goals. That does not mean that over time you will no longer need the assistance of a team of brain injury professionals. It means that the focus changes. As you will see in later chapters, there are many long-term issues that you will need to be on top of—anticipating transitions, making them as smooth as possible, troubleshooting new problems that arise due to ongoing development. Dealing with these issues may require focused intermittent therapy—that is, short-term therapy designed to address a particular issue. However, you are more likely to require advice and occasional assistance when advocating in, and maneuvering through, different systems in the community and school. Consequently, your long-term rehab team may consist of a much smaller group, such as:

- **a physician** who can monitor your child for any secondary complications related to the brain injury and guide the entire rehabilitation process from a medical and rehabilitation perspective;
- **an educator** with expertise in both brain injury rehabilitation and the school systems to help your child obtain an optimal education;

- **a psychologist** who can help identify cognitive issues and provide counseling for behavioral issues; and
- **a social worker** to provide counseling or other assistance coping, as well as help locating financial assistance or other types of support.

So, Does Rehab Work?

We've talked a lot about what "will" and "should" be done for your child, but does it work? Yes, we know that the rehabilitation process works. However, as you can imagine, it is sometimes hard to pinpoint one particular intervention that makes a large difference. What we do know is that patients who are referred early to a rehabilitation hospital spend much less time in rehab than those who are referred later, and do just as well. We also know that if we compare groups of TBI patients with similar degrees of injury who have and have not had rehab, the rehabilitated group functions better, is more successful on the job, requires less daily assistance with their care, and lives more independently.

Even if rehab is not provided until late after the injury, improvements are still possible. When rehab is begun more than twelve months after the injury, gains can still be made in functioning, with improvements in employment, productivity, memory and organizational abilities, and independent living skills. It is clear from these population studies that something in the rehab process works—that it does help improve outcome.

Until recently, we have had to rely on population studies to prove that rehab works. However, now we have new research methods to assess brain function, including functional MRIs or invasive and noninvasive brain mapping techniques (which can determine what area of the cortex is responsible for certain abilities and functions). Through these techniques we are now able to see that therapeutic activities actually alter the cortical map of the brain, and, consequently, alter the recovery process of the brain itself.

Johnny's story illustrates some of the ways that a child with TBI might benefit from different intensities of rehabilitation:

> *On admission to the rehabilitation unit, Johnny was able to localize stimuli (trying to pull out his IVs and tubes). He could not talk or communicate his needs. He was fed through a nasogastric tube (NG tube), through his nose into his stomach.*

He was very weak, especially on the right side of his body, and was unable to roll or sit. He had begun receiving therapies in the ICU. Now, since he wasn't so sick, he could tolerate more intense, frequent therapies. He showed gradual steady improvement. He was able to follow simple commands on day 8. As he "lightened up" [becoming more alert and aware of his surroundings], he became agitated, requiring increased supervision plus environmental and program modification. His period of Post-traumatic Amnesia (PTA) lasted until day 23, when he gradually became more oriented and could remember new things from day to day.

Johnny was discharged on day 38, to the rehabilitation day hospital program (which was structured as an educational classroom). There he continued his rehabilitation and was assisted in making a smooth transition to home, and then eventually to school. At the time of his discharge from the hospital, he was healthy, but he had continuing language and cognitive problems (word finding, memory, attention, and executive function deficits). He required constant adult supervision due to impulsivity, disinhibition, poor judgment, and difficulties with safety awareness. He also needed supervision and cueing to perform activities of daily living (ADLs) such as dressing, grooming, and bathing. He could walk household distances using a right ankle brace (AFO or ankle foot orthosis) and a cane. He used a wheelchair for community distances. (See below for information on these types of adaptive equipment.)

Johnny continued his intense rehabilitation in the day hospital setting for the next four weeks. During this time, his neurologic function continued to improve. Before he was discharged, a transition plan was worked out with the school, so that he could restart his education in his own community school, with added assistance. He was independent in his ADLs. Although he continued to have language and cognitive problems, they had improved and he had also learned to compensate for some of the residual problems. He was still somewhat impulsive and still required adult supervision for safety. He was walking with a slight limp, but without an assistive device.

■ What Are the Medical Issues Related to TBI?

While your child is receiving rehab therapies, it is critical that she also receive expert medical care. This care is needed not only because of the multiple medical issues related to the brain injury itself, but also because there may be medical issues associated with traumatic injuries to other parts of the body.

The type and distribution of immediate injuries to the brain caused by TBI is unique to trauma. No other type of brain injury—including stroke, anoxia, or metabolic or congenital problems—affects the brain in a similar way. Because of this, and because certain parts of the brain are specialized for specific function, the impairments associated with TBI are unique. So, although TBI does not affect any two children in exactly the same way, the same general types of impairments and disability profiles are seen in all children with TBI. This makes it possible to generalize in this section about the types of medical issues your child *may* encounter.

At first, depending on the severity of your child's injury, the brain injury can affect the function of almost every system in the body. This makes sense, given what we know of brain function and its role in modifying or directing function throughout the body. Fortunately, many of the problems in other systems within the body improve as the healing process occurs. As a result, most children will return to a healthy state even after severe TBIs. That is, they will be generally in good health, without ongoing medical problems.

■ Neurological Effects

The most common, persistent, and problematic issues occurring after TBI are learning and behavioral problems directly related to the brain injury. These problems are discussed in great detail in other chapters of this book. The most common long-term *medical* problems that occur as a result of the brain injury are neurological in nature. That is, they are associated with problems with the brain. Types of neurological problems that can result from TBI include postconcussion syndrome, headaches, seizures, hydrocephalus, and motor (movement) impairments.

Postconcussion Syndrome

A concussion is essentially another way of describing a mild head injury, with or without short loss of consciousness. This may be followed by a short period of changes in mental status, but without any focal neurological signs (such as weakness localized to a certain part of the body). As the name implies, postconcussion syndrome occurs after a concussion. It includes symptoms such as:

- headache,
- dizziness,
- memory loss (difficulty remembering new things),
- emotional lability (frequently changing emotions),
- increased sensitivity to sound,
- impaired concentration,
- disinhibition (difficulty not acting on inappropriate thoughts or actions),
- depression, and
- fatigue.

These symptoms usually spontaneously go away, after weeks to months, but in a very small percentage of children some of the symptoms persist.

As you can see, many of the symptoms described above are slightly vague in nature, and could easily be erroneously attributed to malingering. This is, in fact, what used to occur, before postconcussion syndrome was recognized as a true problem occurring after mild TBI. You can imagine how the above symptoms could interfere with the ability to function well in school, at work, and at home. Imagine, your child is trying hard to do her best, the above symptoms are interfering, and on top of that, she's being told that she's just not trying hard enough or that she's making excuses for not doing her work. This is obviously a recipe for potential disaster, leading to a downward spiral of frustration and secondary behavior problems.

One of the most important aspects in managing this syndrome is simply to recognize it when it is present. Then the symptoms can be addressed appropriately:

- Treat medically what can be treated (for example, the headaches).
- Make temporary compensations or adjustments in the daily routine.

- Educate those who are working with your child, so that they don't misinterpret or misunderstand what is going on, and consequently give the wrong messages to your child.

These symptoms usually subside or at least improve. With time and appropriate management, your child should have few or no long-term effects.

Headaches

Headaches can be a significant problem for some children after TBI. It is interesting that headaches are usually less of a problem after very severe TBI than after milder injuries. Many different types of headaches can occur after TBI:

- headaches related to the trauma to the head itself,
- tension headaches,
- head and neck pain associated with whiplash injuries, and
- migraine headaches triggered by head trauma.

Many adults assume incorrectly that migraine headaches occur primarily in adults. In fact, migraines frequently occur in children, and are often triggered or worsened by trauma. It seems that children who have a family history of migraines are more vulnerable. Migraine headaches are severe, usually localized to one side of the head, described as pounding or throbbing, and often associated with nausea, with or without vomiting. There may also be visual symptoms preceding the pain (often described as "looking through wavy water" or flashing lights), and hypersensitivity to light and noise.

Tension headaches can also occur in children. These headaches are less severe than migraines, and are often described as producing a dull, band-like ache. In children with TBI, they can be triggered by stress related to social and academic difficulties when re-entering the school and community.

Headaches can be frightening to parents, who may be wondering whether there is some delayed complication from the head injury. Complications that cause headaches usually occur during the acute hospitalization or immediately after the injury. If headaches begin weeks to months (or even years) later, it is unlikely that they indicate a serious problem.

The general rule is that you should seek emergency care for your child if she is having a very severe headache described as "the very worst one of her life." If headaches are not so severe, but recur, your physician should evaluate your child on a nonemergency basis. Most headaches in children are handled by "symptomatic treatment." That is, when the headache occurs, treatment is provided to try to get rid of it, usually by resting and taking a medication like ibuprofen (Motrin™, Advil™) or acetaminophen (Tylenol™), if necessary.

If the headaches are bad enough and occur often enough, some families give their child medications on a regular basis to try to prevent the headaches. The drawback with this approach is that the medication needs to be taken every day, and, of course, all medications have potential side effects. A variety of medications can be used to prevent headaches, and your physician should determine the best medication for your child.

It is important not to allow headaches to interfere with school. If your child is missing school or spending too much time in the nurse's office due to headaches (and consequently, you're running back and forth to school), something needs to be done. Appropriate medical evaluation and treatment are obviously essential. However, the treatment may not necessarily be medication. Often, the most important treatment is behavioral in nature, or a combination of both medication and behavioral changes. This could involve educating your child, your family, and your child's teacher about:

1. the type of headaches she has,
2. the things to worry about, and more importantly, the things not to worry about,
3. appropriate reactions and responses to the problem, and
4. criteria for appropriate use of medications.

Posttraumatic headaches after a severe brain injury can obviously be very frightening and worrisome to parents. Consequently, it is very important to understand the headaches and develop a plan to manage them. This will help ensure that inappropriate behaviors such as avoiding school are not inadvertently reinforced in your child.

Seizures

A seizure occurs when the normal functioning of the brain is disrupted by disorderly or excessive firing of neurons. This leads to abrupt changes in neurologic function, such as:

- changes in level of alertness (staring, unconsciousness),
- abnormal sensations (such as smelling something that isn't there), or

- abnormal movements (eye fluttering or repetitious jerking of part or all of the body).

Seizures or convulsions are not uncommon after TBI, but repeated posttraumatic seizures (PTS) are uncommon. Early posttraumatic seizures, by definition, occur within the first seven days after the injury. These seizures are relatively common and do not correlate with severity of injury. They also do not predict whether *epilepsy*—seizures that occur on an ongoing basis—will develop.

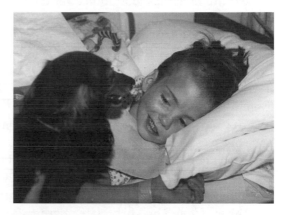

Late seizures, occurring after the first week, are more predictive of the chance of developing posttraumatic epilepsy. Also, the more severe the injury, the more likely epilepsy is to develop.

Overall, the risk for developing posttraumatic epilepsy after a closed head injury is 5 to 7 percent. If your child has a closed head injury with mild TBI, her risk of developing epilepsy is no greater than any other child's. If she has a severe TBI, however, her risk of developing epilepsy climbs to around 11 percent. (In contrast, with penetrating TBI, the risk has been reported as high as 35 to 50 percent.) Your child is most at risk for developing ongoing posttraumatic seizures during the first two years after TBI.

Several risk factors have been reported to increase the chances of developing ongoing PTS. These include:

- focal injuries (such as epidural hematoma, cortical contusion, intracerebral hematoma),
- wounds with penetration of the dura,
- early PTS, and
- factors reflecting increased severity of injury (GCS <10, prolonged coma, prolonged posttraumatic amnesia).

If your child has one of these risk factors, she will probably be started on an antiepileptic drug (AED) during the acute posttraumatic period. This is, in part, to prevent a seizure during the period when she is very sick, because seizures might complicate her care. For example, it might make controlling her intracranial pressure more difficult. After the first week following the injury, your child's AED will probably be discontinued if she has not had any seizures. This is because continuing the medication after the first week to try to prevent (not treat) late PTS has not been shown to be effective in those without early PTS. Guidelines for medication are not as clearly worked out for people at higher risk for developing late PTS (such as those who have had early PTS or open penetrating injuries). However, long-term use of AEDs to prevent late seizures is still usually not recommended, even in children with higher risk factors.

If your child has recurrent late posttraumatic seizures, then you and your physician may choose to treat them. The medication chosen will depend on the type of seizures your child has. Even if your child has had recurrent late PTS, she may eventually be able to discontinue the medications used to treat and prevent seizures.

Now, if your child has a late seizure after her medication is discontinued, it is true that that seizure could cause problems for her. For example, she could have an accidental injury, her self-esteem might suffer, or she might lose driving privileges. Consequently, you may be asking yourself, "Why the big push to get my child off AEDs?" AEDs, like all medications, have potential side effects. Certain AEDs have cosmetic side effects, such as thickening of the gums or increased body hair. There are also other very rare but dangerous side effects, such as liver problems or bone marrow problems (which cause the body to stop making new blood cells). For this reason alone, we like to avoid medications that aren't necessary.

Another important reason to discontinue these medications as soon as possible is that they usually cause undesirable cognitive side effects (such as lethargy and memory problems). These side effects compound the cognitive problems that result from TBI. Theoretically, using certain AEDs during certain periods of recovery may also adversely affect the recovery process itself. It is because of all of these reasons combined that most physicians recommend the early discontinuation of AEDs, when possible.

A word of caution: Never discontinue your child's AEDs on your own. This should *only* be done after careful review with your physician and a discussion about the specific risks for your child. In addition, before AEDs can be discontinued, a careful plan detailing exactly how to wean the medications, and what to do if there are problems, must be developed. Abruptly stopping certain AEDs after prolonged use can be dangerous, so be careful not to run out of these medications, and never stop them on your own.

Types of Seizures

Seizures are classified into several broad categories depending upon the symptoms they cause and the brain wave patterns observed during EEG testing (see below). If the seizure remains focal or localized to a part of the brain, that seizure is referred to as a **focal** or **partial seizure.** If the seizure affects the function of the entire brain, it is called a **generalized seizure.** If it starts as a focal seizure, but then spreads to the entire brain, it is called a **partial complex seizure** (or a partial seizure with secondary generalization).The most common type of seizure associated with TBI is a partial seizure.

What you observe during a seizure and your response will depend on the type of seizure. The seizure may be something as subtle as a staring spell lasting only seconds, with or without some repetitive movement (such as lip smacking or eye fluttering), or it may involve repetitive jerking of part or all of the body, loss of consciousness, and incontinence. Some seizures are preceded by unusual sensations (through any of the senses), called an aura, which may alert the person that she is about to have a seizure. Sometimes rage behavior can be part of a seizure, but this is very rare. If your child is having a true seizure, the behavior you observe will usually be similar each time, you will not be able to interrupt it by talking to or touching your child, and she will usually not remember what happened during the incident.

What to Do If Your Child Has a Seizure

What do you do if you suspect your child is having a seizure? It depends on the type of seizure, of course. But, the first rule is always: DO NO HARM and DON'T PANIC. Children are often injured by well-intentioned bystanders who try to help them during a seizure. The second rule is: Talk to your physician in advance and develop a plan that everyone agrees upon, just in case. A general plan is described below, but depending on your plan and the medical resources in your area, your specific plan may vary from the one described here.

If your child is having a generalized seizure with loss of consciousness and jerking of the arms and legs, first lay her down on her side, if you can do so safely. This will prevent a fall that could cause an injury. Also, if she vomits, it will allow the vomit to come out of her mouth, instead of possibly going down "the wrong way" into the lungs. Next, look at your watch to time the seizure. Seizures always seem at least ten times longer than they really are, and your response is going to depend in part on how long the seizure lasts. Also, observe what your child is actually doing—the way she is posturing or moving, how alert she is, what her eyes are doing—so that you can give this information to your doctor. DO NOT put your finger or anything hard in her mouth. This could result in a broken tooth or a severe bite to your finger. If your child is biting her tongue or lip, you can try to gently slip something soft (like a towel or the hem of a skirt) into her mouth, to block the biting.

Almost all seizures are self-limiting, usually lasting less than two to five minutes. In general, short, self-limited seizures are not felt to cause any additional injury to the brain.

When the seizure stops, your child may or may not be drowsy for a short period of time—this is called the postictal stage. Now is the time to call your doctor, report what has happened, and ask for advice. Your child may need to be seen for evaluation and recommendations, especially if this was the first seizure or an atypical one.

If the seizure does not stop within five minutes, then you should activate your emergency plan. Call your emergency number (911) and arrange transport to the nearest emergency department for medication to break the seizure, if it is still continuing.

Usually when children with TBI have seizures, they are more likely to have a partial seizure instead of the generalized seizure described above. Possibly the seizure will be so subtle that you won't be certain that it is a seizure. Under these circumstances, you should talk to your physician and make an appointment to be seen on a non-emergency basis. In the meantime, you, the teachers, and any other caregivers should observe your child very carefully and keep a log for your doctor with the frequency and types of behaviors that are observed. If your physician feels that these may be seizures, he will most likely recommend an electroencephalogram (EEG) or brainwave test to observe for possible seizure discharges.

An EEG is a noninvasive, painless test. It is done by pasting some small metal disks (electrodes) to your child's scalp. Wires run from the electrodes to a machine that produces a printout of brainwave activity. Your child will need to lie quietly and preferably fall asleep during the test. Possibly other tests will also be recommended, depending on the doctor's evaluation.

Treatment of Seizures

If it is determined that your child is having seizures and that they are interfering with her daily life, an antiepileptic medication (AED) will be recommended. The type recommended will depend on the type of seizure, as well as your child's age and medical history. As mentioned above, all medications have side effects, which you should watch for. Most of the medications may have cognitive or behavioral side effects (some more than others). Since your child may already have cognitive and behavioral problems related to her TBI, it will be important to try to avoid or minimize these side effects as much as possible. Consequently, drugs such as phenobarbital are usually not used in children and adolescents, except in some infants and toddlers. The drugs carbamazepine (Tegretol™) or valproic acid (Depakene™) are currently the most commonly used AEDs. Newer AEDs are now coming on the market, and their role in the treatment of posttraumatic seizures is being explored.

Most PTS can be controlled satisfactorily with medications, without significant side effects. In the rare instances where this is not possible, specialized evaluations such as prolonged EEGs are necessary. Other treatment options can then be considered, including surgery to remove the focus of seizure activity in the brain. Also, if your child is prone to long seizures that require medication to stop them, your physician may give you medication that you can administer on an emergency basis at home. That way you will not have to delay treatment until you can get her to the emergency room for medication.

If your child is placed on one or more AEDs to control seizures, it is possible she may "outgrow" her seizures. She may be able to come off the medications in the future without the seizures returning. The decision to do so is individualized for each child, and depends on a variety of factors, primarily related to the seizure history (type, frequency, length of seizures, complications, difficulty in controlling them, time since last seizure). Ordinarily, your child's doctor should periodically consider having your child try a trial period off medications. He or she might use an EEG to guide this process. If the EEG is significantly abnormal with seizure spikes, it is less likely (though not impossible) that medication can successfully be discontinued.

Hydrocephalus

Hydrocephalus is a condition in which there is too much cerebrospinal fluid (CSF) under too much pressure in the brain, usually within enlarged ventricles. In layman's terms, the condition is often referred to as "water on the brain."

Hydrocephalus is a rare complication, but it can occur if the ventricular system and its canals and openings are scarred or plugged, blocking the normal flow of CSF. It can also occur if the subarachnoid granulations where the CSF should be reabsorbed are not functioning properly.

Although posttraumatic hydrocephalus is unusual, the need to exclude this diagnosis is not. After very severe TBI, the brain shrinks in size due to the loss of some of the neurons. This shrinkage is called "atrophy." Since the size of the head is fixed due to the bony structure of the skull, when the brain shrinks something has to take up the space. This something is CSF. As a result, there will be enlarged ventricles and increased volume of CSF associated with brain atrophy. These changes are permanent in children who have had severe TBI, but do not usually cause any problems in and of themselves.

Usually, the increased CSF is not under increased pressure. If it is, then true hydrocephalus is present and the brain may not function properly. If the pressure is quite elevated, it can cause severe life-threatening problems.

If atrophy is observed in your child's brain, doctors should be asking the question, "Is there increased pressure?" Your child's recovery and progress helps answer this question. If recovery is rapid, it is unlikely that there is hydrocephalus. The neurosurgeon—the doctor who operates on the brain—can also help clarify this question. He or she will do CT or MRI tests to see what is going on in the brain. If there is increased pressure, one or more of the following may be visible in your child's brain:

- There may be changes in the shape of the ventricles.
- The degree of enlargement of the ventricles as compared to the size of the sulci or convolutions on the surface of the brain may not be proportional.
- The brain surrounding the ventricles may be full of fluid, if the fluid in the ventricles is under enough pressure that it tries to flow out of the ventricles directly into the brain tissue (referred to as transependymal edema).

If these findings do not definitely show that your child has hydrocephalus, then measuring the pressure is important. This can usually be done by performing a spinal tap—inserting a needle into the back, below the level of the spinal cord, and drawing out fluid from the space where there is CSF. Since the CSF in the spinal canal connects directly with the CSF space in the head, the pressure will be transmitted throughout the whole space. Occasionally, this procedure requires continuous monitoring through a catheter and needs to be done in the ICU.

Shunts

If your child has hydrocephalus, the neurosurgeon will probably recommend the placement of a shunt—usually a ventriculoperitoneal (VP) shunt. This shunt consists of a catheter inserted into the ventricles, which connects to a length of plastic tubing that runs under the skin and empties into the abdominal space (the space around the stomach and intestines). In between, there is usually a one-way valve within a bulb or reservoir. If the pressure is high enough, this valve allows CSF to flow from the ventricles to the abdominal space. This results in a decreased amount of CSF and pressure within the head.

VP shunts are a blessing for those who need them, as they make it possible to reduce the pressure in the head and avoid its complications. Despite the benefits, VP shunts are obviously a double-edged sword. There are two major potential complications with VP shunts—they may become infected or they may stop working (due to plugging, disconnection, breakage). It is extremely important to know the symptoms of a VP shunt infection or malfunction. A shunt can become infected at any time, but this most often happens within three months of any surgical procedure involving the shunt. It is most likely to become infected with certain types of bacteria that are slow to grow, and consequently may make their presence known only gradually.

Symptoms of a VP Shunt Infection. Symptoms of shunt infections include **unexplained fevers** that tend to recur until diagnosed and treated. Initially, any part of the shunt may be infected. Eventually, if left untreated, the whole system becomes infected. If the infection is in the head, your child may have **changes in mental status,** such as sleepiness and irritability, and a **stiff neck,** in addition to the fevers. If the infection is along the tubing that can be felt under the skin, **redness, swelling, and pain in the skin** surrounding the tubing might occur. If the abdominal end is infected, the symptoms might be **abdominal pain, nausea, vomiting, and loss of appetite.**

Symptoms of a Shunt Malfunction. Other symptoms will develop if the shunt stops working properly, due to infection, plugging, disconnection, or breakage. If a shunt is not functioning properly, the CSF volume and pressure will increase. Depending on what is wrong with the shunt, the malfunction may be partial, intermittent, or complete. If it is an intermittent malfunction, the symptoms can come and go, which can be more confusing and lead to delays in diagnosis. Also, the rate at which pressure rises with a shunt malfunction, and how quickly the child gets into serious danger, can vary considerably. This is because some children are more dependent on shunts than others—some have a total blockage of the flow of CSF out of the ventricles, and others only a partial obstruction or problem with reabsorbing the CSF back into the bloodstream.

If the shunt malfunctions and there is increased intracranial pressure (ICP), symptoms will include **headache, forceful vomiting, and changes in mental status or level of alertness** (e.g., sleepy, lethargic, drowsy, unresponsive). If these symptoms occur, it is considered an emergency. Shunt infection or malfunction needs to be ruled out immediately.

By imaging the brain, the neurosurgeon can tell whether the ventricles have enlarged compared to previous images taken when the shunt was working well. The shunt bulb can also be tapped with a needle. This allows the CSF to be withdrawn for chemical and microscopic analysis (for the presence of red and white blood cells, bacteria, protein, and glucose) and for culture (to see if bacteria can be grown from the CSF). Also, the tap allows the surgeon to tell if the CSF flows out from the ventricles and then down and out of the tubing normally, and if it is under excess pressure. X-rays can also be used to look at the shunt bulb and tubing to make certain that it is hooked up properly. If the shunt is infected or malfunctioning, your child will need emergency medical and/or surgical intervention, with revision or replacement of the system.

Motor Impairment

The brain obviously controls movement and coordination of the body. Fortunately, most children with TBIs, even those with the most severe TBIs, do not have major motor problems. That does not mean there aren't *any* problems. Almost everyone who has a severe TBI will move and react more slowly than they did before the injury. While this may seem like a minor problem given the severity of the problems that could have occurred, it is not an inconsequential problem. These changes may mean that your child no longer has the quickness, speed, or high level coordination to be competitive in activities such as sports or instrumental music. For a young athlete or musician, this can be very distressing, and can require a great deal of emotional adjustment.

A small number of children with severe TBI have more obvious motor impairments. These children often have evidence injury to the deep white and gray matter or brainstem on their exam or neuroimaging (CT scan or MRI). The degree of motor impairment is related to indicators of severity such as length of coma. Essentially all children with prolonged coma (lasting weeks) have some type of obvious motor impairment. As long as the coma lasted less than three months, however, there is a good chance for regaining partial function. Approximately three-quarters of children and adolescents who have been in coma less than three months are eventually able to move around and care for themselves independently in a structured environment.

The types of motor problems that can result from severe TBI include:

- weakness (focal or generalized);
- lack of ability to control or to plan movements;
- abnormal muscle tone;
- loss of postural skills (the ability to hold the head up, to sit, to stand) and balance reactions;
- tremors (usually with movements); and
- lack of coordination.

Children with these types of motor impairments often make rapid gains during rehabilitation. The physical therapist and the occupational therapist are the two members of the team who work most intensively with this part of the rehabilitation. The occupational therapist will focus on your child's arms and hands, helping her to regain as much function as possible. She will help your child relearn to do all the Activities of Daily Living (ADLs)—such as feeding, grooming, dressing, bathing, and writing. The physical therapist will focus on your child's mobility—helping her relearn to roll, sit, stand, and become independent in mobility through walking and/or use of adaptive devices.

Muscle Tone Problems

As described previously, for some children the early stages of rehabilitation are devoted to preventing additional problems. For example, if your child is in coma, she might be *posturing*—assuming abnormal postures that it is difficult for you to move her out of. She might also have *high tone,* or tight muscles. If so, the focus of the therapy will be to prevent any *contracture*—limitations in range of motion of body parts and joints due to shortening of the muscles and soft tissues. A variety of techniques may be used to accomplish this goal, including:

- passive range of motion, in which the therapist stretches your child's limbs for her,
- splints or casts, to hold the body part in a more normal position for a prolonged period of time, and
- positioning in certain ways (in the bed and in an adapted chair).

All of these techniques will stretch certain body parts and help promote relaxation.

There are two basic types of high (increased) muscle tone or muscle tension—spasticity and rigidity.

Spasticity. Spasticity is a "rate dependent" increase in tone. That is, the faster you stretch the muscle by moving the arm or leg, the higher (tighter) the tone becomes. This type of tone is usually present, whether the child is awake or asleep. It is more likely to lead to progressive contracture and is associated with exaggerated reflexes (like the knee jerk). It is also associated with symptoms such as weakness and inability to make fine rapid repetitive movements.

Rigidity. The rigid type of tone is often described as producing the resistance you would feel when bending a lead pipe—constant resistance that does not change when you try to bend it more rapidly. This type of tone often decreases with sleep, and has a lower risk for contracture.

The type of high tone depends on what parts of the brain have been injured. However, due to the diffuse nature of TBI, it is not uncommon for a child to have a mixture of both types, especially during the early phase of recovery. About two-thirds of children with extremely severe injuries have long-term problems with high tone. Muscle tone does improve, however, during recovery.

High tone in and of itself is not bad. Some children with TBI use high tone to help them do certain things. For example, some children who have increased tone in the muscles that extend the hips and legs use this tone to assist them in standing. Consequently, high tone alone is not necessarily an indication for treatment. However, tone may interfere with function. It may make passive or active movement difficult. It may make it hard to find a comfortable position in a bed or in a chair. It may make certain types of nursing care difficult, such as cleaning and changing the diaper area. It may also result in progressive loss of range of motion, which could eventually make it impossible to do things that should be possible due to recovery.

If high tone is a problem, your child may be given medications, in addition to the stretching, splinting, and positioning mentioned above. Medications should always be a supplemental method of managing tone, not the primary mode of treatment. If your child has high tone in a few specific muscles, the possibility of lowering the tone in that specific muscle should be considered. This can be done by injecting botulinum toxin (Botox™) into the specific muscle, or by blocking the nerve to the muscle by injecting alcohol or phenol around the nerve. Both of these techniques will result in reversible muscle weakness. This is ideal during the acute post-injury period, since by the time the effect wears off, the tone may have spontaneously improved.

If high tone is more widespread, your child may need oral medication, which will affect tone throughout the body. The medications that are usually used are baclofen, valium, tizanidine, and dantrolene. If possible, it is a good idea to try to avoid the medications (such as valium) that have the most cognitive side effects.

See the section on "Orthopedic Issues" below for more information on complications of high muscle tone.

Relearning Motor Skills

As your child begins to interact more with the environment, she will be able to actively participate in her therapy and in working toward goals. When this happens, the focus of the therapy will change from preventing problems to relearning skills. Children with the most severe injuries may need to reacquire all of the basic motor skills, starting at head control, and progressing to trunk control, rolling, sitting, standing, and walking. They also need to regain the ability to use their hands and arms to reach, grasp, manipulate objects, and do things for themselves (ADLs.)

The difference in acquiring these motor skills a second time is that the brain has already learned to do these things once before. Even though your child may not appear to be able to do these things, she will have some remaining abilities that can be tapped to assist in reacquiring skills.

While the learning process is modified by previous development, the sequence for acquiring some skills will be similar to the sequence your child followed during her early development. For instance, in order to walk, a child first has to have head control, then trunk control, and then be able to stand.

When your child is learning to do things again, her therapists will insist that she do things with the best form and technique possible. This is to prevent the brain from learning bad habits. During this stage of recovery, your therapist will also tell you that you need to "respect fatigue." Once fatigue occurs, performance deteriorates. This results in doing tasks in less than optimal form, and also can cause safety problems (tripping and falling, or swallowing so that the food goes down the "wrong pipe"). Remember, practice doesn't make perfect, perfect practice makes perfect!

During this recovery period, the therapist will work intensively with your child, helping her practice certain movements or tasks that will build upon each other, improving function. Just as importantly, if not more so, the therapist will set up your child's day and environment so that she can continue practicing skills when the therapist is not there, making the whole day and night therapeutic. For example, the therapist might recommend a wheelchair with a supportive seating system, in which your child can sit and practice head and trunk control. Consequently, you and your child's team will be working intermittently on basic goals throughout the day.

Adaptive Equipment

During this stage of the recovery process, adaptive equipment will no longer be used simply to prevent secondary complications such as contractures. Now it will also begin to be used to help enhance function. The type of equipment and the duration of its use will vary depending on your child's needs and the purpose of the equipment. The basic questions to ask in deciding whether to use a piece of equipment are:

1. Does it enhance function?

2. Does it enhance physical and psychological independence?
3. Does it improve energy efficiency (i.e., make it easier to do something)?
4. Does it make it safer to do something?
5. Does it prevent an unwanted problem?

If the answer to any of these questions is yes, and it fits into your life and budget, then it is reasonable to use it. Here is an example of how a family came up with an adaptation that satisfies all of the requirements above:

My four-year-old, because of his motor impairment, uses a great deal of energy walking, and when he is tired, he trips and falls a lot, which concerns me about his safety. We live on a farm and all the kids like to play in a field that is a long walk from the house. If my son walks to this field, he's too tired to play, and he may hurt fall and hurt himself. Consequently, we hit on the idea of getting him an electric scooter. Now he can ride his scooter to the field, get out and play with his friends until he is too tired to get any more exercise, and then safely come home.
(Comment: this nicely demonstrates the principles of increased function, physical and psychological /independence, safety, and energy efficiency. The child has not gotten any less exercise, yet he has been able to save his energy for what is important to him, and has done it all in a safer manner.)

Some people worry that if their child obtains a piece of equipment, she will become dependent on it, and that will impede further progress or function. If used appropriately, however, this should not happen. Adaptive equipment should be used for specific purposes at specific times.

Let me provide two basic examples of the changing role of equipment.

Wheelchairs. When a severely injured child without head control and with high muscle tone is first able to be out of bed, she will benefit from sitting for a variety of reasons. These include being able to:

- see the world from a vertical instead of a horizontal perspective,
- improve lung function and hygiene,
- more easily go from one place to another,
- decrease the high muscle tone,

- relieve pressure points on the skin that occur while lying down, and
- be in a position in which she can work on relearning head control.

Your child's first chair may be a tilt-in-space wheelchair with a seating system that includes a headrest and side supports and straps to keep the head and trunk upright. It can be tilted backwards, to allow gravity to assist in maintaining the head in the correct position, yet when tilted back, the angle between the back and the seat of the chair remains constant (usually 90 degrees). This usually helps decrease high tone better than if the seat back simply reclined. As head control begins to improve, the chair can be put into a more upright position, forcing your child to work to control her head position. When she is tired and can no longer maintain the head position appropriately, the seat can then be reclined again into a position of rest.

Once head control is good, the tilt-in-space model can be changed to a regular upright model. As trunk control improves, the side supports and straps can gradually be removed. As your child becomes more proficient with her hands, she can begin pushing the wheelchair some herself. This will help improve upper extremity strength and control and general endurance. If your child's legs are working well enough, the footrests can be taken off. With a lower chair, your child can also use her legs to propel and steer the chair.

As walking begins to improve, your child will gradually use walking for mobility instead of the wheelchair. Obviously, the ability to walk short distances comes first. During this period, your child may use the wheelchair only for long distances. For most children with TBI, long-distance ambulation (walking) eventually comes. However, for some children, short-distance ambulation is the long-term goal. These children will use a combination of walking for short distances and a wheelchair or scooter for long distances.

If your child's motor impairment makes it impossible to use her arms for long-distance wheelchair propulsion, then she may want to use an electric wheelchair or scooter for long distances. She would not use the electric wheelchair all the time, however. Instead, she would continue to walk as much as she could in a safe and timely manner, using the power chair only for long distances that would otherwise not be practical or possible for her to do independently. This is in keeping with the idea that adaptive equipment should only be used for specific reasons and at specific times.

Ankle Foot Orthosis (AFO). Another example of an adaptive device with a changing role during rehab is the ankle brace, or AFO. An AFO is a device, usually made of lightweight plastic, that is worn inside the shoe to provide support to the ankle and foot. In the early acute period, in a severely injured child with high tone and minimal active movement, solid AFOs are used. That is, the AFO is all one piece and holds the foot in a fixed position. This type of AFO holds the foot and ankle in a "neutral position" (with the foot at a 90 degree angle to the ankle), prevents deformity and contracture (loss of range of motion), and helps inhibit tone both at the ankle and throughout the legs and body.

As recovery continues, your child starts bearing weight in transfers (when moving from one surface to another, such as from chair to bed) or on a standing board (a positioning device that holds her in an upright position). Later she begins to take a few steps. During this period of recovery, the AFO provides improved lower extremity stability, holding the ankle in a fixed neutral position and indirectly stabilizing the knee. This helps prevent hyperextension or buckling of the knee. As stability and control of the lower extremities continues to improve, it may be possible to wean the brace. However, it may also be necessary to continue using the brace, at least on one side.

As your child's walking abilities improve, the type of brace may need to be changed. For example, your child may need an articulated AFO—one with a hinge at the ankle, allowing the toes and foot to move upward, but not to move downward past the neutral position. Changing the design of the brace decreases the stability provided by the brace, but improves the quality of the gait, smoothing it out.

A problem that commonly indicates the need for long-term use of an AFO is a *foot drop,* or inability to lift the toes and foot up while walking. This impairment causes several problems:

1. stubbing the toes, which may cause tripping and falling; and
2. the need for compensations such as hiking the hip, stepping excessively high with that leg, or swinging the leg out to the side.

These compensations consume more energy per step and make the gait look more abnormal. An AFO in this situation can stabilize the gait, and improve function, safety, and energy efficiency. This can allow your child to walk further and more safely, with a more normal-appearing walk.

Environmental Modification

Your child may also benefit from environmental modification—that is, changes to the physical layout of your home to make it easier for your child to get around and function independently. Your therapists should help with this process, through consultation and possibly a home visit, as your needs dictate. The type of modifications will depend on the physical arrangement of your home, and the type of impairments that your child has.

Whether modifications need to be temporary or permanent will depend on your child's prognosis. For example, if your child has a good prognosis for climbing stairs, but is unable to do so when she first returns home, you may have to make temporary modifications to your home. Modifications might include moving her bed to the first floor, having a bedside commode available, and making alternate arrangements for bathing. However, if long-term wheelchair use is likely, permanent modifications may include building a ramp up to the front door, enlarging doors, and redesigning a bedroom and bathroom.

Whatever you do, don't start any remodeling projects or buy any items without using the expertise of your rehabilitation team. Let them help you make these decisions in a careful and thoughtful manner. Also check your homeowner's insurance to see whether it provides coverage for home modifications necessary to accommodate a newly disabled member of the household.

■ Psychiatric Issues

People who have had brain injuries have a slightly increased risk of developing psychiatric illnesses, including depression and psychoses, for the rest of their lives. In addition, difficulties such as disinhibition, inattention, and impulsivity may lead to behavioral problems. These symptoms can lead to diagnoses such as secondary attention-deficit/hyperactivity disorder (S-AD/HD), and, if behavior spirals out of control, other diagnoses such as conduct disorders.

Chapters 7 and 8 cover behavioral issues following TBI in great detail. This section will take a brief look at the medications that may be needed to help control your child's behavior and/or psychiatric illness.

Attention-Deficit/Hyperactivity Disorder (AD/HD)

Many children who have had a moderate to severe TBI develop secondary attention-deficit/hyperactivity disorder, also known as acquired attention-deficit/hyperactivity disorder. This condition results in a group of behaviors related to inattention and impulsivity, and may or may not include hyperactivity.

Inattention is one of the major problems after moderate and severe TBI. Since inattention can interfere with learning and social interactions, medication is often tried to improve this symptom. Stimulant medications such as Ritalin™ or Dexedrine™ often improve inattention. The goal of these medications is to improve attention, *not* to sedate or "drug" your child. These medications can be extremely useful for some children, improving their performance in school, as well as their ability to interact more appropriately with their friends.

Ritalin and Dexedrine are both extremely safe and do not have severe side effects. These medications may cause side effects such as appetite suppression, insomnia, tics, rebound hyperactivity (when medication is wearing off), and mood swings. However, most of these problems go away with a little time or an adjustment of the dose. In addition, these medications are not known to have any negative effects on the recovery process. In fact, studies

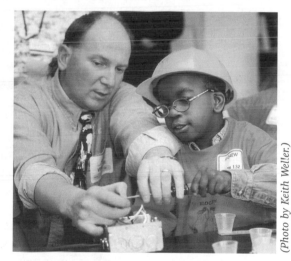

(Photo by Keith Weller.)

suggest that these medication may actually improve neurologic recovery and outcome when given during the subacute period after injury.

Sometimes a child has behaviors such as irritability, aggression, and mood swings in addition to simple inattention. In theses cases, medications that are second or third choices in treating typical AD/HD may need to be tried, and sometimes in combination. If your child needs this type of help, you will need to consult a physician who is skilled in the use of psychiatric medications after TBI.

Some children with TBI outgrow the need for AD/HD medications, but others continue to need medication over the long term. Your child's treatment team should keep track of how your child's behavior is changing with ongoing development and recovery, adjusting or discontinuing medication, if appropriate.

Agitation or Aggression

Children sometimes become agitated and aggressive during the early recovery period. Usually these problems can be controlled without medication. Most often, behavioral techniques (see Chapter 7), one-to-one supervision, and environmental modifications are enough to manage these problems. Rarely, medications are needed to prevent a child from physically harming herself or others. Medications are much more likely to be used for adults following TBI.

During this agitated and/or aggressive stage, it is very important to have your child's mental status (thinking abilities and processes) closely evaluated. Behaviors that appear similar on the surface may be driven by very different problems, and this will change the treatment. For example, usually when a child or adolescent is agitated, there are no psychotic features such as delusions and hallucinations. Rarely, a child may have delusions—false beliefs—and hallucinations— the sensation of hearing or seeing something that is not real. These can feed the agitation and drive the aggressive behaviors. While some benign hallucinations are not unusual during this agitated phase, hallucinations that affect the behavior in such a negative way are unusual. Children with these types of hallucinations usually benefit from treatment with medications.

If medications are used to try to control or modify unwanted behaviors, it is important to reevaluate the need for these medications from time to time. As your child recovers, medications may no longer be needed, or different medications may now be of more benefit. This is a complicated issue. Your child's prognosis will be affected by the type of psychiatric diagnosis and the time at which it occurred in relationship to the injury. In making decisions concerning the use of these medications, it is essential to consult a physician (neurologist, rehab psychiatrist) with expertise in brain injury. Just as with antiepileptic medications, you should never adjust medications without professional advice, since inappropriate or abrupt discontinuation can cause significant problems.

▪ Orthopedic Issues

Bone fractures and other musculoskeletal injuries often occur at the same time as the TBI. Usually these injuries heal well, and do not cause any ongoing problems. Sometimes, however, children with TBI may develop orthopedic problems—problems with the bones, joints, muscles, or other body structures involved in movement and posture. This section looks at the medical treatment of the most common orthopedic problems: injured growth plate, muscle tone problems, and heterotopic ossification.

Injured Growth Plate

The growth plate is the area near the end of a bone where the bone is still growing. If the growth plate of a still-growing bone is injured due to a fracture through it, this can result in progressive deformities of the bone or lack of normal bone growth.

If your child has an injured growth plate, it is very important to consult an orthopedic surgeon, a doctor who specializes in diagnosing and treating orthopedic problems. With long-term follow-up, the orthopedic surgeon can recommend appropriate treatment to correct these problems. Treatment can include surgical procedures, shoe lifts, or braces.

Complications of Muscle Tone Problems

If your child has severe motor impairment with high tone as a result of her injuries, she may be vulnerable to the same types of orthopedic problems as children with cerebral palsy. That is, she can develop problems such as:

1. scoliosis, or curvature of the spine;
2. joint dislocation (out of the socket) or subluxation (partial dislocation) of joints;
3. contracture. See the section on "Muscle Tone Problems" above for an explanation.

These problems are more likely to develop in children who were injured when they were infants or toddlers.

These problems occur when:
1. growing bone is subjected to abnormal, unbalanced muscle pull or tension across joints, and
2. there is a lack of normal movement and weight bearing (such as in a child who is not walking).

Depending on the problem and the severity, these problems may require special therapy, braces, and/or surgery. The rehab doctor, orthopedic surgeon, physical therapist, and occupational therapist on your child's team will let you know which treatment option is best for your child.

Sometimes an injury results in weakened muscles on one side of the body or in one extremity. When this happens, abnormal growth can occur. If one side of the body is weak (hemiparesis), that side may not grow as well as the other side. This results in a short arm and/or leg on that side (limb length discrepancy). The degree of discrepancy, especially in the legs, determines the severity of the problem and also the type of intervention needed, if any. If the weakness begins before age five, we know that the discrepancy will be greater. We also know that the larger the discrepancy, the more problems it causes with walking. If the discrepancy is minor, the shorter side may require a brace because of ankle weakness, with no other treatment required. If the discrepancy becomes larger, a shoe lift may be prescribed. If the discrepancy is still larger or predicted to become larger with growth (something your orthopedist can tell you based on X-rays and tables predicting remaining growth), surgery is sometimes needed. This can involve either operating on the longer leg to slow down its growth rate, or lengthening the shorter leg.

It is obviously important to monitor the growth of your child's arms and legs, especially if she has weakness and/or previous bony injuries. This enables the doctor to identify problems early and treat them appropriately.

Heterotopic Ossification

When new bone forms in abnormal places, such as in the muscles of an arm or a leg, it is referred to as "heterotopic ossification" (HO). HO usually occurs in adults, but can occur in children. When it occurs in children, it is usually in those aged eleven or older, and is associated with greater length of coma. One study found that HO may occur in up to 14 percent of children and adolescents with *severe* TBI. But this study also found that only about one-fourth of the children had residual functional impairments as a result of HO.

HO can be painful, which can limit progress in acute rehabilitation. Any long-term limitations on function, however, are a result of limitation of range of motion. Whether range of motion is limited depends on the extent and location of the new bone. For example, if the HO is close to a joint, it could cause the joint to fuse (join together). If the HO is in a muscle far removed from a joint, this will not happen.

HO is treated with medications to reduce the inflammation and vigorous stretching to maintain range of motion. If HO impairs movement too much, it can be surgically removed when it is "mature"—usually in about a year. If it is removed too early, it is likely to grow back.

∷ Nutritional Issues

Nutrition is yet another area of concern when a child has had a head injury. After TBI, many children have trouble with the mechanics of eating. They also frequently experience changes in calorie needs or in appetite control. These problems can not only threaten your child's good nutrition, but can also make it unsafe for her to eat. Your child's rehab team will therefore spend a considerable amount of time re-teaching her feeding skills.

Swallowing Difficulties

Severe TBI often affects the ability to eat safely. This may be due to difficulty both in the oral and the pharyngeal phases of swallowing. The oral phase consists of moving the food around in the mouth, chewing and preparing the food for swallowing, then gathering it into one clump or "bolus." During the pharyngeal phase, the bolus is transported safely from the mouth through the pharynx (the back of the throat), past the larynx or voice box (the opening into the airway), and into the esophagus (the tube leading from the throat to the stomach). All of this is an active process which takes a lot of fine coordination, under the control of the brain.

After TBI, the muscles used in swallowing may be weak and uncoordinated, just like the muscles of the arms and legs. They can also fatigue with exercise, so that your child's eating abilities may deteriorate during the course of an eating session. Sensation is frequently abnormal as well. Your child may not be able to tell where the food is in her mouth or throat. Even if the food goes "down the wrong way," she may not realize it, and there will be none of the usual coughing when she swallows wrong. This is referred to as "silent" penetration or aspiration.

If your child's control of the oral and pharyngeal phases is abnormal, she may eat inefficiently or be unable to safely prepare the food for swallowing and/or to swallow it. If she eats inefficiently, the process may be so slow and laborious that she cannot eat or drink enough within reasonable amounts of time. There are obviously other things that your child will need and want to do besides spending the day eating.

If your child cannot swallow safely, maintaining an open airway and healthy lungs becomes problematic. If a piece of food is not properly prepared for swallowing, it can slip into the pharynx before it is ready for it. The food then might go down the wrong way into the airway. This has two major potential complications:

1. If the food is solid, it might actually block the airway, with severe consequences. (This is one reason that the texture of foods your child is served will be modified initially, and potentially dangerous solid foods will not be allowed.)
2. Too much food may go down into the lungs, causing possible infections such as pneumonia or symptoms such as wheezing.

Because of these potential problems, your medical rehabilitation team will err on the conservative side in giving recommendations for starting feeding, especially early on. They will evaluate your child to see when she is ready to begin trying to eat again. A program of non-nutritive stimulation may be the first step. That is, her mouth and swallowing will be stimulated, but without using food. Your child is especially likely to begin with such a program if she has the swallowing problems described above or if she is considered not responsive enough or too agitated to eat.

When it is safe to try food, a member of the medical rehabilitation team with expertise in this area will start work with your child. Your child will be given small tastes, usually of pureed foods, because they are usually the easiest to control in the oral and pharyngeal phases of swallowing. Depending on the exam and results of this "bedside clinical swallowing evaluation," your child may be able to begin eating, or she may need further evaluation.

Sometimes a "modified barium swallow" is needed to assess the safety of the pharyngeal phase of swallowing. In this test, done with an X-ray videotape, your child swallows food of different consistencies containing barium—a white contrast substance that allows the food to be seen on X-ray. This makes it possible to see how safely your child is swallowing, and whether safety can be improved with modifications—for example, of food texture, bite size, straw or cup use, and head position.

Just as TBI recovery is a gradual process, so is the recovery of swallowing function in many children with severe injuries. It may take weeks or months before your child can resume a diet that provides all calories, nutrients, and fluids by mouth. Until that goal is reached, feedings and/or water are given through a tube. As your child improves her intake of fluid and calories by mouth, the amount of tube feeding and water will gradually be decreased, making certain that your child stays well hydrated and well nourished.

What about Tubes?

You may hear several different terms used, so let's go over them. A **nasogastric tube (NG tube)** goes through the nose and down the throat into the stomach. It is almost always the kind of tube that is used initially during the acute period. If prolonged use of a tube is anticipated, a **gastrostomy tube (G-tube)** may be recommended. This tube goes into the stomach through a hole or "stoma" in the abdominal wall overlying the stomach. A G-tube may be inserted two different ways:

1. A **surgical G-tube** is inserted by making an incision in the abdominal wall and putting the tube through this incision into the stomach.
2. A **percutaneous endoscopic gastrostomy tube (PEG tube)** is a gastrostomy tube that is inserted down the throat and into the stomach by a physician using an endoscope, which allows him to visually guide the tube.

G-Tubes vs. NG Tubes. There are advantages and disadvantages to each type of tube. If your child is going to use the tube for a short time (days to weeks), doctors may not want to subject her to the discomfort and anaesthesia required for the G-tube. This said, NG tubes have possible disadvantages such as:

- sinusitis (infection of the sinuses);
- incorrect insertion or placement by parents or nurses, which can cause tube feeds to go into the lungs instead of the stomach; and
- increased gastroesophageal reflux (GER), which can cause heartburn, inflammation of the esophagus or esophagitis, and increased chance of stomach contents going up and then down the wrong way into the lungs. (This is much worse than food in the lungs, due to the acidity of the stomach contents.)

G-tubes have the disadvantages related to discomfort and anesthesia mentioned above, although the discomfort is not major and can be controlled by medication. There is also the very low risk of complications such as bleeding or infections, and the occasional risk of the tube migrating into the small intestine. Advantages of G-tubes include: parents do not have to worry about placing tubes themselves, which makes daily and especially home care much easier; improved appearance and relief of having the tube out of the nose; and less chance of reflux and esophagitis.

Children usually tolerate G-tubes very well. After the abdominal incision is well healed, your child can be switched to a low-profile model that looks like a plastic disc on the surface of the abdomen. This makes them well accepted. Also, a G-tube does not restrict activity. Your child can bathe and swim with one. Consequently, if your child is going to need a tube for a longer period of time, a G-tube makes sense.

If your child goes home with either an NG or G-tube, you will need to have spare equipment on hand and know how to replace it, should it come out accidentally. G-tubes need to be replaced immediately, because the stoma or hole in the abdomen will close up very quickly. Certainly this is an advantage if and when the tube is discontinued. The stoma almost always heals quickly and spontaneously once the tube is removed, without need for surgery.

Weight

Weight can definitely be a problem after TBI—in either direction—too much or too little. In the early acute period, weight loss can be significant. This is largely due to a problem with supply and demand. The nutritional and caloric requirements are significantly increased in the first few weeks after TBI, but it is difficult to supply enough nutrients because the stomach does not empty well in the first week. Beginning in the second week, however, the stomach begins to function more normally.

During rehabilitation, one of the goals will be for your child to regain weight, up to her individualized goal. The minimum goal will always be enough weight gain for your child to be well-nourished and to have enough reserves if she becomes sick.

On the other hand, excess weight gain can be, and often is, a significant problem. One contributing factor, not surprisingly, is that children burn fewer calories when they are less mobile than usual. If your child has significant motor impairments, excess weight will make movement more difficult. Consequently, you will likely be told that she should try to maintain her weight at the low end of normal for her age and height. Specifically, you may hear that her weight should be in the 10th percentile on growth charts for children of her height.

Weight gain can also occur due to *posttraumatic hyperphagia,* or excess eating. Rarely, this excess eating can be related to improper functioning of the appetite control center in the brain, as if the thermostat is set wrong. If this happens, your child will not feel full or satisfied after eating, and will be able to go from one large meal to another.

It is much more likely, however, that overeating is behaviorally related. These behaviors are usually influenced by multiple factors. Home cooking (after all that hospital food) may taste so good that your child can't seem to get enough. This, in turn, is flattering to the cook (usually one of you) and satisfying to you, the parents, who like to see your child enjoying something after such a terrible ordeal. Eating may be further complicated by the behavioral changes in your child. If she is now impulsive and disinhibited, she may not be able to squelch the urge to eat something once she's seen it or thought about it.

Whatever the reasons for overeating—whether it's true appetite dysregulation or a behavioral eating problem—the remedy is the same: you need to help your child relearn how to eat a healthy, well-balanced diet in appropriate amounts. Although it is understandable that you will be more lenient with your child when she first arrives home from the hospital, this can't last long. After TBI, what your child needs is a warm, friendly, structured, daily routine with some rules, including scheduled meals and snack times. Amounts eaten should be appropriate and frequency of eating should be regulated, with three meals and appropriate scheduled snacks.

When weight gain is a problem, parents often ask for the help of a nutritionist or dietitian. A dietitian can provide important help, but the best help may come from:

1. knowing the goal for ideal weight and ideal weight gain and growth over time,
2. charting your child's weight weekly on a home scale,
3. getting assistance with the behavioral issues surrounding eating from someone such as a psychologist.

True, your child may be upset with you for putting limits on her eating. In the long run, however, she will be more upset with you if you allow her to quickly gain excess weight that she may have to live with the rest of her life. Be reassured that most behaviors that lead to excessive overeating are temporary, and go away spontaneously in weeks to months. Do what you can to weather this storm—it won't last forever, but the consequences of it can.

■ Other Medical Issues

As Chapter 1 explained, the brain controls everything that goes on in our bodies. Unfortunately, this means TBI will disrupt almost every other system's functioning in some way, during the acute posttraumatic period. Fortunately, most of these problems "resolve" (get better) during the acute period, and your child should not be left with any long-term problems. Let's review a few of the systems that are disrupted, and see how the problems resolve.

Endocrine Problems

The endocrine system includes the glands such as the thyroid, adrenal glands, and ovaries. These glands make and release *hormones*—substances that regulate or control certain important body functions. The endocrine system is in large part under the control of the master gland, the pituitary. In turn, the pituitary gland is directly connected to the hypothalamus, which controls almost all of the function of this master gland.

During the acute period of the brain injury, it is common for the fine tuning of the endocrine system to be subtly out of whack. For example, the thyroid system in general works adequately, but not optimally. Usually no intervention (or investigation) is required. Rarely, a child might have symptoms of thyroid problems that should be investigated, including sluggishness, cold intolerance, dry skin, constipation, and excess weight gain. After the acute period, thyroid functioning usually returns to normal.

Another system that can be disrupted is the menstrual cycle in young women. After a severe injury, it is usual for young women to skip their periods for three to six months, then resume typical menstrual cycles. In the long run, fertility is not affected.

During the acute period, the regulation of the amount of water in the body can also be affected. The pituitary secretes (releases) antidiuretic hormone (ADH), which tells the kidneys to hang on to free water. This is the way the body conserves water when thirsty. When the body doesn't need to conserve water, then the pituitary does not secrete this hormone. The absence of this hormone then allows free water to be excreted into the urine.

In the first week or two after a severe TBI, it is not unusual for too much ADH to be released. This is referred to as Syndrome of Inappropriate ADH (SIADH). SIADH can cause the body to become overloaded with fluid. During this period, the fluids and electrolytes (salts in the blood) will be carefully monitored, in an attempt to keep the body on the "dry" side, because fluid overload may contribute to increased *edema* or swelling of the brain. Consequently, any SIADH should be detected and handled during your child's acute hospital stay. SIADH usually does not occur later. Rarely, mild cases may occur in children who are taking seizure medications such as carbamazepine (Tegretol™).

On the flip side, too little ADH can result in rapid large losses of water in the urine, leading to dehydration. This is called diabetes insipidus or DI (not related to "sugar" diabetes). This rarely occurs after very severe TBI. If your child has diabetes insipidus, it can be controlled by a combination of fluid management and hormone replacement.

Immune System

The immune system ordinarily produces infection-fighting proteins called antibodies and white blood cells to keep the body healthy. The severe trauma of a head injury can temporarily affect this system. As a result, children with TBI sometimes get severe infections such as pneumonia or infections of the blood shortly after their injury. Problems with the immune system may also lead to types of infections that are uncommon in healthy children, such as thrush (a yeast infection in the mouth). These immune system problems are short-lived, with the immune system reverting back to normal within weeks.

■■ Prevention of TBI

As discussed in Chapter 1, once someone has had a head injury, it is very important to avoid another head injury for the rest of that person's life—especially within the first year after injury. Why is it so important to avoid another injury? Soon after the first head injury, the brain is more susceptible to severe injury if there is another blow to the head (even if it is a mild blow). This is of most concern with milder injuries, such as with concussions acquired while playing sports. All too often children ignore the concussion and put themselves in harm's way again too early—for instance, by getting back into the game immediately.

Later, after this period of increased risk is over, a blow to the head may not result in a more severe injury than one would expect. However, the effects of another head injury may be additive or cumulative. For example, the effects of one mild TBI plus one mild TBI may not equal two mild TBIs, but instead might be equivalent to a severe TBI.

After a TBI, the brain has to compensate in order to regain as much function as possible. If this previously injured brain is reinjured, it may not be able to compensate well a second time. As a result, deficits may be more obvious and disabling. For example, someone with mild memory impairment after her first TBI may have learned to compensate and be functioning relatively well. Even if a second TBI only worsens her memory slightly, this slight worsening may tip the person "over the edge" in regard to memory function. She may now act as if severely impaired, and be unable to compensate well in daily life. Because of this additive effect, it is very important for your child to avoid a second head injury, for the rest of her life.

What can you do to help prevent another injury? Let's talk about injury prevention strategies in general first, and then talk about the implications for your child in particular.

The three main principles of brain injury prevention are:
1. Decreasing the amount and rate of energy transfer will decrease the severity of, or prevent, an injury to the brain. For example, a bicycle helmet will absorb some of

the energy during a fall, so that the head doesn't have to absorb it all.

2. "Passive" or automatic strategies to prevent injuries are likely to be more effective than those that depend solely on behavioral changes. For example, a playground designed properly with soft surfaces can absorb some of a child's energy during a fall. These passive strategies are crucial because behavior changes are hardest to achieve in children at most risk (such as children with poor judgment who are disinhibited, such as those with prior TBIs).

3. Strategies and recommendations should be focused and specific. For example: "Be careful" isn't as useful as "Use a car seat," "Buy and use a bike helmet," or "Throw out the baby walker."

What do these general suggestions really mean for your child and your family? Obviously, your child and your family cannot and should not live in a protective bubble. Life is full of risks, and everyone needs to decide what is important in their lives. As a parent, you need to decide what relative risk you (child and family) are willing to take. Below are some guidelines to help you make that decision.

Supervision

One of the most important keys to head injury prevention is making sure that your child has enough supervision. Whoever is supervising your child must be able to make a judgment call as to which activities are unsafe and then restrict them. How much supervision your child needs will depend on her own individual needs and abilities. As your child shows that she can make safe and appropriate decisions, the supervision can gradually be weaned.

For more insight into the reasons your child needs supervision, see Chapter 5, which discusses the learning and behavioral changes that can occur after TBI.

Safe Sports

Sports often present the biggest dilemma to families and their children, although driving *should* be at the top of the list of concerns (see below). Almost all sports involve some risk of head injury, but some obviously have a higher risk than others.

It makes great sense to try to encourage your child's interest and participation in low-risk sports. If she can learn to prefer and excel in low-risk sports, this is clearly to her benefit. Developing this preference may require a behavior change for the entire family, not just your child. For example, if you watch only contact sports on TV, and never watch or participate in low-risk sports with your child, this will probably affect her preference. Try to encourage activities such as swimming, racket sports, dance, noncontact martial arts, and track and field events (minus a few riskier events such as the pole vault and high jump). Try *not* to encourage the more obvious high-risk or contact sports such as football, basketball, baseball, soccer, hockey (ice and field), lacrosse, skating, rugby, and boxing. And make a rule that activities such as riding motorized bikes and three wheelers are simply not allowed.

If your child played on a sports team before her injury, be aware that there are guidelines for athletes and coaches concerning if and when a player can resume play after a concussion. These need to be followed carefully. If your child's coach doesn't know about these guidelines, insist that he or she become familiar with them and use them. You can obtain a copy of the guidelines from the Brain Injury Association, which is listed in the Resource Guide at the end of this book.

Almost any sport can be played safely (with certain modifications), or unsafely. For example, shooting hoops in the backyard can be very safe, while an uncontrolled game of basketball with people crashing the boards and cutting each other's feet out from under them wouldn't be safe.

Whatever sport is being played, it is up to you to ensure it is played as safely as possible. Most likely, you did this when your children were small, only allowing them to do something if they had the ability and judgment to do it safely. This same precaution can help your child with TBI play safely. This means that you will need to help her resume certain activities, supervising and assisting her as indicated, and saying "no" or "not yet" when appropriate.

Rules for certain activities need to be instituted and followed. These may include rules about where and under what circumstances it is safe to play. For example, even if bicycle riding appears safe to you from a judgment, coordination, and balance perspective, you may still make the following rules: ride only in a restricted area (like on a bike path and **never** in traffic); ride only during daylight hours; and always, always, *always* wear a helmet.

Protective equipment, as a rule, should be used when it is indicated and appropriate for everyone else to be wearing it. For example, bike helmets and baseball batting helmets should be used by everyone, not just those with prior TBIs. It is important to choose your battles. Don't insist on equipment that will be overprotective and make your child feel stigmatized. She may have enough problems with social interactions without your insisting that she wear unnecessary protective gear. If it's not indicated for the other children, it's probably not indicated for your child.

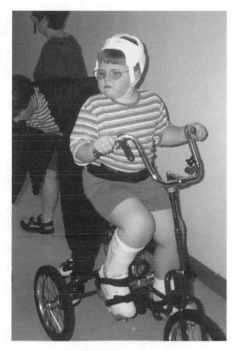

If you make certain that sports and play are appropriately supervised, things won't get out of hand, turning what should be a safe sport into an unsafe sport. If you need a therapist or counselor to help your child accept this guidance, use your therapy time to address these real-life issues. Your child's physical therapist can help you with questions about your child's physical abilities, and your psychologist can help with questions about judgment abilities.

Driving Precautions

Driving is probably the most dangerous thing any of us can decide to do. It requires constant attention, split-second safety judgments and reaction time, and the ability to keep our behavior and emotions under constant control. These essential abilities for safe driving sound like a problem list for many young people after TBI. Consequently, you will need to consider very carefully whether your child should drive, and if so, under what circumstances.

There are rehabilitation professionals who specialize in assessing whether driving is safe for individuals with disabilities, and you should seek their expertise before your child starts or resumes driving. Rarely would it be advisable for someone with a severe TBI to start driving at age sixteen.

The final decision as to whether your child will be able to drive rests with your state Department of Motorized Vehicles, and the laws will vary from state to state. If your child is considering getting a license, she will most likely need to contact the DMV and notify them that she had a TBI in the past. They will then collect information from your child's physicians and others to use in deciding whether to allow your child to drive. If your child previously had a license, it will most likely be invalid after TBI. She will need to notify the DMV about her TBI and reapply.

If everyone agrees that the goal of driving is a reasonable and safe one, your child will most likely need an extended period of supervised driving. She will also need initial restrictions on where driving is allowed. For instance, she might first be allowed only to take an agreed-upon route from home to school and back, which would be the safest route possible, avoiding dangerous intersections and roads with high volume and speed.

If driving is not an option for your child, it may help to point out that many people in our society never learn to drive, relying on alternate means of transportation. Some actually like the fact that they don't have to drive (although this is a fact that's hard to reconcile when you're sixteen).

Making Your Community Safer

If you remember the rules of injury prevention, you will recall that there are other things that need to be done to reduce the risk of TBI, but at a more global or community level. Helpful steps include:

- Be active in your community to make certain that the environment is safe.
- Ensure that injury prevention is a priority in your community, and that there is someone with expertise in injury prevention to help make appropriate decisions and recommendations in your community. Often there will be someone in the local health department or motor vehicle department with this responsibility.
- Do not accept the attitude from your neighbors, local politicians, and news persons that "accidents are un-avoidable." This attitude will only lead to more unneces-

sary suffering. Make certain that the circumstances of "accidents" are examined, and when appropriate, things are changed to prevent another.

Close to home, try these strategies, which will benefit your family *and* community:

- Make certain that playground surfaces are made from materials that will prevent TBI from minor falls.
- Make certain that children in your neighborhood have safe areas to play in, so that they aren't playing on the sidewalks along busy streets.
- If there appears to be a safety hazard in your neighborhood, such as a dangerous intersection for either pedestrians or cars, ensure that someone with injury prevention expertise looks at the problem and comes up with a solution.
- Become active in programs to educate and encourage behaviors that will prevent or lessen the severity of an injury, such as use of seatbelts, appropriate child restraints, and bicycle helmets.

▪▪ Review of the Case History

We've covered a great deal of ground in the first two chapters. Let's look at the sample case story about Johnny that appeared in these two chapters to review some of the things we have learned.

"Johnny is a 13 year old boy."
The fact that he is a boy is usual, considering the 2 to 1 ratio of boys with TBI to girls with TBI.

"He had some mild learning problems and mild attention deficits."
This is also common for those who sustain head injuries. The inattention may have contributed to Johnny's injury in the first place, and certainly the head injury will increase the learning problems and inattention.

"He sustained a Closed Head Injury with Severe Traumatic Brain Injury (TBI) when the bicycle he was riding was struck by a car."

Closed head injury is the most common kind of head injury in civilians, and we know that Johnny's injury included injury to the brain, not just to the head itself. Since the crash involved a car, we know that a great deal of potential force was involved. This increases the potential severity of the injuries, and it also increases his chance of other associated traumatic injuries.

"He was unconscious at the scene of the accident, and was taken by helicopter to the area trauma center. On arrival in the emergency department, he had a Glasgow Coma Scale (GCS) score of 5/15."
The fact that he was unconscious at the scene is not necessarily a bad indicator, although if he hadn't lost consciousness, that would have been a good indicator. However, a GCS of 5/15 does indicate a severe TBI (severe injuries have GCS of 3 to 8 out of a potential 15). It is good that he was quickly transported to a trauma center, because medical attention within the first "golden hour" is very advantageous.

"He was intubated and placed on a ventilator."
This was to protect his airway, so that safe breathing could be maintained, and to assist in controlling his intracranial pressure (ICP) as needed.

"His initial CT scan showed contusions in both frontal lobes, and small punctate hemorrhages in the deep white matter (left more than right), compatible with shearing or diffuse axonal injury (DAI)."
The scan showed physical evidence that the structure of Johnny's brain has been injured in the typical manner of severe TBIs. While structure and function do not always go hand in hand, we would be concerned from this study that Johnny would be at high risk for certain problems. In particular, he would be at high risk for frontal lobe dysfunction, including problems with behavior and executive function. In addition, the control of movement of the right side of the body might be more problematic, at least initially, because of the deep white matter injury more on the left (remember the left side of the brain controls movement on the right side of the body, and vice versa). Because Johnny has visible injury

on the CT scan, we also know that this cannot be a mild
injury—it must be at least a moderate, if not a severe, injury.

"His intracranial pressure (ICP) was normal."
This is good, because it decreases the risk for secondary or
delayed injuries to the brain due to inadequate blood supply
or herniation syndromes.

"He had no significant associated injuries."
Here Johnny was more fortunate than he might have been.
Many people who are riding a bike or walking when they are
struck by a car sustain leg fractures and chest injuries.

*"His initial course was complicated by a pneumonia, which responded to
antibiotics."*
As we have said, infections are fairly common in the acute
period. This is because the instrumentation (tubes, IVs, etc.)
can allow bacteria to enter the body and because the immune
system does not work as well as usual. Eventually these
problems will resolve, and we would expect that he will once
again be healthy.

*"He began opening his eyes and was transferred from the intensive care
unit (ICU) to the rehabilitation unit on day 6."*
It is encouraging that Johnny's neurologic status improved. It
is also good that he was transferred in a timely fashion to the
rehabilitation unit. Early admission to acute rehabilitation
improves a child's outcome and shortens the length of
inpatient rehabilitation required.

*"On admission to the rehabilitation unit, he was able to localize stimuli
(trying to pull out his IVs and tubes)—Rancho Los Amigos (RLA) level
III. He could not talk nor communicate his needs. He was fed through a
nasogastric tube (NG tube), through his nose into his stomach. He was
very weak, especially on the right side of his body, and was unable to roll
or sit. He had begun receiving therapies in the ICU. Now, since he wasn't
so sick, he could tolerate more intense, frequent therapies."*
The RLA levels are a "short hand" way for rehab professionals
to communicate the patient's cognitive and behavioral status

to others. (See the Appendix for more information.) Johnny was totally dependent for his care at this point, and the emphasis of his rehabilitation was to optimize his health and nutrition, and prevent secondary problems or disabilities, such as bed sores and contracture of his joints.

"He showed gradual steady improvement. He was able to follow simple commands on day 8."

Since he had a TBI without obvious secondary or delayed injury to the brain, one would expect that he would improve and make steady progress. Beginning to follow commands on day 8 post-injury would be defined as eight days of coma. Remember, six or more hours of coma is used by many as the cut-off point for classifying the injury as a severe one.

"As he "lightened up" [becoming more alert and aware of his surroundings], he became agitated, requiring increased supervision plus environmental and program modification.

This agitated stage of recovery, RLA IV, is a common one, and is often confusing and frightening to family members. It will end, although the length of Posttraumatic Amnesia (PTA) can be unpredictable. The major rehab emphasis during this time is to keep you, your child, and the rehabilitation staff safe, and to provide an environment that will help your child remain as calm and oriented as possible.

"His period of Posttraumatic Amnesia (PTA) lasted until day 23, when he had gradually become more oriented and could remember new things from day to day."

Some experts believe that PTA lasting longer than twenty-four hours after the injury signifies a severe brain injury; others that PTA longer than seven days indicates a severe injury. By either criterion, Johnny has obviously sustained a severe TBI.

We now have all three major severity indicators—GCS, length of coma, and PTA—indicating that Johnny has sustained a severe TBI. Based on this alone, Johnny would be expected to improve significantly, but to have residual impairments and disabilities, most likely in cognition and behavior.

"He was discharged on day 38, to the rehabilitation day hospital program (which was structured as a classroom), to continue his rehabilitation and to facilitate a smooth transition to home, and then eventually to school. He continued his intense rehabilitation in the day hospital setting for the next four weeks. During this time, his neurologic function continued to improve. Upon discharge, a transition plan had been worked out with the school, so that he could restart his education in his own community school, with added assistance. He was independent in his ADLs. While he continued to have neuropsychological deficits, they had improved and he had also learned to compensate for some of the residual problems. He was still somewhat impulsive, and still required adult supervision for safety. He was walking with a slight limp, but without an assistive device."

As we can see, Johnny did make a great deal of improvement. Still, he had continuing needs and impairments at the end of his acute intense rehabilitation, even though the rehab program had done several important things "right":

- He had been discharged from the hospital as early as possible to receive intense coordinated rehabilitation.
- He had benefited from a rehab model that was functionally oriented. Remember, rehabilitation sometimes doesn't *generalize* well—that is, a child may have difficulty using a skill that she relearned in one setting, such as a hospital, in another setting, such as a school. This makes it important to learn things in a real-life functional environment.
- His rehab program had made certain that the next transition, to the educational system, was well worked out. All the best acute rehab in the world isn't worth much, if the transition to the home and educational system is not well planned and carried out.

It is important to remember that the end of this acute rehabilitation phase does not imply the end of recovery *or* the end of rehab. As noted earlier, recovery occurs for at least the first year after a brain injury, and some subtle but significant recovery can occur for two to five years after the injury. When your child finishes the acute part of her rehabilitation it will mean just that—that your child has now improved enough that she no longer needs it, and is ready to move to the next phase of her rehab. This will include school and some short-term outpatient therapies aimed at achieving certain goals.

■■ Conclusion

You and your child may already be through the acute rehab stage. If so, you are probably saying how glad you are that that stressful period of time is over. If you're still in that acute stage, take comfort in knowing that things should improve and that there is light at the end of the tunnel. To help you get there, make sure that you use the expertise and support of your rehab team. Optimize your communication with them, and make certain that they understand your issues, questions, and concerns.

Remember that all children are unique and that your child is not going to have all of the problems discussed in this chapter. You will have enough to occupy your time and attention without worrying about every potential problem. More importantly, remember that acute rehab is the beginning, not the end of the recovery process. The following chapters will help you on your journey.

■■ Parent Statements

I had to tell myself over and over that today I have to do what needs to be done, and then hope for the best in the future. Even though my heart sank when I thought of my son in a wheelchair with braces on, I knew that he needed it today, and hoped that he wouldn't need it in the future.

❧❦❧

I had to learn to take one day at a time, and worry about the long-term outcome later. I told myself that I could think about that when we got to one year after the injury. That was the only way that I survived.

❧❦❧

Doctors should never take away hope from a patient's family. It's the only thing that keeps us going.

❧❦❧

Once we came back to Kevin's room after he had had another X-ray, and he was counting "… 19, 20, 21…." We asked him, "Why are you counting?" He answered, "I'm seeing how long it takes until they feed me some breakfast."

❦

I feel a lot of discomfort around parents of children who are not recovering as rapidly as my son. It makes me sad.

❦

It would be easier to accept him in a wheelchair than like this. Now he looks just like before, but he's a completely different person. We lost the child that we had.

❦

To get our son to respond, the therapists would sometimes speak loudly to him and pinch him or hit him lightly. I couldn't understand why they were acting this way with someone who had just been hurt so badly.

❦

We couldn't wait for her to come out of coma, but when she did, it was worse than before. She looked at us with her eyes wide open but she didn't know us. That was a low point for me.

❦

We saw amazing progress the first six months or so after the accident, and I thought it would continue like that. The improvements are much fewer and farther between now that it's been over a year, though I still do definitely see some. You have to learn to rejoice in the little things.

❦

The staff at the rehab hospital seems like they're pushing too hard for discharge, and for me to learn how to meet my son's new needs. I need the opportunity to get to know my new son. I need time to attach to this new child. Discharge will happen when I'm ready.

❦

We had one private speech therapist who I could tell was right out of college. She meant well, but she always seemed to be asking Jeanie to do things that were too hard for her.

❦

My daughter had a private physical therapist who had a really upbeat, positive attitude. She always seemed so confident that what she was suggesting would work that her optimism rubbed off on me. She was a huge part of my support system, actually.

❧

The rehab hospital saves lives—lives of families.

3

COPING AS
A FAMILY

Jean Shultz Christianson, M.S.W., LCSW-C

■ Introduction

Just as each child's brain injury is unique, each child's family is like no other.

Each family's responses have much in common with other families' responses, but are still highly individualized. While every family's journey of adaptation usually encompasses certain experiences, feelings, and behaviors, it does not proceed in a set of orderly stages. Instead, it progresses circuitously through a range of states, in no definite sequence. There are universal experiences of vulnerability, uncertainty, "roller coaster" emotions, ambivalence. There are always countless uninvited opportunities for personal and interpersonal growth. In addition, certain inevitable contradictions seem to go hand in hand with recovery from brain injury.

Family responses to a child's brain injury are usually tied to the course of his recovery. That is, certain feelings, experiences, and ways of coping typically coincide with particular stages in the recovery process. For each stage of recovery, we will look at how families often adapt, and discuss frequently experienced contradictions, parents' common feelings, brothers' and sisters' reactions, and specific ways of coping.

For the purposes of this chapter, the stages of recovery will be identified as:

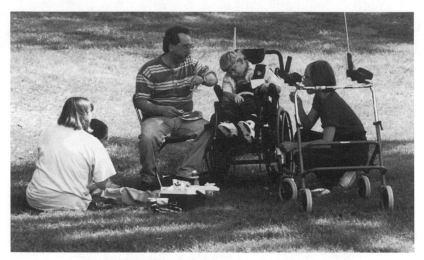

1. the acute phase,
2. the rehabilitation phase, and
3. the back-at-home phase.

Bear in mind, however, that in reality these phases of recovery are never clear-cut, with crisp beginnings and endings. When and how your family experiences the phases of recovery may vary from what is described here. In addition, you may find that feelings you have already experienced will resurface later with changing circumstances.

I. FAMILY RESPONSES TO THE ACUTE PHASE OF RECOVERY

▪▪ Frequently Experienced Contradictions

It seems that life after brain injury is full of contradictions: paradoxes, irreconcilable realities, simultaneously true but mutually exclusive facts, two sides of a coin flipping back and forth. There are certain contradictions frequently experienced by families in the acute phase.

"My Child Did Not Die, But Did Die"

"My child did not die, but did die" is often the very first contradiction you face. When a child is rushed to the hospital from the accident scene, the possibility of death often flashes through a parent's mind. When your child is admitted to the intensive care unit, that prospect becomes more believable. Suddenly, you, the parent, are in the hospital surrounded by children who are fighting for life, in rooms filled with technological equipment and squadrons of specialists. Some of the children around your child do die and parents beside you do lose their children. By some combination of circumstances—often as mysterious as the twist of fate that allowed the accident to occur in the first place—your child lives. In the course of hours, days, or weeks, doctors and nurses will assure you that your child's condition has stabilized, that a corner has been turned.

There is relief and joy. There is hope. And as you caress your child and talk soothingly, other thoughts begin to creep in. "Where is my child—the one I knew until the moment of the injury?" "I miss the little boy I knew just days before this nightmare descended." "The bright eyes familiar to me are gone."

Professionals tell you your child has survived and you believe them—you want to believe them. But that child isn't here right now. In certain ways he has died. The child you knew is missing in physical, behavioral, and emotional ways. You hope the child you knew will return. Your experience of that child as whole and safe, however, has forever changed.

Your previous experience as this child's parent has died. You are now a different parent of a different child, even though your child did not die.

The Need for Grief Work Versus Practical Tasks

In the acute phase, the "emotional roller coaster" takes off, as you come to hang on every positive or negative intonation of staff members and on each breath or blink of your child. You've been thrown into an alternative world and your emotions are in turmoil. You never can quite get your bearings. There have already been losses—your usual routine, casual conversation, confidence, sense of control—but "there's not time to think about that." There is a new contradiction at work. You have grief work to begin but you cannot address it because there are so many practical daily tasks to accomplish.

It is hard to carry out the necessary, practical chores because you are consumed by your child's great need and uncertain condition. "I don't have time to deal emotionally with what's happening," you feel. "It's all I can do to grab a snack from the vending machine, make sure someone takes the mail into the house, see that the laundry gets done, complete the hospital paperwork, figure out how many vacation days I still have left at work. . . ."

Social Support Versus Social Stress

Early on, it becomes clear that your family's social network is being put to a test. Whether relatives and friends are few or many, their reactions to your crisis can have a big impact. Sometimes people come through for you in ways you never expected. Neighbors or co-workers you barely know appear to offer assistance. Sometimes friends or family let you down, disappear, or are so emotional they make matters worse. Often social contact is simultaneously a support and a source of stress—another contradiction. "I just can't bear telling one more person how he's doing." The strain of recounting "the event," keeping your feelings in check, responding to other people's emotions can be very taxing.

The near death of a child reactivates relationships from the past. It often brings forth a parent who has been minimally involved or intensifies the need for cooperation between parents or between parents and grandparents who already have difficulty getting along. Delicate decisions are required: Who can visit? Who gets information? Who attends family meetings with medical staff? At what point should your child's friends see him? What's good for him? What's good for them? The fact that human beings are social beings is very apparent when a child is seriously injured.

▪▪ Parents' Common Feelings

Much has been written about adaptation to death and loss. A unique aspect of adapting to traumatic brain injury, though, is that family members must simultaneously come to terms with their losses while meeting their injured loved one's new needs. Adaptation is further complicated by the ongoing nature of the recovery process (often over years) and the uncertainty of outcome. Your child's needs change with time and no one can tell you for sure when or if the problems will resolve.

Shock, Numbness, Disbelief

In the acute phase, your initial reactions to your child's injury are likely to be shock, numbness, and disbelief. The information being forced upon you simply does not compute. You may not hear what is said to you, in the sense that you are not processing what is said. Things don't "sink in" and you forget what you've been told.

Loss of Control

Loss of control is another typical feeling early on. The sense of order or predictability in life vanishes. A parent can easily feel overwhelmed. It seems that most matters are out of your hands—you did not prevent the injury, professionals are in charge of your child's life, most of the variables in the situation are beyond your influence, with only fragments of a daily routine remaining. Even your own emotional responses—tears of sorrow or joy, anger, laughter—can be difficult to predict and modulate.

Anxiety and Fear

Anxiety and fear usually quickly flood through a parent's being and can be pervasive in the early days of the crisis. Uncertainty, more questions than answers, and an unfamiliar new reality trigger feelings of panic, hyper-vigilance, agitation, and emotional discomfort. It can be hard to concentrate and to eat or sleep.

Remorse, Guilt, Blame

Embedded in this mix of feelings, parents often find remorse or guilt, sometimes blame. These feelings surface as it becomes clear that your child is badly hurt, is suffering, and will have difficulties to face for some time to come. Remorse, deep sadness over the turn events took, can well up. Thoughts like "if only we had not taken that ride in the car" or, "I wish I had said 'no' instead of 'yes' that night" hover in your consciousness.

You can feel guilty when there is no conceivable way you could have prevented the injury. As a parent, a basic task is to protect your child from harm. The feeling of failure can be immense, even if it does not match the objective reality.

Sometimes parents do regret certain decisions, actions taken or not taken, or mistakes made. There can be terrible pain. It can be all-consuming. You can feel overpowering blame toward yourself or others. Somehow you must put this aside.

Parents have found that if they try to focus on the present circumstances and keep in mind how much their child needs them now—

no matter what their own pain or regret—they can go on in spite of negative feelings. They have found, too, that they may need to go outside of themselves or their usual circle of family and friends for help in struggling with remorse, guilt, and blame.

A member of the clergy, the clinical social worker or psychologist at the hospital, a psychotherapist in the community can provide support and direction. If you are able to find it in your heart to forgive, your child's recovery and your family's well-being will be enhanced.

▪▪ Sisters and Brothers

As parents are responding to their child's injury, survival, and beginning recovery, sisters and brothers are often going through parallel experiences. Often they feel much of what their parents do, but their ages and developmental stages color their understanding of events and shape their reactions. In the midst of the crisis, siblings' needs can be overlooked. Their concerns can seem the least problematic ones on a parent's endless list of exhausting worries. Some of these concerns correspond to the injured child's stage of recovery. Like their parents, siblings will find that some issues persist over time or reoccur periodically. Below are some questions that readily come to a sister's or brother's mind in the acute phase.

"'In-a-Coma': Where's That?"

First of all, siblings have the challenge of understanding what is happening. Initially, much is literally taking place behind closed doors. Events are also occurring in a foreign language: medical terminology. "'In-a-coma': where's that?" a child may wonder. "Why won't he talk to me?" "What are those tubes for?" These and hundreds of other questions are probably swirling in a child's mind, often unasked. Sometimes the child's imagined answers are even more frightening than reality.

"Why Did It Happen to Him and Not to Me?"

Other questions that can exist openly or under the surface have to do with feelings. "Why did it happen to HIM and not to ME?" "Was the crash my fault, somehow?" "I was mad at him before he got hurt—did I cause this?"

"I'm Scared."

"I'm scared" is an inevitable reaction for brothers and sisters, just as it is for parents. They suffer the intense emotions characteristic of this early phase and often face these feelings with diminished support and guidance. Still immature, they try to interpret events without an adult's cognitive tools and with limited life experience. They are likely to be overwhelmed emotionally even if they manage to succeed at the routines of daily life. For siblings, many problems at home or school—crying easily, failing to follow rules, getting into fights, skipping chores, forgetting homework—can indicate the inability to cope.

"Where Are Mom and Dad?"

An underlying question for siblings often is, "Where are Mom and Dad?" The demands of the acute phase of the injured child's recovery typically rob sisters and brothers of a parent when they too are especially vulnerable and in need of a parent's dependable support.

■■ Ways of Coping

When your child is hurt, you are suddenly whisked to an alien planet, assigned to a journey you did not choose to take, and pointed toward an unknown destination. You are in risky, foreign territory.

The ability of individuals and families to respond to difficult, almost unbearable challenges sometimes defies comprehension. Family members of a child with a brain injury often bring impressive strengths and develop new skills as they adapt. At times you feel the world will end. At times you discover and tap astonishing resilience.

This section describes some coping strategies that other families have developed, used, and shared. No one solution fits every family, but some of the following ideas may help you cope. Some strategies are uniquely applicable to the time period soon after your child's injury. Some techniques will continue to make sense over the long haul. Choose the techniques that you think will maximize your family's chances for future well-being.

1. Get Information

There is a lot to learn. Ask questions. Ask again if you forget an answer. Be honest when you do not understand. Write down what you are told. Write down names and numbers of people with whom you talk. Ask for written materials from professionals serving your child and you. Talk with other families in the hospital. Always remember that your child, your child's injury, and your family's circumstances are unique. No information you are given will definitely apply to you, but it will help you get your bearings on your journey.

2. Start a Journal

It is important to organize and safeguard the information you gather. Many parents find an ongoing log of information, events, observations, thoughts, and feelings to be an indispensable tool. A spiral-bound tablet or loose-leaf notebook with pockets can work well. So, too, can a journal kept on a computer. Be sure to date and label each entry and each volume of the journal as it expands. This can help you keep track of current happenings.

Your journal can be a vehicle for sharing experiences among family members. It can serve as an outlet for thoughts and feelings, especially during the long periods of waiting and uncertainty that can be part of acute care. Later, it can be a valuable source for forgotten facts or feelings. This journal also gives a message to staff treating your child: you are organized, tuned in, documenting your observations. Often your journal tracks information that helps the professionals helping you.

3. Find Listening Ears

Your child's trauma is yours, too. You must identify a few family members, friends, and/or professionals who can listen to you, no matter what you need to express. The emotional turmoil of a child's near death and uncertain recovery evokes strong emotions. The very process of being heard, of sharing feelings with a listener who is empathic and nonjudgmental, is healing. Often you do not seek advice; you just need to have someone present for you in the midst of your anguish. A concerned friend who can be calm under pressure is a good choice. An extended family member who wants to be helpful and is slightly less immersed in the situation can sometimes meet this need. A member of the clergy, hospital social worker, or another hospital staff member can also help fill this important role. If you have used counseling in the past, you might want to return to that therapist now, if he or she is someone you know and trust.

4. Do Talk with Loved Ones

Your "listening ear" may be someone who is not emotionally close to you. Sometimes it is painful to pour out your heartfelt sorrow or bitter anger to the spouse or partner or family member suffering beside you. You may also find it hard to listen to your companion's grief. Sometimes it feels like your hurt is magnified when the process of sharing it further pains the listener. Nevertheless, it is crucial to keep communication, and, if possible, emotional support, flowing between your partner and you.

Following a child's brain injury, there are many forces pulling parents in separate directions. Survival often dictates specialization: one parent stays at the bedside while the other tries to work so a paycheck is coming in; one parent pays the bills while the other calls relatives to provide updates. In the new split routine, the two of you can lose contact and closeness.

This is a life-changing time when important decisions are made and new patterns are established. In a two-parent household, parents need to be available to each other somehow. You may want to plan supper together in the hospital cafeteria; spend weekends together, partly at home, partly at the hospital; set up planned, routine phone appointments (not just for emergencies); strive for at least one overnight home together each week.

Sometimes aunts, uncles, grandparents, significant dating partners, or parent figures to your children have been active participants in your family's daily life before your child's brain injury. As part of the household, or an extension of it, these loved ones also need direct communication, painful as it may be.

By sharing the crisis and joining together to face the challenge, new bonds are forged and emotional links strengthened. These ties are needed so you can shoulder future burdens and celebrate future triumphs together. To the extent that loved ones can support each other, your injured child's needs will be better met in the short run and in the long run.

5. Include Sisters and Brothers

Siblings are full of questions and concerns. The adults in the family must reach out to provide them honest information, opportunities to visit their injured brother or sister, and time to spend alone with parents. Adult relatives, teachers, and close friends can be asked to supplement parents' efforts. It helps if they reach out, express concern, and provide extra support and supervision.

Brothers and sisters who write can be encouraged to keep a diary of their thoughts and questions, to be shared with adults at special times. Younger children can be encouraged to make and keep drawings depicting their experiences. Siblings of all ages can make cards and letters to be taken to the hospital. Special preparation can be made with hospital staff for a visit by siblings when a nurse, child life specialist, social worker, doctor, or other staff person can be available for support.

As a parent, you may feel relieved if your noninjured children don't give you any trouble when the rest of life feels out of control. You may feel angry if they are adding to your stress. Try to take advantage of every possible opportunity to include them in matters related to your child with TBI. If you routinely provide your noninjured children information and support, it can minimize their hidden suffering. It can also decrease problem behaviors and emotional difficulties over time.

6. Respond to Inquisitive Well-Wishers

Social support is a mixed blessing. During a crisis, you need and want the support of those close to you. Your child is injured and the whole family is hurting and vulnerable. You need help for practical and emotional reasons. If relatives and friends do not come forth, you can feel isolated, alone, angry. If they do appear, you have the challenge of figuring out how and when to respond to their questions and offers of help.

It can help if you as parents, or you as a single parent, decide who needs to know what and how they will find out. In the very beginning, identify a family spokesperson (usually a parent or immediate care giver) who will be the primary contact person for hospital staff and the conduit for key information back and forth. Also decide which family members or friends you want to provide with detailed information. That is, which people do you want to tell when your child emerges from coma, and what that means; why your child went in for another surgery; when transfer from acute care is approaching; and so forth. They, in turn, can relay information to others if you want them to, so that you are not the hub of all communications.

If your child is in school, you may want someone to be a liaison with classmates and teachers. Consider ahead of time how much information you want to share. Also decide whether there are certain acquaintances with whom you do not want to share information and certain potential visitors you want to exclude from the hospital.

Use technology creatively. Instead of worrying about not returning concerned friends' calls, try taping a message like this on your answering machine:

"Thanks for your care and concern about (child's name). We are caught up for now in (child's name)'s recovery and may not be able to get back to you. We are glad to tell you that (child's name) got out of intensive care (or equivalent update) on (the date). We so appreciate your messages. Feel free to leave one at the sound of the tone."

You can change this message weekly or whenever you feel a need to update the information. If you have select family and friends with whom you communicate by e-mail you could use a similar strategy, sending updates to the e-mail group and providing an easy way for recipients to respond to you.

Another way to manage concerned or curious questioners is to rehearse what you might want to say to them. (This works in the earlier stages and later when strangers may ask you or your child awkward questions.) A face-to-face or voice-to-voice encounter can be easier if you practice your answers ahead of time. Sometimes parents want to be honest but still pretty vague. "How is he doing?" a co-worker asks. You might reply, "He's making slow, but steady progress. He's starting to move his arms and legs." Or, "He's having his ups and downs but we are confident in his doctors and he's getting great nursing care." Or, "It's been a hard week. We really need your thoughts and prayers."

Expressions of concern by others may trigger your own emotions, sometimes tears. Though this can be embarrassing, *there is no need to apologize.* Just try saying, "I really appreciate your concern; it means a lot to our family," and keep tissues on hand for yourself and your friends.

7. Accept Help

Accepting help is tricky business, but you will have to learn to do so when your child has a brain injury. You simply cannot manage alone and your child deserves every possible resource. The private trauma of a family is somehow a public event because news travels fast and a child is part of a community. He is part of the fabric of others' lives, beyond the boundary of his family.

Those who wonder, "How's he doing?" may also ask, "What can I do to help?" This may startle or embarrass or anger you. Sometimes the genuine and best answer is simply, "Thanks a lot, but I can't think of anything right now." But sometimes there are small things that would be helpful and an automatic "no, thank you" may be a missed opportunity for a benefit to your child and family and a lost opportunity for that person. Often those who offer help need to give it. They have their own fears, grief, and helplessness and want to do something tangible. Your acceptance can help their adaptation and yours.

There are many ways that acquaintances, friends, and family can assist during your child's earliest recovery. Consider developing a mental or written list. It could include schoolmates sending a cheerful card or a group letter, a neighbor walking your dog, church members praying, friends preparing casseroles, family members checking your answering machine, parents of your children's friends supervising your children after school. Your own list will be unique to your family. At times you also may need to initiate a request for help. The challenge of coping with your child's brain injury could certainly justify such a request.

Sometimes professional help is offered. You have perhaps never needed counseling. You wonder why the hospital social worker or psychologist would stop in to see you. You need not always say "yes" to their offers of help, but try to rule out the automatic "no" that might restrict certain opportunities for your child or family. Realize, too, that hospital professionals are there for you. Even if you are just curious about how they might assist, try asking about what they do. You might discover a new resource for your child. You are in a serious situation and unusual measures may be warranted.

8. Eat and Sleep

When your child is acutely injured, he becomes the center of your universe and his needs are like a strong magnet pulling you. Your immediate reaction is to put your own needs aside and to focus wholly on his fragile life. This works for a brief time; however, adaptation following brain injury is often more like a marathon than a short sprint.

Neglecting your own needs will soon translate into decreased ability to respond effectively on your child's behalf. "I cannot leave his bedside" is an understandable reaction when your son's intracranial pressure increased suddenly just hours earlier. That response will not work weeks into the hospitalization when your own unmet physical needs for adequate nourishment and rest will interfere with your ability to observe your child and to participate effectively in decisions on his behalf.

Meeting your needs is not always incompatible with meeting your child's needs. Meeting your own needs can actually help you meet his needs. Taking care of yourself helps you care for your child.

II. FAMILY RESPONSES IN THE REHABILITATION PHASE

:: Frequently Experienced Contradictions

There are contradictions in the rehabilitation phase of your child's recovery, as there were immediately after the injury. Some contradictions continue from that earlier period; some new conflicting realities emerge. As the medical crises subside and your child progresses to the point where constant, intense scrutiny by doctors is not needed, the term "rehabilitation" is introduced. A welcome shift from the medical focus occurs. You know it is a good sign. But this idea of other kinds of problems is worrisome. It is not just that a sickness goes away and life returns to normal. There are new issues requiring new kinds of treatment: motor problems, cognitive deficits, difficulties with speech and language, unusual behavior, dependence in self-care skills. There is more work to be done by a new team of specialists. You begin to think about recovery in a different way. Recovery is not an endpoint; it is a process.

"My Child Is Recovering but May Not Recover"

A new contradiction presents itself: "My child is recovering but may not recover." At the beginning of rehabilitation, many families realize that, while things are looking better for their injured child, their child's life and theirs may never be "normal" again. As a parent,

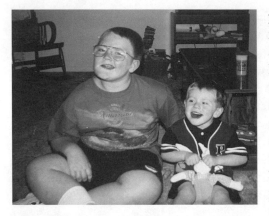

you usually remain hopeful that everything will be all right in the end. You hold firmly to the faith that this will be so, knowing that your child has already beaten the odds and has proven many of the professionals wrong. You also may feel that your positive attitude is the most potent force your child has in his favor and be reluctant to abandon hope for 100 percent recovery for fear you will sell your child short.

Part of this contradiction is that while you feel some underlying sadness about what your child cannot do and may never do, you do not know for certain what your child may have lost because of the brain injury. It is hard to mourn—though you may feel mournful—because you do not know what is lost. As one mother put it, "I don't know how much of my child I'll get back."

During this rehabilitation phase, while the focus is on making the most of every strength your child has, there is a shadow of fear that all of the problems will not disappear. Your child is definitely recovering but may not fully recover.

The Need for Flexibility Versus Structure

The uncertainty that is inherent in a child's brain injury demands enormous flexibility from parents. During this rehabilitation phase, you see inklings of your child's next ability . . . then nothing. His spoken "yes/no" is emerging. It seemed reliable last night, but this morning he nods "yes" to everything. He smiles and gives you a big kiss; a minute later he cries and screams and doesn't seem to recognize you. Your ability to "flow with it," to be in the moment without knowing how what happened an hour ago will connect with events in the hour ahead, is essential, the most valuable trait, it seems.

You are also learning, however, that "structure" and "consistency" are magic words in the world of brain injury rehabilitation. Being flexible as a parent is necessary but not sufficient to help your child to recover optimally. Flexibility requires the counterbalance of structure.

A key to recovery is providing a highly structured environment: surroundings where time, space, and the responses of family, friends, and staff are as organized, predictable, and consistent as possible. Routines are necessary.

The requirement of being simultaneously "loose" and highly organized can be daunting. Parents who can tolerate a great deal of ambiguity are often disinclined to structure and systematize the world around them. Parents who excel at creating order out of chaos are often less flexible and have trouble with uncertainty. The person with strengths in both arenas is rare. Dealing with a child's brain injury requires both types of strengths.

In a two-parent household, the mother and father sometimes have complementary coping styles. This can benefit their child with TBI. If parents do have differing coping styles, it is important that the differences be recognized and respected. Both flexibility and structure are needed for optimal recovery and effective family functioning.

Patient Focus Versus Family Focus

As time passes, there are new skills for parents to learn. Now that your child is increasingly responsive, your own reactions must be carefully matched to his level of recovery. Rehabilitation professionals have a lot to teach you and they look for as much family participation as possible. Your child may now actively demand your presence, cry when you leave, and forget that you have been with him all day. Everything seems to point to the need for you to stay in the rehabilitation setting with your injured child.

On the other hand, days, weeks, or perhaps months have elapsed since this crisis began and the needs of the rest of the family have been put aside. Your spouse, your other children, perhaps your own parents have been in the background instead of the foreground long enough to need you badly. They have their own problems; they miss you, and you them. Your other relationships clearly need tending.

This tension of being drawn in two directions (and more) at once is especially hard because by now you are tired and the end is not in sight.

"I'm a Member of the Rehabilitation Team and I'm Not"

In the acute care setting, medical issues dominated and you sometimes felt helpless, on the outside looking in. Treatment was primarily manipulation of surgical instruments, medicines, and tubes. In contrast, rehabilitation is primarily manipulation of the environment surrounding your child. Treatment includes subtle incremental changes in physical surroundings, social responses, and expectations. As a parent, your therapeutic value is especially potent, making you potentially the most valuable participant in your child's rehabilitation. No one knows your child like you do and no one has your emotional impact.

You get this message when rehabilitation begins: your goals, expectations, needs at discharge are sought out from the start. You are part of the rehab team. At the same time, the professional members of the team approach your child with a perspective all their own. They sometimes make decisions without you; they have preconceived notions about "independence" and "safety"; they have criteria that you and your child must meet in order to share a snack or enjoy a visit home. You are a member of the team and you are not.

:: Parents' Common Feelings

Anger

Anger is a feeling that can surface during the rehabilitation phase. Emergencies are less frequent now and the demands, though still relentless, are less urgent. You have time to think. Feelings submerged before can now surface. You may feel angry at your child, other family members, rehabilitation staff, even yourself.

"I can't believe the driver that hit Joe has never called ONCE to see how he's doing." "Why can't you think about someone else's needs? Your sister's in the hospital and all you care about is getting to a party." "How do you expect me to get time off work AGAIN? If the rehab team thinks I'm so important, then you can adjust to MY schedule." "If for once in your life you had done what I told you, you wouldn't have BEEN in that car and we wouldn't be IN this mess."

Relief

Many parents experience great relief when the "ups and downs" of the early days have subsided and they see a steadier course of improvement. Having almost lost their child and now seeing much of the child they know back again, they think of how much worse things could have been and are thankful for the child they have.

You may feel, "When you think about how he looked in the intensive care unit—just one month ago—and see him now, you have to believe in miracles."

Sadness

Sometimes you may look at your child and think, "He was such a perfect child; everything going for him. He has quite a struggle ahead. It makes me cry when I see he can just barely tie his shoe now."

It hurts to see your child suffer and to consider the challenges ahead. As a parent, you feel sorrow for your child and for yourself. This is not the life you planned.

▪▪ Sisters and Brothers

"When Will This Be Over?"

Often the siblings of the injured child are feeling much of what their parents experience. Sometimes they say what parents hardly dare to think, and they ask unspoken questions, such as "When will this be over?" Like you, the parents, they are tired of this troublesome interruption of normal life and are ready to get on with things as before. Rehabilitation can seem to drag on forever and "getting better" does not seem to end.

"What's 'Rehab'?"

If your brother is "getting better" but isn't like he was, what are they doing in that rehab hospital? Rehabilitation can be mysterious to a brother or sister. It is hard to understand why someone who walks and talks needs a wheelchair to travel the length of the hallway and sometimes speaks nonsense. Hospitals are supposed to fix people so that "getting better" means everything is OK. Understandably, siblings may wonder if rehab means doing the best you can with something bad, and not REALLY making things completely better.

"Why Can't We Do What We Used to Do?"

As parents, you feel the tension of being pulled in competing directions. Your noninjured children know that you've pulled away from them. Things they used to count on aren't happening—repeatedly—now. Going clothes shopping, discussing homework, eating a home-cooked meal have become rare events. They probably feel jealous of the time you devote to your child with TBI, even resentful sometimes.

"Where is the Family?"

"Where is the FAMILY?" is the big question that emerges during rehabilitation. If parents and children are rarely experiencing life in the same place and time, the children at home can feel disconnected. Depending on their ages, they may try to create a substitute form of family life where they help each other and rely on outsiders to fill unmet needs. Sometimes they turn to their parents in new ways. Dad, instead of Mom, prepares school lunches; Mom, instead of Dad, picks them up after ball practice. The family as they knew it is missing right now.

■■ Ways of Coping

Caught up in the demands of rehabilitation, you can be totally absorbed in the details of your child's stages of recovery, the conflicts of where to spend your precious time, the worry that life may never be the same. There are, however, things you can do that other parents have found helpful. These include strategies that were useful earlier as well as some new ones.

1. Keep Track of How Far You Have Come

The journey ahead can look very long during rehabilitation. Be sure to look back as well as ahead. Usually you can identify insurmountable odds that were overcome, as well as gradual long-term gains that have been achieved. It is vital to give yourself and your loved ones credit for how far you have already come. Be sure to recognize the individual and family strengths that have already produced unexpected achievements.

2. "One Day at a Time"

"One day at a time" is probably the phrase most frequently verbalized by parents successfully coping with their child's rehabilitation. The ability to narrow your focus to current challenges makes it possible to expend emotional, mental, and physical energy where it is most needed. Focusing on today instead of stewing over the past or brooding about the future gives you the best chance of having a positive impact now. These daily positives add up to a more promising future.

3. Be Honest with Yourself and Others

When your child with TBI is weeks or months into the recovery process, the shock has probably worn off. Now the stresses of reality weigh upon you and basic existential questions about values and meaning and why bad things happen cannot be avoided. Your life is very much different from before. You and your family need to openly consider these things and decide how to manage in new ways.

What is most important for your injured child and for the whole family? What do you relinquish? What do you hold on to? Here's an example:

You have planned a special summer vacation for a long time. Should the vacation be postponed due to all the uncertainties? Could your child with TBI tolerate it? Would it be enjoyable? Is it extravagant, given recent unexpected expenses? Could it be carried off in a different way? Are you too exhausted to plan a break? Can you take additional time away from work? Is it too painful to tell the children it won't happen? Is it compatible with recommended therapies? Is a shared experience like this just what the family needs right now?

Here's another example:

Honor roll grades are important in your family. Your children have always done well in school. High academic achievement is expected and your family takes pride in this. The injured child's teenaged sister wants to take a week off school to spend time in the rehabilitation hospital. She is asking to participate in her brother's therapies. She has not been studying much and her grades have been low. The end of the term is approaching and she needs to focus on her work or will do poorly. Is this a time to lower the family standard? Is she taking advantage of you? Will you set a precedent that will create problems later? Will she be better able to return her attention to school if she has a better understanding of her brother's condition? Would spending time at the hospital be more beneficial closer to discharge? What will her teachers think? Would it be good to have her with you for a stretch of time like this? Would this be an opportunity for you to leave the hospital for awhile each day?

Each family's answers to questions like these will be unique. There will be many choices to make as the impact of the one family member's brain injury is realized. Friends and acquaintances, too, need to learn that things are different for your family. Protecting them from the truth is no service to your child, your family, or them.

Being honest includes careful self-assessment and recognition of when to say "no" rather than "yes." You are at a point where you have to take stock of what you can and cannot do. Immediately after the injury you were probably on "automatic pilot." Now, in this middle phase, you have to consciously address reality, recognize that the challenge is a marathon—not a sprint—and plan accordingly. In some ways this can be more painful than the initial crisis, because the shock and numbness are wearing off. You can no longer believe that everything will be back to normal soon.

You must evaluate your present situation: What are you doing that you need to stop? What are you not doing that you need to resume or begin? What have you considered doing that you may have to give up for now? For example, if you have been rooming in or spending most of your waking time with your child with TBI, you will need to consider changing this pattern when he begins inpatient rehabilitation. It can be very difficult, even frightening. Can you now trust staff to care for your child? Are there ways you can stay on top of what's happening without staying in the hospital so much? Are there others who could regularly visit in your stead? If you do limit your time at the hospital, what can you say "yes" to?

Usually, "neglected" areas include roles and responsibilities separate from attention to the injured child, such as return to work or school, resumption of household chores, attention to financial matters, time with spouse and/or other children, interaction with extended family or friends. You probably also need to say "yes" to your own self-care—exercise, sleep, balanced meals. Are there other plans or activities that you now may need to cancel or postpone, such as the extra class you were going to take, the volunteer work you had agreed to do, the push for a promotion at work? Again, there is no one correct answer to any of these questions. There is just the suggestion that you seriously examine what you can and cannot do at this point in your journey with your child with TBI. Get support from hospital professionals and other families as you examine your family's new situation.

4. Involve Brothers and Sisters

Part of facing a new reality is including siblings in decisions about the family. The strategies from the acute phase continue to make sense in the midst of rehabilitation. But sisters and brothers now need help coming to terms with changes that won't be over quickly.

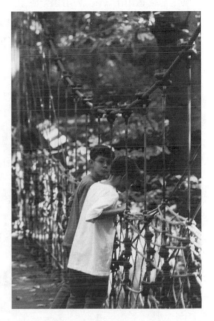

If at all possible, arrange regular family meetings between parents and noninjured siblings. In time, your child with a brain injury can be included, but probably not yet. Adjust information to your children's ages, and systematically discuss progress, disappointments, plans for the week ahead. Give the children the chance to ask questions and to offer insights and opinions. Really listen. Find out what matters most to different family members. Begin to plan together for a sibling visit to the rehabilitation program, for an initial visit home by your child with TBI, and for discharge. If you have a hard time talking about these difficult things, ask the rehabilitation social worker or psychologist for help.

Give sisters and brothers an opportunity to observe therapy sessions. Participation in occupational, physical, or speech-language therapy makes rehabilitation real and concrete. With the assistance of these professionals, identify specific things siblings can do to help, such as speak slowly and only ask one thing at a time; play catch gently with a bean bag; or leave certain foods at home if they are forbidden to your child with TBI.

5. Begin to Refocus on Home

Part of the routine in this phase is for parents to resume some of the roles and responsibilities that have been put on hold. The overall goal of your child's inpatient rehabilitation is to return home. While therapists work to maximize your child's function and independence and arrange for any necessary equipment, they teach you skills needed to manage your child in the community. The day your child starts rehabilitation, all steps are directed toward discharge. This means you as a family, too, need to switch your focus away from a "sick" child toward a child who will have the most normal life possible at home and in the community. It may be hard to imagine that it might not be your "old child" who is discharged. It may help you to remember that recovery and rehabilitation will continue after that day.

6. Rediscover Humor

Your child's condition and treatment are serious matters to be taken seriously. Along the way, though, funny things happen and it is OK to laugh. While it is never good to make fun of your child, it is normal to see humor in life's difficult moments. It is an important aspect of coping and it can release pent-up emotion. Regaining the ability to smile and laugh also signals that you believe life will go on.

III. FAMILY RESPONSES TO THEIR CHILD'S HOMECOMING

:: Frequently Experienced Contradictions

Risk Versus Safety

Contradictions continue, some old, some new, when your child with TBI is back home with the family. A big one is the need to encourage your child's independence, which involves some risk, while you keep him secure and safe. The balancing act between risk and security is a theme from your child's earliest acute care—to perform a risky procedure, or not; to discontinue a medication, or not.

At home, you are in authority and your child probably has little awareness of the dangers at hand or of his limitations. Your child probably wants to do what he did before. You want him to have as many normal experiences as possible and you DON'T want another injury. You also feel he's lost a lot and feel guilty depriving him of any positive experience. "Tom is determined to ride his bike again, even though he still gets confused just finding his way back to the house from the mailbox." "Jenny's friends want to take her to the mall. I can't bear to let her out of my sight, but one girl in particular has a good head on her shoulders and seems to recognize the changes in Jenny."

Medical Miracles and Societal Inadequacies

"They did a great job saving Sam—actually brought him back to life. But now he's been home awhile and insurance has stopped covering therapies; my family leave is used up; his friends have fallen away; education funds were cut, so there's no summer school program." With your child back home, you may experience discrepancies between the resources poured into the technology that saved him and the resources now available to maximize his quality of life. Your child was saved—usually not cured—and now you need to work to sensitize those around you to your child's and family's needs.

Old Child and New Child

The child back at home with you is both familiar and different. As time passes, more of his "old self" emerges. It is a relief. There are also traits that catch you by surprise—he may be more outgoing, funnier—and new qualities that disturb you—he may have a quick temper or dislike reading.

Let Go of the Past and Hold onto the Past

You know you cannot spend the rest of your days dwelling on what life was like before your child's brain injury. In time that event recedes. You need to move on, concentrating on life's current achievements and challenges, regardless of how they might have been different without the injury. On the other hand, the history of your child and family before the injury remains as much at the core of your family's identity as the traumatic event imposed upon it. The dreams and goals remain, stated and unstated, and shape how you experience reality now. Your awareness of what has been lost and gained depends on your ability to look back, to see where you and your child have come from.

■■ Parents' Common Feelings

Exhilaration

Exhilaration often accompanies discharge. Your child is elated to "get out of this place" at last and you have the thrill of achieving this long-awaited goal. The scene is triumphal, even if your child uses canes or is unable to clearly say, "Good-bye!" Your child and family have earned a celebration.

Fear

Most parents welcome discharge, but worry as the reins are placed in their hands. Some of this fear will subside as you establish a new family routine and fine tune the management techniques you have learned so they will work better at home. You will probably gain confidence as your experience at home lengthens. Through practice, you will learn who and when to call about concerns you cannot manage alone.

You may always be a little bit afraid that something bad will happen again, either to this child, yourself, or someone else. Experience has taught you that the unexpected *can* happen in your family and in dozens of families you have met while your child was recovering.

Life Will Never Again Be the Same

Most families feel changed forever by their child's brain injury. No matter how perfect the recovery, how strong the supports, how excellent the treatment, they and their child are different because of the injury. In fact, everyone closely attached to them is changed. The experiences of loss, of gain, of helplessness, of meeting a challenge, of asking for help, of facing disappointment, of receiving the care and concern of others, of learning what is most important—these experiences change people.

Reconciliation

In time, over years, most families reach a point where they are reconciled to what has happened. They hold onto their dreams, they mourn their losses, and they move ahead. Family members have good times and bad. They have moments "out of the blue" when they re-experience intense sadness or anger or fear, when they are catapulted back to the earliest events and feelings following the brain injury. But life does go on. The children become adults, achieving some goals and failing at others. The parents have varying degrees of burden. The siblings mature, indelibly marked by the experience of one family member's injury, but able to achieve their own developmental tasks. Usually, the child's injury is one important part of a large, full life. Individual family members and families as a whole are forever changed, but they come to terms with what life has been and move forward to make it the very best it can be now.

▪ Sisters and Brothers

"Who Is This Person Who Came Home?"

Brothers and sisters are acutely attuned to changes in their injured sibling. At discharge, their dreams of life getting immediately back to normal are dashed. Differences in their sibling with TBI are usually obvious, and it is clear that he will still absorb a lot of attention and require sacrifices on their part.

"How Old *Am* I, Anyway?"

The return of your child with TBI may force siblings to re-examine their understandings about age, appropriate responsibility, and expectations. A younger sibling can be baffled by the experience of seeing an older sister behave like a baby. An older sibling can feel weighed down by increased responsibilities for a younger brother with poor memory. The predictable, ordering factor of age loses meaning.

"What Do I Tell My Friends?"

School-aged sisters and brothers are very conscious that their sibling with TBI does not blend right back into the social group. Usually, there has been much community attention during the whole course of his recovery. The return home rarely escapes notice and may even be chronicled in the local paper.

Siblings have usually been asked questions all along. Now, the changed behavior, odd gait, or diminished social skills are visible to the world. Sisters or brothers can be embarrassed, torn between loyalty to their sibling and the desire to be accepted by peers, freshly aware of how different their sibling still is, in spite of dramatic gains and hard work on everyone's part. Siblings may feel like hiding. They may be able to say, "He's my brother. His brain was hurt. It controls everything so it's hard for him to do some things. He is still healing. Sometimes he needs our help."

"I Like the Way Life Used to Be."

It is natural for brothers and sisters to miss the way life was before their sibling's brain injury. It is important that they have opportunities to say this aloud to their parents. It is also important that they learn not to say it in front of their injured sibling. They need to explore with adults what they miss and how some of those experiences can resume. It is important for parents not to label these, or other feelings, as bad or unacceptable. This does not make them disappear. These feelings are real and deserve consideration in a deliberate manner.

"What about *Me?*"

Sisters and brothers usually make a lot of sacrifices in the course of their sibling's trauma and recovery. Although your child's discharge to home centralizes the family under one roof again, it does not necessarily rebalance the attention equation. The consequences of the injury may actually be more obvious and have more impact when your child returns home. Siblings need:

- reassurance about their importance,
- protection of their boundaries,
- encouragement to keep sharing their feelings,
- acknowledgment of their contributions to the family, and
- guidance on how to learn and grow under these new circumstances.

You will need to make a conscious effort to provide your other children with these things. Some ways to do this include:

- **Provide concrete evidence of your interest in them:** share activities that are important to them, such as hobbies or sports events; discuss how school is going; ask questions about their friends; celebrate their accomplishments and special events.
- **Ask about their feelings and set aside time to talk.** When their feelings emerge unsolicited, try to respond at that moment and then find a time to follow up in more depth. Your children need the message that negative as well as positive feelings can be shared, even though you may find it hard to hear their sadness or anger.
- **Acknowledge the sacrifices and contributions they are making.** Parents often emphasize the suffering and losses of the child with TBI. From a sister's or brother's viewpoint, however, it seems that he is getting constant attention. The other siblings need any recognition possible for their efforts, from parents as well as others outside the immediate family.

■ *Help them find ways to use your family's challenges for their own maturation.* Depending on their developmental stages, they might be asked to help their sibling with his range of motion exercises, to supervise him as he sets the table, or to play a memory game with him. This kind of involvement and responsibility can help sisters and brothers grow in competence and confidence.

∷ Ways of Coping

1. Find Others Who Understand

You may have mixed feelings about leaving the hospital for home. In inpatient rehabilitation your child fit in, you were surrounded by people who needed no explanations, you were not alone. That support is needed now as much as ever. There may be a few families you "clicked" with before in inpatient or outpatient rehabilitation settings. Do not hesitate to stay in touch with them by phone or e-mail. Think about getting together with them.

Join your local Brain Injury Association. (See the Resource Guide at the back of the book.) The Brain Injury Association is a source of information, advocacy opportunities, social activities, and support groups for survivors, siblings, and/or parents. Even if you are not ready to get involved (and many parents are not, initially) you can learn about what is happening and can know that others share your experiences. You are not alone. Your anger, which will inevitably surge forth at times, can be harnessed and directed positively with the help of others who truly understand.

The Internet offers families direct access to a wide range of information, organizations, and resources. An excellent starting point is the Brain Injury USA Home Page, found at http://www.biausa.org.

Stay in contact with your rehabilitation setting even if treatment officially ends. Staff members are a resource for you and can be a link to compatible families if you let them know of your interest.

Mental health professionals familiar with brain injury can also be of direct support as your child makes the transition to home or when you face challenges requiring special expertise. If you find you simply cannot function, are unable to carry out your roles, struggle to meet your responsibilities, or do not find enjoyment in life, be sure to seek professional help. Your rehabilitation setting, local Brain Injury Association, or family physician can direct you to a clinical social worker, behavioral psychologist, neuropsychologist, or psychiatrist qualified to address your concerns. Sometimes a combination of professionals is best for understanding and alleviating family members' problems related to a child's brain injury.

2. Go with Your Strengths

No one person has the range of talents to meet all of the needs of a child with traumatic brain injury. You did not ask for this assignment and you are not superhuman. The parenting tasks can be intimidating. Early on, identify the skills you bring to the situation. Your spouse, a close friend, a trusted relative, or a mental health professional can assist in this self-assessment. Recognize your abilities and figure out how you can use them on your child's and family's behalf. Do you keep excellent records? Are you a good listener? Maybe you are an assertive advocate or unusually patient or able to use your sense of humor to ease family tensions. Use and develop your gifts.

3. Admit Your Weaknesses

Not every parent is cut out to manage every parenting task. It helps to identify your weaker points so those liabilities do not hinder your child's progress and your family's development. Do you talk too much, so others don't get much chance to express themselves? Are you inflexible? Maybe you have difficulty saying, "No?" Again, it can be useful to reflect on this with a trusted, more objective observer.

Once you have identified your weaknesses, you can make a concerted effort to improve them or find other ways to fill these gaps. If you are part of a two-parent family, you and your spouse can develop complementary abilities. For example, one of you may be skilled at organizing and submitting health insurance paperwork, while the other is gifted in explaining your child's learning difficulties to professionals. One parent may be a natural at diffusing sibling conflicts, while the other easily masters the schedule for administering medication.

Specialization is fine. It's not necessary that both of you know everything equally well. Sometimes you discover your own and each other's strengths. Sometimes you also realize weaknesses. Inadequacies that have previously been a source of conflict may resurface or seem more significant. It is important to openly discuss them. If you are unable to resolve conflicts yourselves, it's important to look beyond yourselves for assistance, including help from professionals, if needed.

If you are a single parent, extended family or friends may be able to help in your areas of weakness. In any situation, creative solutions can grow out of honest self-appraisal.

There can be a temptation to rely on the noninjured children in the family to fill the gaps. A little of this is fine and can promote new competencies and a sense of responsibility. The children's develop mental needs and abilities must always be taken into account. For example, a six-year-old brother or sister might be able to make sure there's always a supply of diapers in the cabinet by the bedside; a twelve-year-old might routinely pack lunch bags for school; a fifteen-year-old might be capable of providing supervision while a parent runs errands.

Although siblings can offer valuable assistance under some circumstances, remember that their main job is to be children, not parents. If you take steps now to preserve their healthy development, it will enhance their future ability to have a positive, productive relationship with their brother or sister with TBI.

4. Do Not Dwell on the Past or Live in the Future

One key to successful coping is to focus on the present. When your child has been badly hurt and still has problems as a result of that event, it can be hard not to concentrate on that event or what life was like before that defining moment. Likewise, you carry worries about what the future will bring. "He always wanted to be a veterinarian. Every day I wonder if he'll ever achieve that goal."

These thoughts are unavoidable. But you can best influence the future by focusing today on the values and skills that will keep your child's future options as open as possible. Does he still want to be a vet? Which school courses most relate to that goal? Can he handle them? Is there an animal-related volunteer experience or job opportunity available? Can he achieve some of these tasks? All of them? Does he like doing them?

Current choices and actions can link past and future. If you are suspended anywhere but in the present, you are helpless to shape your child's future. If you are immobilized and cannot concentrate on today, you may need the advice and support of mental health professionals.

5. Consciously Rebuild Your Family

Reorganization of your family is best accomplished through a thoughtful, gradual process. All family members have been changed by one member's injury. The trauma has been the whole family's trauma. This does not mean everyone or everything is totally changed, just that there has been some impact.

Usually the emotional bond between one parent (often the mother) and the child with TBI has intensified. The feelings are not all positive, but there can be an especially strong connection now, related to the time and energy that parent has invested. One consequence is that less energy is expended on other family relationships.

In a two-parent household, the marriage has often been neglected. Sometimes wife and husband have been alternating duties for months, and when their paths do cross, they are tired. Precious moments together are used to solve the most pressing problems. Time as a couple is unusual; opportunities for intimacy and sexual expression are rare. Also, siblings have usually missed out on much family interaction while events in the hospital absorbed their parents and their sibling with TBI.

With everyone back at home now, it is time to restore some balance in family patterns. This benefits the whole family, not just the child with TBI. In two-parent families, set aside **couple time.** You may need to establish a "date night" when you go out alone, even if it is just to take a ride. The children need to know that this is a priority. If you are a single parent, it is also important to get out for a break.

It can be very hard to get out of the house for many reasons. The first obstacle is often obtaining care for your child with TBI. If there are no family members or friends who can help, look for leads about respite through parents of other children with special needs, your child's school, the local Brain Injury Association, or the state agency serving children with developmental disabilities. Most states have respite care programs with care providers trained to meet the needs of children with disabilities. Services are usually available on a sliding scale, depending on your ability to pay.

If it is hard for you to entrust your child to anyone else's care, start small. Leave for a short length of time at first, and don't go far if it makes you too anxious. Have modest expectations for yourself and your spouse or companion when you first go out. You will inevitably spend some of the time talking about your child with TBI. Gradually make yourself venture on to other topics and ask your partner to help you think about other things. This may be very uncomfortable, perhaps because it's been so long since you tried to change focus. You might feel guilty trying to enjoy yourself. You might find it hard to face issues you have avoided in the hurry and distraction of day-to-day living.

Resume some regular activity as a family or establish a family activity that all can enjoy. Maybe you can still have picnics at the park, with some modifications. A trip to the mall might work out if you keep it brief and take a wheelchair for now. It might make more sense to have a home video night because your injured child's attention span is shorter and the movie theater is too distracting.

Take turns letting family members select preferred activities. Not everyone will always get top priority, including your child with TBI. Recognize that some previous favorite family activities might now have to be shared by some, not all. Sometimes there are ways to modify a favorite activity. Be sure to openly acknowledge changes and compromises. If it seems that these are temporary, say so. As much as possible, ask your children to share in the problem solving that goes into modifying activities.

Create opportunities for one-on-one parent-child time with the various parent-child combinations (for example, older brother and Mom, younger brother and Mom, older brother and Dad, younger brother and Dad). It does not have to be elaborate, just individualized and predictable. Perhaps Dad and younger sister or brother can routinely wash the car together, visit the pet store, or play catch. Maybe Mom and teenaged brother or sister can garden, practice for a driver's license, or go to the library. The idea is to structure time together in a way that doesn't overly burden anyone and allows natural opportunities to talk and re-experience each other.

Share family meals. Eating together establishes regular times to talk about daily events. In a way, you all need to get to know each other again. It's usually good to turn off the television and limit distractions, for everyone's sakes. You may choose to turn off the telephone as well. You are trying to establish an environment that encourages family interaction and gives the message that family is indeed important.

Share responsibilities. Structure is vital to successful coping with brain injury. Along with routines for recreation together, rou-

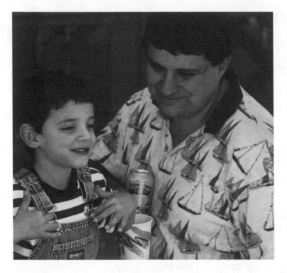

tines for the chores that keep a household running need to be established or re-established. The abilities of all family members must be taken into account. Under most circumstances, however, all of your children can be expected to do chores on a regular basis. Working together is as important as playing together. As the inevitable conflicts arise, they can be used as problem-solving opportunities.

Sometimes rebuilding the family requires professional help. Family difficulties that were present before the brain injury may predispose you to difficulties now. In addition, if any family member had mental health problems before your child's injury, they may be exacerbated by this trauma. The injury-related problems of your child with TBI may also pose major challenges, making it hard for family members to communicate and cooperate. You may feel stuck as you try to adjust and restore family life. Family therapy with a qualified mental health professional familiar with brain injury can help get you on track as a family. Be sure also to read the suggestions in Chapters 7 and 8 for dealing with behavior problems.

▪▪ Mysteries of Time

A family's experience of traumatic brain injury changes over time. The event can also change the experience of time. Parents talk about how, "in an instant, life is changed forever." One moment's happening immediately demands change and alters perceptions about life. Adaptability becomes a trait worth gold.

On the other hand, it can feel like recovery "takes an eternity." Some experiences can feel stretched out, elongated, painfully slow. Patience becomes a priceless treasure.

Then, again, "there are not enough minutes in the day." Time plays tricks. The tasks of family members seem to multiply and time shrinks. There is never enough of it.

A child's traumatic brain injury and subsequent recovery process can also provide a new slant on the present. Parents talk about how they learn to deeply appreciate "the moment." The capacity for joy and thankfulness in the present can grow dramatically.

Is it true that "time heals?" In a literal sense, time allows the opportunity for biological healing. The passage of time also provides a chance for psychological and social changes in individuals, families, and those around them so they can develop responses appropriate to new conditions. With the passage of time, new perspectives can emerge. Priorities often shift. Values come into the foreground as hard decisions are faced. Time itself does not heal, but its passage is like the paper of a scroll unrolling, providing the backdrop on which new understandings and gradual realizations can be recorded.

▪▪ Conclusion

No two brain injuries are alike and no two families react in the same way. There are, however, experiences that many families have in common. Certain sets of contradictions appear frequently in the course of recovery. Families often feel specific emotions in response to a child's brain injury. Sisters and brothers have typical questions. There are strategies for coping that work successfully for many families.

Life is never the same after a child's brain injury, even though recovery may be superb and family adaptation may be exemplary. There is suffering. Something is always lost. Sometimes there are new burdens. Often, too, there are unexpected opportunities for growth and transformation.

Many families travel ahead of you on this uncertain journey. Professionals walk beside you. The world around us is becoming more and more aware of the "silent epidemic" of brain injury, increasingly attuned to the challenges your child and your family face.

Families have taught us much in our work with children with brain injuries. We hope that the ideas gathered here will ease your journey through this new, uncertain territory.

■ Parent Statements

It has been hard on her brothers and sisters, especially the little ones. For one thing, she gets all of our attention and they resent it. The older one is embarrassed to have friends over or to go anywhere in public with the family.

❦

I have to admit, my husband and I were embarrassed by her behavior at first, but the therapists said it would be good for her to get out. So, we go out, and if strangers have a problem with it, I can't worry about them. My family comes first.

❦

I'm so embarrassed to go anywhere with him. He acts too weird and everyone looks at us. (Sister of a teenaged boy with TBI)

❦

I'm not sad about the way Robbie is now. I'm sad for the way he used to be. (Seven-year-old sibling of a child with TBI)

❦

All my friends are telling me that I should be able to move beyond this. It has been two years since the car accident. What they don't realize is that brain injuries don't ever heal.

❦

It's been literally years since my husband and I have been out by ourselves. I couldn't tell you the last movie we went to see.

❦

We've become a real solid unit, my husband and I. There are so many important things going on in our lives, it's as if we have to just laugh off the little irritants that we would have been arguing about in the past. We are just always so focused on doing what's right for every member of our family.

❦

Sometimes I am so mad at him for doing this to us, to me. What was he thinking, being so careless? Now our lives will never, ever be the same.

❦

Everybody thinks that my child is fine because he looks so good and is walking and talking. Only I seem to understand that he is not the same as he was before his accident.

❦

I have learned that I have the capacity to love my child as he is and to see the value in him as a person. I feel very good about myself for that. It helps me put everything in life in perspective.

HELPING YOUR CHILD ADJUST

Cynthia H. Bonner, M.S.W., LCSW-C

■ Introduction

Although no two children or their brain injuries are alike, many children struggle with similar emotions and challenges after TBI. These include:

- denial that the injury will have a long-term impact,
- grief over their loss of function and skill,
- changes in how they relate to others,
- frustration with the recovery process, and
- limited awareness of the differences in themselves.

Your child's ability to cope with or develop strategies for dealing with these changes will vary depending on many factors. Some of these may include your child's previous coping skills, her intellect and personality, the support available from friends and family, her emotional health, the strength of her relationships, the stage of development she was in when injured, and the extent of the injury.

As a parent, you will play a key role in helping others understand your child. Thanks to your unique experience parenting your child, you will be able to provide professionals with valuable information and insight into your child's individual traits. During the rehabilitation process, parents' involvement and commitment are often seen as pivotal to their child's recovery and return to home and school.

To help you better help your child, this chapter will examine some of the changes that children with TBI commonly face during the acute, rehabilitation, and back-at-home phases of the recovery process. It will also offer suggestions for helping your child cope with and adjust to these changes.

■■ Your Child During the Acute Phase

Once your child's condition is stabilizing and she is beginning to emerge from coma, you feel some reassurance. There is joy, relief, and hope but still uncertainty. You try not to be overjoyed, as the road ahead is still uncertain, but you experience some slight relief, a small lift of the burden. This was the small step, the sign that everyone has been waiting for. From this moment forward, your experience of parenting your child is changed forever.

In the acute phase, as you are trying to manage your emotional roller coaster, you find yourself asking, "What should I be doing for my child?" Below are some suggestions for supporting your child as she emerges from coma.

Emerging from Coma

Emerging from a coma is a frightening experience for a child. One child recalled the experience this way: "I remember being scared and wondering where I was. I remember there were doctors and nurses and I saw my mom sitting by the side of my bed." Each child's beginning steps of recovery are unique and marked by varying memories. The environment is unfamiliar and your child's memories leading up to the injury may be unclear and uncertain. Usually, there is no memory of the actual injury. Uncertainty and unfamiliarity mark the beginning of the road ahead that your child now faces in coping with the changes in herself.

When your child is emerging from coma, there will be times when she is not alert or responsive. Providing stimulation, support, voice, and touch can be helpful to your child. Even if your child is not responsive, providing this support can help *you* feel connected to your child. If possible, surround your child with familiar items, including pictures of family members and friends, mementos from home, and familiar music. Try to create a familiar environment within the unfamiliar hospital room. When you are ready, encourage close family members to visit your child. You and your family members should keep talking to your child, providing those familiar voices and reassuring words of love and support.

■ Your Child During the Rehabilitation Phase

The work begins. Your child may be faced with many physical, cognitive, and emotional challenges. As a parent, you are constantly observing and encouraging your child, hoping for changes, slight improvements that might ultimately lead to larger accomplishments. Your child may experience difficulty walking, managing personal care, expressing wants and needs, and remembering: things that she once did without any thought or effort. Now is the time in the recovery phase where the effort to regain previously mastered skills begins. Demands are placed and goals are set, as a variety of specialists begin challenging your child to reach her potential. Your child begins making small, slow steps toward larger accomplishments.

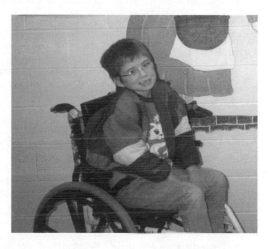

During the rehabilitation phase, your child may have difficulties with memory, self-awareness, and problem solving. She may have sudden changes in her emotions (emotional lability) or show no emotions at all (flat affect). She may also become easily frustrated, fatigued, and irritable, and have changes in her behavior and personality. These changes often lead to poor social behavior and interactions with others.

Confronted with Changes

Recovery is a gradual and challenging process with no clear endpoint. It varies depending on the injury and the child. As your child begins to slowly emerge and progress, deficits become more apparent. Your child may be discouraged by the slowness of progress and the ups and downs that come with recovery. Seemingly simple activities may now by difficult to perform. She may also be faced with accepting changes in her physical appearance. Often there are healing wounds that are difficult for a child to accept. Hair may have been shaved immediately following the injury. Your child may not be comfortable with changes in her appearance. Additionally, she may be frustrated by her new physical limitations. For instance, a once very active 14-year-old basketball player with artistic talents was very frustrated by the difficulties he experienced in walking, and in using his dominant hand to eat, care for personal needs, and draw as he used to.

Difficulties with Insight and Awareness

Sometimes children are not aware of other emerging differences aside from the physical differences. They may not agree that their academic performance, memory, language skills, behavior, personality, or social behavior have changed. Often children lack insight into their cognitive deficits, as it is easier to see, understand, and focus on rehabilitation of the physical differences. This can be particularly challenging for family members who are able to observe both the physical and cognitive difficulties their child is facing.

Developmental Stages

During the rehabilitation phase your child is working hard to regain a multitude of lost skills. Your child has experienced a tremendous amount of change in herself in a very short period of time. How your child views those changes will likely depend on her stage of development. For instance, an infant or toddler will have little understanding of her differences. Older children and adolescents have more capacity to understand these changes in self that can affect identity, self-perception, peer relations, previously mastered skills, and goals for the future.

Often children and adolescents experience grief, anger, a decrease in self-esteem, and depression, as the loss of skills and changes in personality, social behavior, academic performance, communication, language skills, and appearance become more apparent. During adolescence, children normally struggle with the formation of their identity and have often formulated negative attitudes toward those who are different, less capable, and less "cool." The discrepancy between an adolescent's former and current self can be problematic.

▪▪ What You Can Do for Your Child during the Rehabilitation Phase

During this rehabilitation phase, your family will become central to recovery and the primary support for your child. You can provide professionals with specific information that can't be gleaned by testing, serving as a window into your child. You know your child best, and have the commitment to become her lifelong advocate. Below are some suggestions that will help you and other family members support your child.

Focus on Daily Successes

During the rehabilitation phase, your child may be discouraged by the slow process of recovery, experiencing periods of ups and downs. Help her to see recovery as a long process by focusing on the daily positives and progress already made. You can compare specific challenges to other times in life when accomplishing a goal took time and was challenging. For example, you might remind her of the time when she practiced her flute every day and took private lessons to prepare for her audition for the school orchestra. Praise your child for her accomplishments since the injury. Be supportive and encouraging while maintaining realistic goals. Try not to evoke additional frustration by focusing on the negative, putting extra pressure on your child to perform, or setting goals that she is not ready for.

It may be difficult to see your child struggle with physical needs as well as cognitive demands. You can help, however, by reinstilling confidence while she is relearning and regaining skills. When appropriate, encouraging her to be independent can help your child feel a sense of self-worth.

Your child's feelings and motivation may fluctuate as she faces numerous changes during the recovery period. Family members can help by providing consistency, support, and encouragement. Focus on the positive, and minimize critical feedback. Again, you know your child best—what motivates her, her personality, her previous coping style, and her level of acceptance. Communicate this knowledge to professionals who work with your child.

Your role in supporting your child in her daily coping may seem like a high-wire balancing act, but remember that your family is her primary source of support. It is well worth your efforts to do whatever it takes to help your child regain her participation in the outside world.

Managing Changes in Appearance

How much of an emotional impact your child's physical changes have on her will depend on her age and stage of development. Your child may not like the way she now appears to others and may therefore be uncomfortable with visits by friends and family members. Helping your child understand the importance of family and friends in her life may help to ease her discomfort. In the meantime, it is fine to respect her wishes and minimize the number of visitors until she feels more comfortable.

Help your child feel as comfortable as possible with her appearance. For example, allow her to wear a baseball cap or clothing that covers her injuries if it makes her feel more secure.

If your child feels comfortable discussing her differences (for example, hair, stitches, cuts, scars, braces/splints), encourage her to talk about them and how they affect how she perceives herself. Discuss how these physical changes also take time to heal. Hair grows back and some cuts and scars will fade over time. It may help your child to see photographs of herself before the injury and during the course of recovery so that together you can observe and realistically discuss changes.

If your child does not seem comfortable discussing her appearance, take her lead. Minimizing the attention placed on physical appearance may reduce the importance of this in your child's mind. Listen to your child if she wishes to talk about her appearance, but do not keep bringing up the topic if it seems to be a sore subject for her. Once again, you know your child best.

Understanding Cognitive Changes

It is often difficult for a child to conceptualize the magnitude of a brain injury and its effects on memory, problem-solving ability, language, and personality. With the assistance of professionals, you can help your child to understand all that the brain controls, while emphasizing the importance of, and length of time for, recovery. Tell your child that just like an injured arm or leg, the brain needs time to heal and to be exercised. Be sensitive to your child's reaction to these deficits and changes. Allow her to express thoughts and feelings associated with the anger and grief surrounding the loss of skills. Seek the assistance of professionals to help your child feel that it is OK to have such difficult feelings about deficits, the recovery process, and thoughts about the future.

Your injured child's lack of insight into her actions and behaviors and recently acquired limitations will present new challenges for your family. Where you may have once felt comfortable with your child out of your sight, you may now feel just the opposite. This can be particularly difficult with teens and children with active lifestyles. Again, you are balancing on the high wire. One of the greatest challenges is for you to reinstill a sense of responsibility in your child while providing what may now be a greater level of safety and supervision than ever before.

Without insight and awareness into the reasons for heightened supervision, your child may feel mistrusted. It's best to continually discuss this issue and help her achieve a sense of responsibility in other, possibly new and creative ways. For example, find things for your child to do around the home where she can feel a sense of responsibility within a safe environment. If it was previously your child's responsibility to mow the lawn, you might change her responsibility to the equally important chore of getting the mail.

To balance your child's desire to regain her previous autonomy and freedom around the neighborhood with the need to keep her safe, you may consider asking for help from trusted friends and neighbors. Talk to adults and responsible children in the neighborhood about your child's limitations and the importance of safety while she is recovering. Ask adult neighbors and friends' parents to help supervise and monitor the safety of your child's activities. Maintain open communication throughout the recovery process and continually focus on the length of the recovery process in working toward future progress.

The Peer Network

When a friend suffers a brain injury, peers often struggle with the same emotions that parents and family members experience, including guilt, fear, anger, sorrow, and concern. Your family will need to decide which peers need to know what and who will be the one to share this information with them.

While your child is beginning the recovery process, it is important to involve peers who are responsible and close to your child. Like your family, your child's friends are wondering if your child will ever be the same and need to learn to accept some of the obvious and more subtle differences. Peers need to be educated about brain injury and recovery . . . to relearn and readjust to your child, their friend.

When it is comfortable for your family, involve peers in the rehabilitation process. How much peers are involved may vary depending on your child's age and comfort level, as well as distance/accessibility of the rehab facility. Identify a handful of responsible and devoted friends whom you know and trust, and whom you can envision being your child's eyes and ears once she returns to school. Encourage peers to contact your child in the hospital through phone calls, letters, cards, and face-to-face visits when the time is appropriate. This will help friends to cope with the changes in your child and adjust to and understand her new needs. It will also help your child begin to accept the changes in herself. Educating and exposing peers along the way will help with the inevitable transition to home and school, and with the understanding of differences, limitations, and changes in personality and behavior. If supportive peers understand your child's needs, this will hopefully lead to a positive and accepting transition back into the community.

Changes in Self-Esteem

As your child becomes more involved in the rehabilitation phase, her self-esteem can suffer. The noticeable changes in herself and her skills, as well as differences in behavior, moods, cognition, and personality, can challenge your child's self-esteem. For example, this is how one parent described the changes in her child:

"Before his injury, Tom was so positive and confident. He was always the first to try something and most things came easily for him, be it school work, sports, artistic endeavors. Since his injury, he no longer has the use of his right arm and hand and requires a cane to help with walking. It takes him longer to process information, and math, which was once easy, is now a chore. He is a different person now, ashamed of what his friends might think of him, frustrated that he can no longer do things the way he used to, and unwilling to try new things. You see, Tom wanted to be an electrical engineer and play

basketball in high school and college. I know that when he thinks about his future now it scares him."

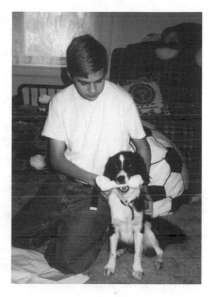

The evolution of such changes, coupled with the uncertainty of recovery, is extremely frustrating for a child with TBI and can cloud a previously favorable and confident self-perception.

As a parent, watching your child struggle with the emotional impact of the injury can be very painful and difficult. Often you have shared the same hopes and aspirations for your child. You may feel as if you want to take this struggle away, since your child already has so much to manage.

Again, encouraging and rewarding progress while remaining sensitive to the length of the recovery process will help your child feel supported and recognize her accomplishments. Be patient and communicate with your child. Help her to know that it is OK to talk about her feelings and experiences, and allow frustrations to be expressed. Never try to talk your child out of her feelings. Your child's feelings are what she feels—they are neither right or wrong. The losses that your child is experiencing are real and will inevitably be accompanied by a variety of emotional expressions and reactions. The support and strength provided by your family will help your child through all stages of the recovery process.

If your child seems to need more emotional support than your family can provide, do not hesitate to seek supportive therapy for her, as well as your family, from psychologists, social workers, or counselors experienced with traumatic brain injury.

▪▪ Your Child Back at Home

After weeks, possibly months, of recovery in the hospital setting, your child is now ready to transfer her recovery process to the home and community. As a parent, you may feel both positive and negative emotions about this step. On the one hand, you know that your child has made progress and that there is hope for continued success once your child returns home. You will probably become more confident as time at home increases, experiencing some relief and hope. You will also probably welcome the longed-for semblance of normalcy in your life, with your family again reunited at home.

On the other hand, you may feel ambivalent, scared, and worried about how this transition home will play itself out. You know there may need to be physical changes made to your home as well as changes in roles and expectations. You have been part of the team process, working and training closely with professionals who have provided care for your child twenty-four hours a day. You have come to rely on the support of professionals, and now your family is expected to carry out this lifetime mission back at home.

With practice and experience, families can learn to adjust to the changes at home *and* continue to support their child. This section details some of the changes to expect.

Changes in Family Roles and Responsibilities

When your child returns home, many of the physical and cognitive difficulties that she experienced during the rehabilitation phase will continue, only now these issues will play themselves out in your family's everyday life experiences. You may find that the demands and challenges increase and that roles within the family shift. For example, younger siblings may take on more of a big brother or big sister role in the family, with greater responsibilities. Siblings may assist your injured child with her homework or daily care routines. Or they may take on chores and responsibilities for their recovering brother or sister.

I'm Home, I'm OK

Depending on the injury and level of recovery, children with TBI often feel that they have returned to preinjury life once they are home. Now, more than ever, parents will struggle to balance their instincts to overprotect their child with the need to allow for some independence within the constraints of safety and supervision. Your child may not value or understand the need and importance of safety and close supervision, particularly if she is an older child or adolescent who has previously been granted some independence and freedom. Often when children return home, they feel that this is the permission they have been waiting for to resume previously enjoyed social activities. "I'm out of the hospital, so now I'm better and I can do what I want," they may think.

For children who do not show any physical signs of a traumatic brain injury, yet have cognitive challenges, restrictions on activities may be difficult to adjust to and understand. The reaction of this six-teen-year-old who was struck by a car while crossing the street is typical: "Since I've been home from the hospital, my mom won't let me out of her sight. She won't even let me ride my bike or go swimming unless she is watching me. She says she's worried that I may injure my brain again." It is difficult for children who previously had very active lifestyles and enjoyed such activities as football, soccer, roller-blading, skateboarding, or swimming to now see these activities as risky and potentially dangerous.

In short, although the return home is a positive and significant step in recovery, it often exposes your child to more restrictions and limitations than could be imagined while hospitalized. As your child re-enters her life at home and in school, the discrepancies between what she could do before and what she can do now become more evident.

Your Child's Losses

As your child adjusts to home, losses that were beginning to be apparent during the rehabilitation phase may intensify and become more real. In addition to the previously discussed cognitive and physical losses, additional losses may begin to surface once at home. These may include the loss of roles and responsibilities within the family, changes in friendships and social groups, and adaptations to goals and dreams for the future.

Once home, the emotions associated with loss will resurface throughout your child's and your family's life cycle, depending on the specific loss and how it affects your child and family at a specific point in time. For example, as your child reaches the age when milestones often occur—learning to drive, high school graduation, college accep-tance—your child and family may feel a sense of loss if those mile-stones aren't reached on schedule.

Peer Involvement and Response

With the early and timely involvement of close friends, these friends will hopefully become an integral piece of your child's transition back to home and school. Many times, peers are able to cope with the changes in their friend and can provide the support and understanding that your child will need. Other times, friends can become less supportive, unsure how to respond to the numerous changes they see. Often the injured child's social behavior may be inappropriate or disruptive, or seem immature and even embarrassing to friends. They may think, "Before her injury she was quieter and liked to do different things. Now she is always embarrassing me with her comments and never invites me to do anything." It is often difficult for peers to understand that these changes in their friend are the result of the brain injury and that behaviors, emotions, personality, and moods may now be very different.

Returning to School

Preparing to return to school is yet another milestone in the recovery process that evokes a variety of emotions for children with TBI and their families. Again, there may be positive feelings about this transition, yet, it can be another time of ambivalence and concern. Depending on what kinds of extra help your child will need and what is specifically provided by the school, your child may be better served at a different school. (See Chapter 9 for a thorough discussion of these issues.)

Whether your child returns to her school or transfers to another school, there will be challenges to face. If your child now requires special education services, becoming involved with the special education system may be a new experience for your family. Children often perceive that there is a stigma attached to special education services that reinforces the permanence of differences in themselves, causing a change in identity. Whether or not your child needs special education services, she may be worried about changes in academic performance and about how peers may respond to physical and cognitive changes. On the other hand, your child may not have the insight into her differences, and may view herself as unchanged, believing that everything will be the same. Regardless of your child's level of insight and understanding into the complexity of such changes, educational services and supports need to be designed for her specific needs.

Social Behavior

As your child rejoins the community, social situations that once seemed natural and appropriate to your child's development may now present challenges. For example, your once outgoing, social child may now be quiet and withdrawn and appear confused at birthday parties. Or she may be disinhibited and impulsive, blurting out comments without thinking and engaging in risky behavior. Adolescents may struggle with

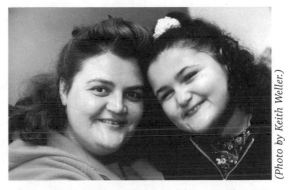

(Photo by Keith Weller.)

peer interactions, requiring the re-teaching and rehearsing of social skills. Sometimes this can result in social isolation, and a growing distance between your child and her peers.

▪▪ What You Can Do for Your Child at Home

As described above, returning home presents its own set of challenges for your family and your child. Over time your family will gradually adjust its life to address these changes. This section describes things you can do for your child to help with this transition back to the home and community.

Encouraging Family Communication

One of the most critical steps you can take to help your family weather your child's transition back home is to facilitate and encourage open dialogue between family members as to how these changes are affecting each individual. Important issues to discuss include:

- Feelings about changes in household roles, routines, and responsibilities;
- Siblings' feelings about your injured child's new behaviors and how they are managing at school and in the neighborhood;
- Feelings your injured child has about her siblings being allowed to do things that she is not.

Consider holding regular family meetings to gather feedback from family members. Set a time during the week when all family members are expected to attend and discuss what is and is not working within the home. Ongoing open communication within your family will help to establish a foundation for solving problems, alleviating stress, and strengthening relationships within the family.

Setting Limits and Encouraging Other Activities

There are ways to provide safety and supervision for your child while enabling her to have some sense of control and responsibility. First, encourage activities to take place in your home or the home of a trusted adult so that supervision can be unobtrusively provided. Second, set limits with siblings, friends, and your child regarding activities that are safe and appropriate so that your child does not feel pressured or confused in social situations. Third, schedule time together as a family to explore and encourage new activities or interests that present less of a risk for reinjury. Fourth, continue to communicate openly with your child, allowing her to express her frustrations with restrictions. Lastly, educate and inform others as you learn new ways of keeping your child safe. The more people know about the importance of providing a safe environment for your child, the less likely your child is to be put in compromising social situations.

One mother of a sixteen-year-old sat down with her son and his friends and listed activities that Jimmy was allowed to participate in, activities that would require adult supervision, and activities that were completely off limits. This particular mother developed valuable relationships with friends and neighbors early on in her son's recovery process through educating and informing. Several months following her son's return home, she felt comfortable with a handful of trusted friends who understood the importance of safety and were willing to look after her son in social situations.

Managing Losses

Helping your child to manage losses can be a challenging and difficult task, especially when you are likely experiencing and managing your own losses. Establishing a strong support network of family, neighbors, friends, members of religious and community institutions, school personnel, and other professionals is critical. When comfortable, encourage your child to express herself to you and other people in her life.

As mentioned above, there are many times when support from outside professionals can be very helpful. It is worth getting outside help whenever your family does not seem to be coping well, and the neutral, objective perspective and support from a professional might help you over a hump. Additionally, you should seek professional assistance if your child is feeling very distressed, angry, overwhelmed, stressed out, frustrated, depressed, or isolated from peers. In these instances, it is likely that your child's emotional struggles are affecting the whole family.

One way to seek out professional help is to utilize school resources, including school social workers, guidance counselors, and psychologists. Your child may also benefit from counseling services provided by a professional who is experienced with traumatic brain injury. Additionally, family counseling or support groups may help all family members, as issues of loss and change cycle throughout one's life and will likely need to be revisited.

Memory Book

Many families use memory books as a tool to help their child understand what has happened to her from the point of injury through the recovery process. Often these books include:

- photographs of the child taken at different points during recovery;
- significant dates, times, and events during recovery; and
- pictures and comments of professionals who have helped the child and family along the way.

By providing a chronology of the events that happened, the memory book can reinforce the seriousness of the injury to your child, let your child see that she is recovering, and help her integrate this trauma into her lifetime experiences. This tool can also be used to encourage conversation with your child and help in educating others.

Some families reserve a section of the memory book or make a separate memory book to help their child remember information needed for day-to-day life. For example, as an aid to remembering, they list names, dates, times, phone numbers, school schedules, and the steps needed to complete daily living tasks or routines within the classroom or home.

Managing Social Situations

As discussed above, children with TBI often experience social isolation as a result of changes in behavior, personality, mood, and awareness. This can be extremely difficult for your child if she has previously had solid peer relationships. If your child struggled with relationships before her injury, making and keeping friends will probably be even more challenging now. In addition, difficulties with insight, good judgment, and social awareness could place your child in vulnerable situations. For example, your child might be pressured to do something that could place her at risk for another injury. If she is feeling anxious to be liked and accepted by the group, she might take the risk.

Again, help your child by educating her friends and school personnel about recovering from, and long-term effects of, a brain injury.

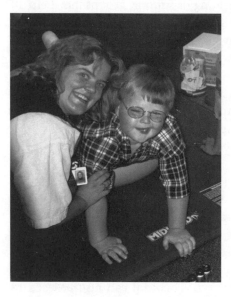

If your child's friends seem to be backing away from her, try offering them more information about your child's condition to help them understand the changes in her. It may help to talk to the parents of your child's friends to better understand the friends' perspectives.

Listen to your child's frustrations about social situations. With the assistance of professionals specializing in traumatic brain injury, you may need to reteach and rehearse social skills with your child by role playing or by practicing responses to scenarios that your child may be confronted with. Encourage your child to initiate social activities and conversations with her friends, serving as a role model for appropriate behavior.

Returning to School

Returning to school can be a difficult yet positive experience for you and your child. It will be very important to establish close and frequent communication between your family and school personnel (social workers, guidance counselor, teacher). Communication is the key to better understanding and helping your child. Often a communication log or notebook that travels between home and school is the easiest way for the school and family to communicate and is helpful in tracking and planning for the needs of your child. Parents can ask questions about what is happening at school and write about progress and difficulties that their child is having related to school. Likewise, teachers can use the notebook to record what they observe, respond to questions, and have an ongoing dialog with parents.

Your child may feel anxious about returning to school or beginning a new school. Anxiety could be the result of insight into changes in herself, concerns with changes in academic performance or physical appearance, concerns about peer reactions and acceptance, or worries about being placed in special education or the amount of time missed from school.

It is natural and appropriate for your child to worry about returning to school, yet there are some ways to help to ease this process for your child. First, professionals who are experienced with traumatic brain injury can help by educating peers and school personnel before your child's first day at school. Professionals can educate staff and students through in-services to help others less familiar with brain injury to better understand your child. Second, your child should have access to a school professional, such as a social worker, guidance counselor, or nurse, who is available to discuss her concerns about returning to school. Third, as a parent, you can ask to meet with school personnel to discuss your child's educational needs at any time. In fact, you will probably find that advocating for your child will be critical to your own well-being. And finally, it may help for your child to be paired with a "buddy," a trusted and responsible peer who can look out for your child and help to guide her during the school day. Your child may be able to help choose this buddy. Ultimately, however, the buddy should be a responsible student with whom both your family and school are comfortable.

If your child is placed in special education, she may worry about the perceived stigma. Be available to talk with your child regarding the unfairness and unkindness of this stigma and help her to understand the purpose of special education services. In addition, make sure that school personnel are attuned to this issue and available for your child during the transition period. Maintaining frequent contact with your child's school prior to her return, at the time of re-entry, and throughout the school year will help you help your child adjust to the changes in herself and her school program.

Community Resources

Community resources can be vital in helping your family and child adjust to your new way of life. Become connected with support groups and organizations where you can share your experiences and learn from others. Become active in your local chapter of the National Brain Injury Association, groups and organizations involved with special needs, and the local educational system. Use the supports of church and community members in bringing understanding and awareness to others. Go online and get virtual support and real information from some of the Internet resources listed in the Resource Guide. Most importantly, establish connections with others who have shared similar experiences. This will open doors for extended emotional support while acquainting you with other families who have faced, problem-solved, and made it through varying phases along this lifelong process. See the Resource Guide at the back of this book for organizations that can help you get started in seeking support.

▪▪ General Guidelines

Below is a collection of basic guidelines for helping your child adjust following a traumatic brain injury:

1. Encourage and praise progress.
2. Involve peers, school, and the community when the time is right for your family.
3. Listen to your child and provide support.
4. Serve as a role model for social behavior.
5. Encourage your child to have relationships with friends.
6. Explore finding a counselor experienced with traumatic brain injury for your child and the family.
7. Consider family counseling to address role changes, sibling issues, understanding of differences, and the impact of this trauma on the family life cycle and development.
8. Encourage your child to focus on one day at a time by setting small goals as steps toward accomplishing larger ones.
9. Encourage independence with supervision. Be creative with this!

10. Seek the support and services of community members (professionals, church members, support groups).
11. Communicate (with your child, family members, neighbors, friends, professionals, and the school)!
12. Help your child understand her injury and recovery. (Let her know that the brain needs time to heal like other body parts.)
13. Instill confidence in creative ways—draw on previous skills and interests, applied in new ways.
14. Create a Memory Book. (Memory difficulties are often frustrating. This will also help to document events and reinforce progress.)
15. Encourage a normal lifestyle, predictability, and routine as much as possible.

Above all, remember that this is challenging and a lifelong process!

:: Parent Statements

I prayed to the good Lord to bring her back to me. He didn't say how she would be. Now I've got to deal with what I've got.

❧

We've got this huge modified, accessible bathroom and a tiny laundry room. The bathroom is like the part of my life devoted to my child's needs and the rest of my life is like the laundry room—squeezed into a very small space.

❧

Joe has done some things that have my heart floating—like walking to our neighbor's house independently!

❧

Tommy's friends were really supportive when he went back to school after his bicycle accident, but now they seem to have moved on. He can't understand why they don't want to spend time with him anymore.

❧

Sometimes I wish she could just see her problems so she would accept the fact that she needs help, but most of the time I'm glad she doesn't see.

❧

The social worker has been the constant, predictable factor in a situation where nothing is predictable. When I'm in her office, I can pause and think and be myself.

❧

He is doing really well now. When other kids ask him why he walks that way or why he can't use his right arm, he tells them "Somebody very bad hurt me once, but he is in jail now." Then he says, "Let's play." Because he handles it so calmly, other kids handle it well too. Sometimes he still is upset or confused about it, so we talk and practice ways he can respond to other kids' questions. He really is a terrific kid and everybody loves him.

How TBI Affects Learning and Thinking

Kathleen D. Brady, Ph.D.

At the instant Johnny's head struck the pavement, a series of mechanical and chemical changes were set into motion. These changes would drastically disrupt normal brain cell activity, not just at the point of impact, but diffusely, throughout the brain. Johnny's injury was severe enough that the disruption reached the deep structures of the brain responsible for arousal. Though brain functions necessary for survival continued, all awareness of external and internal events, as well as all voluntary activity, virtually ceased. Johnny has entered a state of coma.

Johnny's parents soon learned that resolution of coma is not the "all or nothing," sudden and dramatic return to normalcy sometimes depicted on television. By eight days after the injury, their son was able to respond appropriately to a very simple verbal command ("squeeze my hand"). This meant he was out of coma, but cognitive functions—his abilities to perceive, understand, think, remember, and speak—were far from restored. Their worry shaped itself into a new question: not, "Will he live?" but, "Will he be the same?" The ICU staff *and the rehab team were unable to make long-term predictions at this early stage. However, as the coma extended past a week, the social worker and others gently suggested that complete recovery of cognitive ability after this length of unconsciousness was "very unlikely."*

By the time Johnny was discharged from day-hospital rehabilitation, approximately ten weeks after the accident, his parents had seen dramatic improvement in his cognitive status. They were therefore dismayed to read the long litany of continuing "deficits," "impairments," "weaknesses," and "disabilities" described in the neuropsychological report. The jargon was confusing: "VIQ-PIQ discrepancy," "expressive language disorder," "retrieval deficits," "executive dysfunction." Over the next year, though, they gradually learned to recognize these cognitive problems as they were reflected in real-world difficulties. Johnny's verbal thinking skills were in the average range for his age, but his visual-spatial problem-solving was much weaker—in the range they called "borderline." He had trouble finding the words he wanted to say, and his voice was usually "flat" and expressionless. His response time, in general, seemed to be in slow motion. He was able to learn, but then seemed unable to remember what he had learned after even a short delay. His written work was so sloppy as to be almost unreadable. He couldn't seem to stay on the lines or even form the letters correctly.

Of greatest concern were Johnny's distractibility and restlessness. He had shown these tendencies before the accident, but his teachers had been able to deal with them within the regular classroom. They were much worse now. He responded impulsively, without taking time to think. He was unable to focus on important information and filter out the irrelevant. He couldn't seem to keep track of an idea or a simple set of directions long enough to carry on a conversation or play a game with friends. He had trouble formulating a plan for anything from getting dressed in the morning to figuring out what to do at his birthday party. When he got stuck, instead of trying something new, he just sat and did nothing, or repeated the same thing he had been doing, even though it didn't work any more. It was hard to explain to people how these little things we take for granted could have such a big impact on everyday life at school and at home.

*Now, five years postinjury, small gains continue to occur—
mostly as Johnny, his family, and the school learn new ways to
compensate for his difficulties. On the other hand, adolescence
is presenting new concerns. As demands for independent
judgment and abstract thinking increase, some previously
unrecognized limitations are becoming apparent. A new set of
adjustments are needed, and the family is finding it useful to
resume contact with their previous support system through the
rehab follow-up clinic.*

■■ Introduction

Every thought and action we produce, every memory evoked,
every mood experienced—in short, all that we are—is the product of
brain cell activity. Even a simple "automatic" behavior, such as a swallow or a step, requires the coordinated and precisely timed interaction of millions of cells located throughout the brain.

As described in Chapter 1, traumatic brain injury, particularly
closed-head TBI, typically results in two types of damage: focal and
diffuse. Focal or localized damage occurs as a result of the mechanical
forces of impact or pressure from a blood clot, and is most frequently
seen in the frontal and temporal lobes. More diffuse (widespread) damage throughout the brain results from stretching and tearing of fibers as
the brain moves and twists within the skull on impact. Diffuse damage
also results from swelling, oxygen-deprivation, and poisoning from the
release of toxic levels of neurochemicals. It is not surprising, then, that
any TBI severe enough to produce even a brief loss of consciousness can
result in alterations in thinking and behavior.

When loss of consciousness persists for more than seven days or
so, it is very likely that some of these changes will be permanent and
disabling to some extent. For parents, it is these changes in cognition
(thinking) and in behavior, rather than motor disabilities, that most
disrupt the family and interfere with the return to a normal life.

In this chapter, we will discuss the effects of TBI on the major
domains of cognitive function, including general intelligence, memory,
attention, visual processing, and self-regulation or "executive" functions.
Changes in other important cognitive domains—language and academic
achievement—as well as behavioral changes are discussed in other chapters. As you read this material, remember that your child's individual

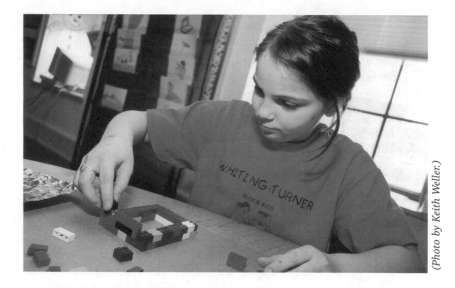

(Photo by Keith Weller.)

outcome will be influenced by many factors, including age at injury, preinjury ability and personality, the nature and severity of the injury, any medical complications, rehabilitation and educational experiences after the injury, and family resources and adjustment. In general, however, traumatic brain injuries result in specific types of cognitive difficulties. Every child who has had a brain injury with coma (and many who do not experience coma) will demonstrate one or more of the problems described in this chapter, at least for a period of time.

■■ How Is the Brain Organized?

Before discussing the changes in thinking and learning that you may see in your child after TBI, it will be useful to briefly review what is known about the functions of different brain regions. It is also important to explain some general principles that describe how these areas work together in an organized way. You may not need to read this section if the discussion of brain function in Chapter 1 is still fresh in your mind, although this section offers additional detail about cognitive functions of particular parts of the brain.

Parts of the Brain

In very broad terms, the brain can be divided into three regions: the cerebrum, the brainstem, and the cerebellum. (See Figure 2, page

6.) We will be discussing primarily the cerebrum and brainstem, since these areas are crucial to cognition and are the areas most frequently affected by TBI.

The **cerebrum** is divided anatomically and functionally into two hemispheres:

- The **left hemisphere** is known to be responsible for verbal functions, including producing and understanding spoken language, reading, writing, and verbal memory.
- The **right hemisphere** is best suited to the processing of information that cannot readily be verbalized or that is best processed all at once, such as perception and memory of shape, texture, pattern, and three-dimensional spatial relationships; construction, such as copying, drawing and putting things together; and the understanding and expression of emotion.

The important thing to remember is that nearly every cognitive act is the product of coordination between both hemispheres. Math, for example, places demands on both hemispheres, since it involves both spatial processing (such as alignment of columns for calculations) and linear, sequential processes that can be verbalized (such as $a + b = c$).

In addition to their left/right separation, the cerebral hemispheres are divided roughly front to back into four lobes: the frontal, temporal, parietal, and occipital. Each lobe is primarily responsible for a particular type of cognitive processing. One, the **frontal lobe,** is the brain's *output* center. That is, it is responsible for the preparation and execution of all voluntary activity. The other three lobes are specialized *input* centers. The **temporal lobe** receives and processes auditory information. It is essential for hearing, as well as for understanding and remembering what is heard. The **parietal lobe** is the destination for sensors in the skin and joints that convey information regarding touch and position. The **occipital lobe,** located at the back of the brain, is the receiving area for all nerve cell activity in the retinas of the eyes and thus is essential for vision.

Receiving incoming sensory signals is just the beginning of the brain's work. What the brain does with the information it receives is what determines the quality of thought and behavior. These more complex aspects of processing cannot be precisely localized to single areas, or even to single lobes. To understand brain function beyond the level of sensation, we need to depart from schemes of anatomical divisions and consider the *functional* organization of the brain. How do these areas work together to produce what we know of as thinking and learning?

How the Parts of the Brain Work Together

One important theory proposes that we think of the brain in terms of three functional units. Two of these—the sensory input unit (temporal, parietal, and occipital lobes) and the response programming and output unit (frontal lobe)—have already been described. The third unit regulates level of *arousal*—the general state of alertness, ranging from coma to hypersensitivity. The arousal unit consists primarily of the brainstem.

Each functional unit can, in turn, be divided into three zones: the primary, secondary, and tertiary. Primary zones are the smallest and most specific, consisting (in the sensory input unit) of areas where auditory, visual, and tactile sensations are initially registered. Secondary zones are adjacent to primary zones. In secondary zones, separate bits of information from primary areas are combined to build up a perception. Tertiary zones fan out from secondary zones, overlapping and merging together the borders of temporal, parietal, and occipital lobes (and become one large, unified tertiary zone). The job of the tertiary zone is *sensory integration.*

Sensory integration allows us to combine information from different sensory systems into a unified, multidimensional experience. Sensory integration makes it possible for us not only to know what something looks like, but to simultaneously associate a particular touch, smell, sound, and an emotional quality with it.

We learn, for example, that a particular small, furry animal is called "dog." Because of sensory integration, we come to understand a great deal about what a dog is and is not. Eventually, we learn that the visual pattern consisting of the letters DOG can represent the small furry animal, and has the same meaning as the sound "dog." We then are able to begin to read with comprehension.

Sensory integration is also essential for "higher-level" abstract thinking. For example, as we repeatedly see and touch round objects, we build up a concept of "roundness" that is separate from either vision or touch.

As sensations move through the primary, secondary, then tertiary zones, they are processed in hierarchical fashion—from simple to complex, from isolated to integrated. Some of the implications of this type of organization are:

1. Complete loss of sensory function (for example blindness or deafness) seldom occurs in closed head TBI. This is because complete, focal destruction of primary zones—which are responsible for receiving sensations—is rare.

2. The tertiary zone is most vulnerable because it occupies the largest area and because small, diffuse injuries throughout the hierarchy will have a cumulative effect at the highest (tertiary) level.

3. Damage in tertiary areas can affect a wide range of abilities.

What happens, then, when a traumatic brain injury intrudes upon this very intricately balanced, complexly integrated system?

If the injury is focal, or localized to a specific region, such as occurs in some gunshot wounds or in stroke or tumor, the effects may be quite localized as well. They may be limited to the specific function controlled by the affected tissue, often with no loss of consciousness. This is not, however, the type of brain injury typically seen in children. In children, brain injuries usually result from motor vehicle or sports accidents, or from falls. As explained in Chapter 1, these events tend to create violent movement of the brain within a closed skull, resulting in both focal *and* diffuse damage. It is this type of damage (a combination of focal and diffuse) that is likely to produce the cognitive problems described below.

∷ General Intellectual Ability

One question parents understandably have is, "Will my child recover to the same level of intelligence as before the injury?" This is a difficult question to answer, as this section will explain.

At some point in recovery, most children who have had a TBI will be given a standardized IQ test by a psychologist. This is an important part of an evaluation, but *not* because of the particular IQ scores it generates. Instead, it is important because in provides an opportunity to observe the child performing a variety of cognitive tasks. The profile of cognitive strengths and weaknesses that emerges will be useful to the psychologist, both in identifying areas that need further assessment and in making recommendations for rehabilitation and/or educational programming.

There are two very important things to remember about IQ tests following TBI:

1. Results can only describe status around the time of testing. Changes may be expected to occur within the first year after the injury and beyond.

2. IQ tests tell us how a child performed compared to children without TBI of the same age, on an IQ test. These numbers alone, however, cannot tell us important information such as the impact of the injury on future development, or on the child's ability to function in the "real world." These issues, as we will see, are affected by many factors that influence learning and behavior, but that IQ tests are not designed to assess.

For these reasons, it is difficult to give a meaningful answer to the question posed at the beginning of this section. More fruitful questions might be: "What are my child's cognitive strengths and weaknesses (including but not limited to IQ)? How will these abilities and disabilities work together to influence everyday function? What can be done to optimize my child's outcome?" With these "qualifiers" in mind, let's briefly describe what you can expect in terms of I.Q. scores after TBI.

Intelligence Testing

The most frequently used individual test of intelligence for children is the Wechsler Intelligence Scale for Children-Third Edition (WISC-III). It consists of ten to thirteen (three are optional) subtests, which in turn cluster into two broad domains of ability. The six Verbal Scale subtests require the understanding and use of oral language for various types of thinking and reasoning. Results of these subtests are weighted and combined to come up with the Verbal IQ (VIQ). The seven Performance Scale subtests require perceptual analysis and manual manipulation of visually presented materials. Results of these subtests make up the Performance IQ (PIQ). Together, the VIQ and PIQ yield an estimate of overall intellectual ability called the Full Scale IQ (FSIQ).

The VIQ, PIQ, and FSIQ are standardized, or mathematically adjusted, so that a score of 100 is considered exactly average when compared to a large group of children of the same age who were given the test when it was developed. Scores of 90 to 109 are "within the average range," while 80 to 89 is "low average" and 110 to 119 is "high average." Scores from 70 to 79 are considered "borderline." A score below 70 is labeled as "deficient," since only a very few children (fewer than 2 percent) scored in that range when the test was standardized.

Children who obtain scores below 70 because of an inborn condition are said to have an "intellectual deficiency" or "mental retardation." This term may also be applied to children who *acquire* an intellectual deficiency through TBI. This is not the usual practice, however, because of possible cognitive changes during recovery and because of the variability or "scatter" in subtest scores (patterns of strengths and weaknesses). This is often seen in children with TBI, but not those with mental retardation. That is, children with mental retardation typically have very low scores in all subtests, whereas children with TBI often do significantly better in some areas than others.

In most children without TBI, the VIQ and PIQ are within a few points of each other. Early in recovery after severe TBI, however, both VIQ and PIQ will probably be lower than they were before your child's injury. In addition, there may be a wide discrepancy between VIQ and PIQ scores. If the discrepancy is more than fifteen points or so, the psychologist may choose not to report the FSIQ because your child's cognitive profile is too uneven to be validly summarized in a single, overall measure. In most cases, the PIQ will be lower than the VIQ. This is thought to reflect the remarkably stable nature of "old" previously well-learned factual knowledge that your child has stored in long-term memory, and that is tapped by the Verbal Scale subtests. PIQ subtests, in contrast, are timed and require rapid inspection and manipulation of unfamiliar materials.

The decline in PIQ after TBI may be due to a number of factors, including:

- difficulty making sense of visual information because of gaps in sensory integration;
- difficulty using visual imagery for problem solving;
- overall slowing of the rate of information processing;
- slowed motor responses;
- difficulty organizing a response in new and unfamiliar situations.

Further evaluation will be needed to identify your child's key difficulties.

Usually, IQ scores continue to increase up to a year or two following a brain injury, then appear to plateau. Often the VIQ returns to the level (known or estimated) of preinjury ability. The PIQ may also improve, though generally not as strongly as the VIQ. As noted earlier, however, many other important domains of cognitive function, over and above IQ scores, also affect how much of his cognitive abilities your child regains. These include memory and attention. How well your child's memory and attention are functioning will determine the rate of intellectual progress *after* the injury, and thus will affect future IQ scores. For example, scores may decline again after the initial increase and plateau, if difficulties in memory and attention interfere with continued development. In other words, it is premature to assume that the injury has not had a significant effect on your child's general intellectual ability because he initially recovers his preinjury verbal ability. We will turn our attention to these other cognitive areas in the section below.

▪▪ Memory and New Learning

Memory problems have been identified as the most common and most persistent consequence of TBI. Memory is essential to our sense of continuity of self, to an appreciation of cause-and-effect relationships, and to the acquisition of new knowledge. Learning, particularly academic learning, consists in its most basic sense of improvements in memory for particular information over repeated exposure. Memory, then, is one (though not the only) important determinant of your child's ability to learn.

Old vs. New Memories

It is the process of establishing memories for *new* information that is most frequently disrupted after TBI. "New information" refers to factual material or events that have occurred since the injury. Memory or recall of "old," previously well-learned or *consolidated* information is often well-preserved, even after severe brain injury. For example, a young child will remember his name and age and recognize his parents. An adolescent may be able to describe his daily preinjury routine very accurately. Though there may be scattered "gaps" in your child's old or "remote" memory, a complete loss of past knowledge is extremely rare. He may, however, not remember the few minutes, hours, or days immediately preceding the injury, which presumably had not yet been consolidated in memory at the time of the injury. This period of preinjury memory loss is sometimes referred to as "retrograde amnesia."

Retrograde amnesia tends to "shrink" with time as your child remembers more and more events leading up to the injury. However, your child will *never* remember the actual injury itself, as well as the period of time before his post-traumatic amnesia (see below) resolved. This is not because the event was so emotionally traumatic, or because your child has consciously or subconsciously "repressed" the unpleasant event. Rather, it is assumed that the brain's memory "machinery" abruptly stops at the time of injury and does not resume operation for a period of time. The silver lining here is that you do not need to worry that your child will "relive" those frightening moments in his mind. He will not relive them because they simply never registered in the first place!

Though certainly cause for celebration, your child's preservation of preinjury memories may be misleading. Testing prior to return to school, for example, may indicate that your child has lost few academic skills. This could lead to the possibly erroneous assumption that your child is ready to return to his preinjury classroom and "pick up where he left off." If he has memory problems, the education specialists that work with you (in the hospital, rehabilitation program, or local school) will recommend a special placement, program, or system of accommodations in the classroom to ensure that he will continue to make progress. It is better to take these steps early, gradually returning your child to a regular program as warranted, rather than to place your child in a situation where he may experience tremendous frustration and discouragement.

The Different Memory Systems

In trying to understand memory function after TBI, one of the most important issues to grasp is this: there is not a single, unitary memory "storage vault," located in a specific area of the brain, which is the repository of all memories. Memory is a *process* rather than a *place* in the brain.

As human behavior and thinking have become more complex over the course of evolution, more complex memory systems have developed. These newer systems have been added to, but have not necessarily replaced, older systems. For example, *procedural memory* refers to motor skills, conditioning, and other types of memory that can be stored and retrieved without apparent conscious awareness or effort. Knowing how to ride a bicycle and unlock a door are examples of complex procedural memories. Memory for facts and episodes of personal experience, on the other hand, is referred to as *declarative memory*. Some memory systems are more vulnerable to disruption than others.

Declarative memory is much more likely to be impaired after TBI than is procedural memory. For example, your child may readily learn a new motor activity, such as removing a leg splint—a skill that depends on procedural memory. This may give you the mistaken impression that he "is not trying hard enough" to learn other types of new information, such as the names of therapists. He may be able to remember and learn specific facts and personal experiences, but only after many repetitions. For example, your child may gradually learn the names of therapists but be unable to tell you the morning's events. Sometimes the additional step of attaching "tags" to a declarative memory to identify the source, time, place, and sequence of events may be omitted. As a result of this kind of memory glitch, your child might report that he visited Disney World yesterday instead of three years ago. He may even report as fact something that he merely thought or heard or read about. This is because that important "context label" telling when and how that event was experienced was not encoded along with the event. This kind of false memory, or "confabulation," is *not* intentional lying, though it may be mistaken as such.

Now that we have established that declarative memory is likely to be impaired after TBI, we will discuss the organization of declarative memory and where breakdowns in the system tend to occur.

Short-Term vs. Long-Term Memory

Declarative memory is generally divided into two distinct stages: short-term memory and long-term memory. (Sometimes there are considered to be three stages if initial attention and sensory registration are considered.) These stages differ in terms of capacity, format or code used for storage, duration, and cognitive processes involved.

Short-term memories are thought to exist as patterns of electrical signals among neurons. Long-term memory takes a more permanent form, most likely as actual changes in the physical connections among neurons. What the brain does with the information when it is in short-term memory determines whether it becomes part of long-term memory. Both the process of transfer from short-term to long-term memory and the process of retrieval from long-term memory may be disrupted by TBI. Often, when a child with TBI is said to have short-term memory problems but no long-term memory problems, what is meant is that the child has more difficulty with *recent* (new) than *remote* (old) information.

Short-term memory is not permanent. It lasts just a few seconds, though it can be extended indefinitely with *rehearsal* (repeating the information such as a telephone number mentally or out loud). The contents of short-term memory are lost if a distraction occurs before they are transferred into permanent storage in long-term memory.

How much information we can hold in short-term memory increases with age. Most adults can hold seven (plus or minus two) items in short-term memory, though functional capacity can also be increased, through *chunking* bits of related information together. For example, you may remember more than seven items from your grocery list if you mentally group them in categories such as produce, canned goods, etc., both as you store them and as you later try to retrieve them. Rehearsal and chunking are cognitive processes that increase the likelihood that information in short-term memory will be encoded into long-term memory.

The actual capacity of short-term memory is often found to be within normal limits for age soon after TBI. This may be measured, for example, by determining the number of digits that your child can recite immediately after seeing or hearing them. However, short-term memory seems to be very unstable after TBI, so that the contents vanish rapidly with the slightest distraction. For example, a child who is given a simple instruction to "Get out your math book and open it to page 19" may have forgotten what book he is looking for by the time he gets his backpack open.

In addition, children who have had a TBI have difficulty using processes such as rehearsal and chunking on their own. Even if they are taught to use these strategies, they may not be able to apply them before their fragile short-term memory is overwhelmed by distractions. As a result, a reduced amount of information finds its way into permanent storage (long-term memory). Failure to chunk or organize new information as it is stored may interfere with ability to retrieve it later, just as putting library books back on shelves in a haphazard manner interferes with locating them later. Before discussing retrieval difficulties, however, it is important to mention a specific type of injury that can prevent storage of new information no matter how effectively it is processed in the short-term stage.

Encoding Failure

Deep in the temporal lobes, near the center of the brain, is a cluster of structures called the limbic system that is absolutely essential to the transfer of information from short-term memory to long-term memory. If certain of these structures, particularly the hippocampus, are completely destroyed in both the left and right hemispheres, no new declarative memories can be formed. As a result, there is a very rapid rate of forgetting, with little benefit obtained from cues or hints. This problem is sometimes referred to as *amnesia,* or *amnestic syndrome.*

This syndrome is extremely rare. It may happen in some types of focal brain damage, such as from a stroke, tumor, infection, or severe oxygen deprivation. It does not typically occur after a traumatic brain injury. In TBI, the limbic system more often remains functional, but is less efficient. As a consequence, the rate of learning is slow and many extra repetitions of new material are needed, but new learning can and does occur.

Difficulties in Retrieving Memories

The most common type of memory problem following TBI is impaired *retrieval,* or inability to gain access to information that has been encoded into storage. That is, your child will recognize that information presented for a second time is familiar, but will be unable to spontaneously recall it on his own. Inability to retrieve stored information may occur because of factors operating at the time of storage or at the time of retrieval. Children with retrieval failure problems often benefit from prompts and cues, such as the beginning sound of a word.

Retrieval failure may result from disorganized or haphazard storage of information, making it hard to "find" later by way of any logical path. This situation can be compared to a library where books are placed on shelves in random fashion. This type of retrieval impairment may occur if rehearsal and chunking in short-term memory are used ineffectively. That is, the injured brain does not process new information "deeply" enough so that it becomes embedded in a meaningful network or web of related information. Instead, it allows information to be placed haphazardly "onto the shelves," based on some random, often superficial association. As a result, information cannot be located later except by chance.

Another common reason for retrieval failure after TBI is due to an inability to *plan* and *execute* an organized search. This situation is analogous to a well-organized library where information nevertheless cannot be found because the child has no idea how to use the card catalogue to organize a search. Memory retrieval, even for the most familiar of information, is an *active* cognitive

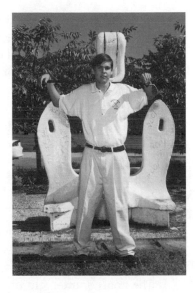

process. It requires: first, a motive to recall, then the planning and execution of a logical system of searching, and finally comparison of the results of the search with the original goal, with adjustments and "updates" of the search plan being made constantly as the process proceeds. In fact, although difficulties with this process result in failure to remember, this complex type of processing is usually thought of as falling within the self-regulatory or "executive" function domain. In other words, sometimes what appear to be memory problems may actually be due, at least in part, to problems with executive functioning, which is discussed below.

There are other cognitive problems that may mimic problems with memory. For example, a child who fails to attend to information in the first place or has impairments in perceptual processing can appear to have problems with memory. If your child has an observed memory problem, it is important to have a careful neuropsychological evaluation. This will help to identify which cognitive processes are contributing to your child's memory problem, so that the most appropriate compensatory techniques can be implemented.

Help for Children with Memory Problems

There are many common-sense strategies that can help children with memory problems. In the classroom, new material to be learned should be broken into smaller units, and presented over numerous, spaced repetitions. Some children benefit if new information is presented within a meaningful context, such as a story, rather than as a set of isolated facts. New material should be "chained" to previously learned information when possible. (For example: "Last week we talked about the land and weather in Egypt. Now we are going to talk about the kinds of things that can grow there.") Previewing and preorganizing (such as providing an outline in advance of a lecture) are helpful for older children, as are graphic organizers such as timelines and charts.

Your child should be given active instruction in techniques such as rehearsal, chunking, and visual imagery. Both at school and at home, external aids such as notes, pictures, written instructions, appointment/assignment books, and calculators should become part of everyday routine. Your child should be provided liberal cueing and prompting, such as the beginning sound of a word, a sentence stem, a multiple-choice "menu," or a context cue ("Who did we see today—we were at the mall?").

The goals of intervention for memory problems are:
- to reduce frustration;
- to provide the information needed to allow your child to continue to participate in life and learning;
- to promote the independent use of techniques to compensate for difficulties.

There is no danger that your child will become "lazy" or dependent on external help. These supports cannot interfere with the recovery process, and in fact, will facilitate it.

■■ Attention

Like memory problems, attention problems occur almost universally after closed head TBI, and are among the most persistent of post-TBI symptoms. This makes it vital for parents to understand what is meant by the term "attention."

Attention is a prerequisite to all other conscious and voluntary cognitive activity. Before we can perceive, remember, or manipulate information, we must attend to it, at least on some level. Different types and locations of brain injury will result in different manifestations of attention problems:

1. Injury to the brainstem (which is responsible for arousal) results in the most basic dysfunction of attention, known as coma.

2. Injury to the sensory input unit (the temporal, parietal, and occipital lobes) results in omissions and errors in the processing and integration of incoming signals. These errors may range from failing to notice when signs change from plus to minus on a math worksheet to complete unawareness of one side of space or one side of the body.

3. Injury to the frontal output system (the frontal lobe) interferes with the ability to manage, allocate, and direct attention in a purposeful and productive fashion.

In severe TBI, where both focal and diffuse injury is present, all of these aspects of attention will be affected to a greater or lesser degree.

Attention Problems Related to Altered Consciousness

Coma

Coma is defined as a state of decreased responsiveness to external or internal stimuli following injury to the brain. It is characterized by:

▪ lack of voluntary eye opening,
▪ lack of response to simple commands, such as "squeeze my hand," and
▪ lack of comprehensible speech.

Contrary to popular misconception, a coma is *not* a state of deep sleep. Sleep is a highly active state. During sleep, the brain uses oxygen at the same rate as in the awake state. In coma, however, the rate of oxygen uptake is always lower than during the normal resting state. Coma involves both failure of arousal and absence of awareness. In contrast, sleep is a state of decreased but not absent arousal with lack of awareness. Very rarely, massive destruction of the cerebral hemispheres may destroy the capacity for awareness, while preserving some degree of arousal, resulting in sleep/wake cycles. This condition is referred to as a "vegetative state" and may be considered irreversible. Coma, on the other hand, usually resolves over time. Only when a child begins to regain some arousal can the extent of his problems in awareness or higher level cerebral activity begin to be assessed.

Coma results if the normal function of the upper portion of the brainstem is disrupted by either swelling or by stretching or tearing of nerve fibers. If swelling of the cerebral hemispheres is severe and prolonged, it can actually cause the hemispheres to push down upon and compress the brainstem. This may be what has occurred if your child initially seems lucid after TBI, but then enters coma. More often in TBI, however, the violent forces of impact cause the hemispheres to rotate around the brainstem, resulting in stretching and shearing injury to upper brainstem pathways. This results in immediate loss of consciousness. The most basic functions necessary for life—breathing and heartbeat—are controlled by the lower brainstem and will continue, but both arousal and higher level awareness will cease for a time.

As your child's upper brainstem function resumes, he regains a minimal level of arousal. His awareness of internal and external events also increases, as brainstem activation awakens higher cerebral areas as well. Once your child's motor, eye-opening, and vocal responses begin to be somewhat purposeful and selective, coma is said to have terminated.

Post-Traumatic Amnesia (PTA)

Now your child will pass through a period of confusion in which no new memories are being laid down. He will respond to simple commands and other stimuli, but will be unable to remember from moment to moment where he is, why he is there, what time it is, who all the busy strangers around him are, and what they are doing to him. This interval, called the period of Post-Traumatic Amnesia or PTA, may last from a few hours to many weeks.

Early in PTA, possibly because recovery of awareness lags behind increased arousal, your child may be overwhelmed by confusion and become quite agitated, fearful, combative, and aggressive. After waiting anxiously for your child to speak, the first words you hear may be profanities or other bizarre language. This can be alarming, even embarrassing to parents, but be assured that staff are familiar with this transitional behavior and view it as a positive sign of recovery. The best approach is to reduce stimulation, maintain sameness, and frequently repeat information that will help your child understand what is going on. As PTA resolves and your child begins to retain new information, active rehabilitation efforts can begin. (See Chapter 7 for more information on handling your child's behaviors during PTA.)

Attention Problems Related to Sensory Input Problems

Clearly, the arousal unit (brainstem) has an important role in maintaining consciousness, thus setting the stage for more complex aspects of attention. However, attention problems related to brainstem injuries (coma, PTA) are not usually what we are referring to when we talk about "attention problems" in children recovering from TBI. As discussed above, the sensory input and response output units also play important roles in attention, at higher levels of information processing. Knowledge of this area of brain/behavior relationships is still limited, but some generalizations can be made.

At any particular moment, *millions* of bits of sensory information—visual, auditory, tactile—find their way to the primary zones of the brain, but only a small fraction of this information ever enters conscious awareness. That is, we only pay attention to some of it. How does this happen?

As soon as sensory impulses enter the primary zones (actually, well before that point), they begin to undergo a process of selection. Some features are filtered out early in the process, while others that are particularly important to identification (such as angles, certain sounds, etc.) are actually enhanced and made more prominent in our awareness. The filtering process at this early stage is mostly automatic, based on internal wiring we are born with. It is an actual physical process performed by our brain cells, not something we have any voluntary control over. Some types of information, such as faces, seem to get preferential treatment right from birth.

As information proceeds through secondary zones, it is further selected, now based on more learned criteria such as, "Is this something new that I haven't seen (heard, etc.) before?" Something new perks up the neurons, while old, familiar stuff, after many repetitions, gets a weaker and weaker response. It becomes just "background." Even at this stage, the process is not usually under voluntary control. An exciting new event can "grab" our attention easily, no matter what we are *supposed* to be paying attention to. But overall, the system protects us from being overwhelmed by a flood of irrelevant stimulation. Imagine what it might be like if this selective attentional system was impaired! Nothing would be "just background" anymore.

Since the sensory input unit occupies a very large region of the cerebral hemispheres, it almost always suffers some damage in closed head TBI, either through focal or diffuse types of injury. Without this natural attention regulator, your child may alternate between states of oversensitivity to stimulation and apparent shutting down or "zoning out," accompanied by blank staring. You can help by maintaining a calm, quiet environment. As much as you want your child to see his friends again, it may be best to limit the number of visitors and length of visits, until you see what your child is ready to handle.

Attention Problems Related to Response Output Problems

There are still more reasons for the attentional problems following TBI. A crucial component of attention is contributed by the response output unit. As you will recall, this unit is composed of the frontal lobes of the brain, which we have already said are the most frequent location for focal injury in closed head TBI.

With age, the frontal lobes become increasingly important in directing and focusing a child's attention. This is because the process of selective attention becomes less and less automatic as we grow older, and is driven more by our important goals and plans. Selection of some stimuli over others is no longer automatic, but voluntary and purposeful. The frontal lobes achieve this complex task through their neural connections with the sensory input unit. The frontal lobes are able to maintain a working memory of a goal and use it to decide what to attend to in the environment and what to disregard. Thus, with age and with development of the frontal lobes, children generally gain the ability to actively manage their attention, to direct attention to goal-relevant information, and to resist extraneous distractions.

If your child's frontal lobes are injured, he loses some ability to voluntarily direct his attention. As difficulties with purposeful, goal-related behavior are among the most disruptive and persistent problems after TBI, we will return to the subject in the section entitled "Executive Functions."

Some of the specific components of attention that may come up in discussions of your child's cognitive status after TBI include sustained, selective, divided, and alternating attention. These are described below.

Difficulties with Sustained Attention

Sustained attention, sometimes referred to as span of attention or concentration, refers to the ability to keep responding consistently for the amount of time needed to complete an age-appropriate task. Both the length of time and the consistency of the response that can be maintained over time are important aspects of sustained attention. Children with difficulties in sustaining attention are unable to stick with even a nondemanding activity, such as a meal or a TV program, but will move restlessly from one thing to the next. Problems in sustained attention are often seen early in recovery, but greatly improve over time in many children with TBI.

Difficulties with Selective Attention

Selective attention is a much more complex form of cognitive activity, and is what we usually think of when we consider the topic of attention. It is what we are requesting when we direct someone to "Pay attention." To be precise, it is the ability to keep focusing on relevant stimuli *in the presence of a distraction.* It is sometimes referred to as "freedom from distractibility." Children who have problems in selective attention are easily drawn off-task by any passing sight, sound, or touch, or even by their own thoughts and internal events (such as stomach growling).

Selective attention is the form of attention that is most needed in the busy real-world environment of home, school, and community. Unfortunately, deficits in selective attention are very common after TBI. Though improvements occur with time, difficulties in this area tend to be quite persistent. Without the frontal lobes to set priorities, it is as if every possible bit of incoming information has equal access to your child's attention. The younger child with TBI may be unable to tolerate a scratchy clothing label, while the school-age child may have difficulty picking out the teacher's voice in a full classroom. Music from a teenaged sibling's room or a baby's cries, once part of the normal household background noise, may become sources of great irritation to children who have had brain injuries.

Difficulties with Alternating Attention

Alternating attention refers to the ability to shift focus from one task to another. It involves a complex series of cognitive activities, including disengaging from one "set" of demands and smoothly shifting the focus of attention to a new set of processing demands. Management of attention in this way is sometimes referred to as mental or cognitive flexibility. Children with problems in alternating their attention may have great difficulty making a transition from one activity to another, or in beginning a new activity on their own. They tend to benefit from preparation or advance warning that a transition time is coming up. They often require very direct instructions on how to start a new activity, in order to be able to make a shift in focus.

Sometimes problems with this form of attention are not apparent in a young child with TBI, but may emerge with age. This is because the complex management skills needed for alternating attention do not usually develop until school age and continue to develop over several years. For example, older children might be expected to be able to take notes while listening to a lecture, or to quickly shift attention from talking with friends to checking for traffic when crossing a street. Younger children are generally not expected to be able to make several shifts back and forth among different mental activities of this nature. As a result, problems might not become apparent until children are older and encounter situations calling for alternating attention.

Difficulties with Divided Attention

Finally, divided attention refers to the ability to attend to multiple tasks, or multiple different components of a task, simultaneously. Examples include talking on the phone while microwaving a snack, watching TV while doing homework, and reading music while watching what the band conductor is doing. What appears to be divided attention may actually be the ability to rapidly alternate attention. Again, this type of complex achievement is generally not expected until late in development and thus may appear as a "delayed" effect of TBI.

Help for Children with Attention Problems

Helping your child with the attention problems that result from TBI can be a great challenge. Fortunately, many teachers are familiar with the skills and techniques that will benefit your child in the classroom, since they are the same measures that would be recommended for a child with attention-deficit/hyperactivity disorder (AD/HD). (AD/HD is the term for developmental— rather than acquired—attention deficits.) Often the single most helpful thing the school can do is to place your child, at least for a time, in a small (six to eight students), self-contained classroom where individual instruction is available. Many other techniques, such as reducing distractions when selective attention is required, maintaining structure and routine, and keeping instructions clear and simple, are useful both at home and at school.

As a parent, one key to helping your child with attention problems is to understand which behaviors are under his control. Some behaviors attributed to attention problems are similar to those that would be considered normal at a younger age. So, parents sometimes feel that their child is just "acting silly" in order to gain attention from others. In addition, it is very common for these problems to appear intermittently, even within a single day, and in connection with some activities but not others. Parents often report, for example, that, "It seems like he can pay attention when he wants to." They wonder if symptoms may actually be occurring because their child was a bit "spoiled" in the hospital, and they worry that they may actually interfere with recovery by making accommodations and lowering expectations.

Actually, variations in your child's behavior are more likely due to fluctuations in energy level, other competing demands on his limited attentional resources, or the appeal of a particular sound or sight. Even children with significant attention impairments can sustain attention in *some* situations. It is the ability to generate attention from within when an activity is *not* appealing that is impaired after TBI.

Rehabilitation professionals would be quick to reassure parents that the vast majority of children want to do their best. They want to be competent and independent, and they need and deserve our trust and confidence.

Books and organizations for parents of children with AD/HD are good sources of support and information. Since difficulties with purposeful, goal-related behavior, including management of attention, are among the most disruptive and persistent problems after TBI, we will return to this subject in the section entitled "Executive Functions." Chapters 7, 8, and 9 offer additional guidance in helping your child with attention problems.

∷ Visual Processing

The sense of hearing, because of its role in language and communication, is considered to be our "most essential" sense. Disorders that affect how the brain processes auditory information—particularly *ver-*

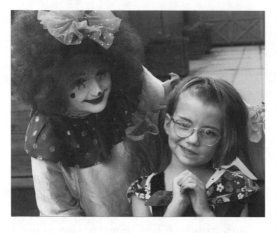

bal auditory information (language)—, often occur after TBI, and are discussed in Chapter 6.

Next to hearing, we obtain most of our information about the world through our sense of vision. Visual processing plays a key role in self-care, leisure, work, and school activities. The visual system is very complex, and is widely distributed throughout the brain. Disruptions of visual processing often occur with TBI, but are not as obvious to the observer as are disruptions of language. Consequently, their impact on an injured child's functioning is not always fully appreciated.

Difficulties with the Visual System

To help you understand the visual processing problems that can occur after TBI, we need to continue the discussion of the functional organization of the brain begun earlier in this chapter.

Light entering the eye stimulates receptor cells in the *retina*—the membrane at the back of the eyeball. Fibers from each retina travel into the brain in separate bundles called optic nerves. At a place near the center of the brain called the optic chiasm, fibers from the inside (next to the nose) halves of each retina cross over and join with fibers from the outer half of the opposite retina. These "mixed" bundles, called optic tracts, fan out and travel backward until they reach their destination in the brain—the primary zone for visual input, called the visual or occipital cortex. At this point, the complex process that converts light energy into something meaningful begins. Before discussing ways in which this process might be disrupted by TBI, however, we need to briefly consider things that can go wrong before information ever reaches the visual cortex.

Cranial Nerve Problems

All the muscles of the head—including the muscles responsible for eye movements—are controlled by nerves located in the brainstem.

These ten brainstem nerves (plus two that do not travel to the brainstem) are called the cranial nerves. Cranial nerve dysfunction occurs frequently after TBI, generally due to swelling, bleeding, or other sources of pressure. Three of the cranial nerves, the oculomotor (III), the trochlear (IV), and the abducens (VI), are involved in movements of the eyeball and pupil. Injury to these nerves can result in a number of problems, including:

- *ptosis*—drooping of the eyelid (the effects are primarily cosmetic).
- *dilation of the pupil*—inability of the pupil to get smaller in response to light. When this happens, the lens cannot focus on near objects, so that acuity, or the ability to see things clearly, is reduced.
- *strabismus*—a condition in which both eyes cannot focus on the same point because one eye is deviated outward, inward, and/or upward. This results in double vision.

These problems tend to get better without treatment as swelling subsides in the first days or weeks after injury.

Optic Nerve and Tract Problems

As we noted above, the optic nerve carries fibers from the retina to the visual cortex. It is also considered a cranial nerve, although it does not enter the brainstem. Compression of the optic nerve can cause decreased acuity (ability to see clearly) or even loss of vision. If the optic nerve is ruptured or cut, there will be permanent loss of vision in a particular portion of the *visual field*—the total area that can be seen without moving the eyes or head.

How the visual field is affected depends on the location of the injury. If the optic nerve is completely severed or *sectioned* before it reaches the optic chiasm, blindness in the same-side eye will result. A cut or injury past the level of the chiasm will interrupt fibers coming from the opposite visual field, resulting in blindness in each eye for that portion of the visual field when the eyes are stationary. This condition is called right or left homonymous hemianopsia or quadrantic field defect.

Though visual field cuts are often seen following focal injury, such as from stroke or tumor, they are not common in TBI. When they do occur, they are usually temporary and disappear as swelling subsides. If not, children usually readily learn to turn their head so that images fall on the "good" portions of the retina. If your child seems to be holding his head at an odd angle in relation to what he is viewing, he needs further visual evaluation. If your child has persistent visual field cuts, rehab staff will recommend ways to position materials to help your child see them best.

A Note about Blindsight

As noted previously, most visual information travels from the retina to the occipital lobe, where complex processing begins. However, some impulses do not make it that far but take a detour, ending instead in a structure located in the upper brainstem. This pathway is referred to as the "second" visual system. The role of this system in vision is not completely understood. However, it appears to provide information about the *presence and location* of an object, while giving no information about the specific features or identity of the item, or even any awareness that something is being "seen." This apparent perception without awareness has been termed "blindsight."

Damage to this system can result in difficulties in shifting gaze, and in orienting to, tracking, and localizing objects in the environment. A child with these problems may be confused and have vague complaints of visual problems, even when no problems can be detected in acuity, eye movements, or ability to identify visual stimuli. On the other hand, a child with an intact blindsight system may be able to respond to a moving target, navigate around obstacles, and reach accurately. This may be the case even if he has severe visual field cuts or destruction of the visual cortex resulting in an inability to identify anything by sight or even to have conscious awareness of vision. This child may unfairly be assumed to be "faking" or at least exaggerating his visual difficulties, when in reality he is using information supplied by this "second" visual system.

Visual Perceptual Problems

At last we are ready to consider higher-level visual perceptual problems following TBI—that is, difficulties in *interpreting* the visual signal that reaches the occipital cortex. These problems vary, depending on whether damage has occurred in the primary, secondary, or tertiary zone of the occipital cortex.

Problems in the Primary Zone

The primary zone of the visual system is located at the back of the brain. It is where electrical signals traveling from the retina by way of the optic nerve terminate.

Blind Spots. Localized injury to the visual primary zone is rare in TBI. When it does occur, it results in problems similar to those caused by optic nerve damage. That is, it causes loss of vision in the specific area of the retina that is connected to the damaged area in the brain. This area of loss is known as a *scotoma* or *blind spot*. The brain is very clever about "filling in" such blind spots, either by learning to turn the eye to use functional portions of the visual cortex, or by using experience to make a "best guess" estimate of what should be in the missing spot.

Problems in the Secondary Zone

The story is quite different, however, as information continues on to the secondary zone of the visual cortex. It is here that the isolated sensations of lines or flashes of color received in the primary zone are built up into unified images of whole objects or scenes that correspond to something in the external world. Cells in this region combine the input of cells from different parts of the primary zone that happen to be activated at the same time that an individual looks at a particular object. After the same group of cells has repeatedly fired together, that group tends to be linked in some way so that they fire together more easily. When the brain recognizes a pattern as having fired in synchrony before, a visual memory has been formed. This is what enables us to recognize a horse as a horse, or a particular face as belonging to a particular person.

Damage to these secondary areas makes it more difficult to make sense of the visual world than damage to primary areas does. It is difficult for us to imagine or describe what this type of visual experience must be like. Someone who has this problem himself is unable to pinpoint the problem. He is not blind in the usual sense of the word. He perceives individual features quite well, but does not reliably combine them into recognizable wholes. He may guess the identity of an object based on a few prominent features. For example, he may see a yellow marker as a banana. He may be unable to recognize items that are partially hidden or that are seen in silhouette or at an unfamiliar angle. He may be unable to judge where one item ends and another begins.

Ability to detect patterns, to discriminate subtle differences, and to match items by sight alone may be impaired. He may have great difficulty appreciating the overall meaning of a picture or series of pictures, focusing instead on isolated details. He may have trouble with particular kinds of stimuli, such as letters or faces. Facial expressions and other types of "body language" may no longer carry clear meanings for him.

The more complex the visual environment, the more confusing it is for someone with damage to the secondary areas. In settings such as a busy classroom or city street, your child may have to expend a great deal of mental energy and processing time simply trying to determine the identity of everyday objects. As a result, it may seem as if he has a general slowness of thinking, rather than a visual deficit per se. At this stage of processing, however, his difficulties will be restricted to visual material only. Your child will still be able to recognize complex sounds or identify objects by touch, for example.

If your child has these types of visual-perceptual problems, he will benefit from the simplification of visual materials. For instance, a page of math problems might be divided into quarters with only one problem per quarter and a box to indicate where to put the answer. Enlarged and darkened print might also be helpful.

Problems in the Tertiary Zone

As visual information proceeds to the tertiary zone of the sensory unit, it is linked to many different types of input, including auditory, touch, and body-sense (position of joints and muscles). Injury in this area is not reflected by an impairment in any specific sensory domain, such as vision. Instead, it results in more subtle difficulties in complex processes of thinking and understanding.

The tertiary cortex is unique to humans, and doesn't reach maturity until a child is around six or seven. As noted earlier in this chapter, the tertiary cortex occupies a very large region of the brain. It is at the "top" of the hierarchy of information processing, and thus "accumulates" errors from lower levels of processing. For these reasons, deficits in one or more aspects of tertiary zone function frequently occur in children with TBI. Although we will discuss these difficulties from the perspective of their visual components, bear in mind that none of the tertiary zone functions affect vision alone.

As the visual pathways continue beyond the secondary occipital cortex and into the tertiary association cortex, they can be divided into two main "streams," each of which participates in different cognitive functions. One pathway leads into the temporal lobe and forms connections primarily with auditory/verbal representations of information. This pathway is sometimes called the "what" system of vision, since it allows us to label and describe what we see in words. The other pathway extends into the parietal lobe. Its major role is the combination of visual, touch, and position information, which allows us to understand spatial relationships and to perform movements guided by our vision. This system is sometimes called the "where" system.

Visual-Auditory Integration Problems. When areas devoted to visual-auditory integration (the "what" system) are disrupted, it interferes with many types of naming activities. Your child may have difficulties naming pictures or actual things, recognizing and naming letters and words (reading), recognizing the meaning of symbols such as mathematical signs and punctuation marks, spelling and writing, and connecting names with faces.

Unilateral Neglect. One rather extreme phenomenon that can occur with extensive damage to the tertiary zone, particularly if the damage is on the right side of the brain, is called unilateral neglect. It consists of inattention to, or failure to respond to, anything that is presented to the child's left side. Neglect may be accompanied by an actual visual field loss. (This situation occurs due to involvement of primary visual pathways, as described above.) But it can also occur despite completely intact vision. Neglect is considered a failure of *attention,* due to loss of spatial awareness.

Children with this problem are not aware that they are not attending to part of the environment. They may bump into walls, furniture, etc. to their left. It is as if they do not perceive that part of space as real, even though they can see it. In extreme cases, they may fail to wash or dress the left side of the body, even though they can clearly see it, because it does not "feel like" it is a part of them. More frequently, the problems are more subtle. Your child may fail to return to the left margin in reading, so that a passage becomes nonsensical. Or he may start in the middle of the page when writing, or fail to look to the left when crossing the street.

Even though obvious forms of neglect tend to get better over time, subtle signs may remain. For example, your child may have a tendency to overlook things to the left, or to make more errors with items on the left side of the page. Some helpful compensatory techniques include reminding your child to scan by turning his head through the full range of motion, and providing some kind of left-margin signal for printed material, such as a dark line, or a number. Sometimes placing items in a vertical rather than a horizontal array is helpful.

Difficulties Interpreting Spatial Information. Even if your child is aware of, and responsive to, the full range of visual space, he may not fully appreciate or comprehend the spatial information that is normally conveyed through visual experience. This might mean, for example, that he no longer knows the location of your home in relation to a familiar visual cue. Even if he was previously independent in your neighborhood, he may suddenly find himself easily lost and disoriented. He may have great difficulty learning and remembering new routes, such as the way to math class in middle school, or the way back to the car at the mall. He may have significant problems using a map or telling time on a clock with hands. Knowing how to turn and manipulate two objects to make them fit together may be a complete puzzle to him, only accomplished after painful trial and error instead of visual inspection.

A broad range of activities depend upon processing of spatial information, including things such as making a bed, putting clothes on correctly, and making a fort out of blocks. With repeated experiences moving, turning, and looking *right* or *left,* we build up an internal sense of the part of space that those words refer to. But with damage to the tertiary zone, this ability to "feel" the difference between left and right may be impaired, so that those words alone no longer tell your child how to move or where to look.

Other words with visual-spatial meanings, such as "over," "behind," "inside," etc. become confusing. (Imagine the plight of the third grader who is told to "Put your paper inside your book and put your book under your desk, then line up to the right of the door." He may be able to comply by verbally thinking through each move, but by then his class will be long gone!) Besides following directions, these problems will interfere with many visual activities in the classroom, such as interpreting pictures, graphs, or charts.

Difficulties with Abstract Concepts. When children have difficulties understanding and using concrete space, they may also have problems understanding and using conceptual or abstract space. As a result, children who have had TBI may find it especially challenging to grasp concepts that require understanding a spatial relationship.

For example, they may have trouble with numerical reasoning, logic, time, and complex grammatical constructions such as passive voice or embedded clauses.

Difficulties with Visual-Motor Integration. The ability to use vision to guide movement is called visual-motor integration. It involves mentally converting information received through the eyes into a plan for motor output. It is involved in every act of moving the body through visual space (such as maneuvering a wheelchair through a doorway or reaching for something seen), as well as in copying, drawing, and writing.

Though other areas of the brain are also essential to planned motor output, the tertiary zone is thought to contain the internalized "map" of external space used for planning movement. Without access to this integrated "visual-motor plan book," many complex tasks that were once almost automatic become agonizingly laborious and frustrating. For example, your child will have great difficulty using fine motor skills to copy shapes or a homework assignment on the blackboard, or using visual memory to form letters (written expression).

Help for Children with Visual Processing Problems

At some point in recovery, your child should have a complete visual examination. Ideally, this should take place after he is medically stable but before he returns to school. If this is not done as a part of inpatient rehabilitation, you can ask hospital staff or your pediatrician to recommend an ophthalmologist who is familiar with traumatic brain injury.

An occupational therapist can also provide excellent guidance in helping your child make the most of his visual function. For example, the OT might suggest ways to help your child maintain proper positioning, whether in a chair, a school desk, or a wheelchair. He or she can also recommend ways to properly position materials on a work surface, perhaps with a slantboard or other assistive device. The OT evaluation can take place in a rehabilitation or through the school.

At home, your child will benefit from simplification of the visual environment. It will help to reduce visual distractions or "clutter," and to keep household items in familiar places. To help your child participate in meals and dressing, you may need to set up or arrange utensils, food containers, and clothing in a way that makes it easier for him to perceive them. You may also need to give your child reminders to search intentionally and systematically for needed objects. And you will definitely need to be ready to provide your child with extra supervision for safety.

There are many strategies that can help your child in the classroom. Fortunately, many school staff are familiar with visual processing problems because they have encountered them in children with developmental learning disorders. For example, usually, it is very helpful to reduce the amount of written work required. For example, your child might write just the assigned spelling word on a test, rather than a complete sentence. Children with visual perceptual and visual-motor problems also need extra time to complete written work. Other accommodations that might help your child include:

- Minimize copying from the blackboard or book.
- Provide a printed copy of homework assignments.
- Use dark-lined paper, bold and/or enlarged type, and clearly marked answer boxes.
- Put a dark line on the left margin of the page to help cue your child to pay attention to that side of the page.
- Attach an alphabet strip and number line to the desktop for reference.
- Use a straight-edge or "window" cut-out on the page to reduce visual distractions during reading.
- Consider using computers and other technology. The selection of assistive technology devices and training in their use is usually a collaborative effort by professionals in the rehabilitation or school setting.

:: Executive Functions

Executive functions is an umbrella term for the cluster of cognitive processes that are needed for organized, goal-directed behavior. Executive functions are involved in any cognitive activity requiring us to mentally manipulate information not immediately present to our senses. They are also involved in any decision or activity requiring anything more than an automatic or habitual response. Executive function deficits are very common after closed head TBI, and you may see this term in reports or hear it frequently from your child's treatment team.

How Executive Function Works

You will recall that, earlier in this chapter, we divided the brain into three functional units. We have discussed the effects of TBI in two of these units: the brainstem arousal unit and the sensory reception, processing, and storage unit. What remains is the unit that is specialized for *response output*—that is, for sending out messages that result in the performance of some action. Centers for selecting, sequencing, and initiating responses are contained in the frontal lobes. As you know, the frontal lobes are almost always injured in closed head TBI. In addition, pathways connect the frontal lobes to nearly every other area of the brain. These pathways are often disrupted by widespread stretching and tearing.

We also noted earlier that each of the three functional units can be divided into three levels of complexity—primary, secondary, and tertiary. The primary division of the frontal cortex consists of a "motor strip." Impulses arising in the motor strip result directly in particular actions. In lower species, the motor strip has close connections with sensory processing areas. Much of behavior, then, is determined by particular sensory input. That is, it is set into action by a particular sensory stimulus and is fairly automatic and invariable. This is an effective system for insuring the fulfillment of basic needs (like eating) and the survival of the animal.

With evolution, humans have acquired the ability to control "automatic" responding. Consequently, our behavior is not "driven" by stimuli in the environment as animal behavior is. We are able to combine bits and pieces of motor patterns to produce entirely new responses to meet the demands of new circumstances. We are able to keep working on a solution, even if the original stimulus is no longer present. These abilities (and others we will discuss below) are absolutely essential for appropriate, effective functioning in our complex world. They have been made possible by development of secondary and tertiary frontal regions which do more than simply initiate automatic responses. These regions are able to plan both complex motor patterns (for example, a slam-dunk) and complex behavior sequences that are completed over time (for example, writing a term paper). But before these more complex behavior patterns can have a chance to be expressed, automatic responses must somehow be blocked.

Inhibition

One key executive function controlled by the frontal lobes is inhibition. The frontal lobes make it possible for us to pursue these longer-term plans and goals by *inhibiting* impulsive, automatic responses to stimuli—whether external stimuli, such as a comment from a friend, or internal stimuli, such as hunger or fear. The frontal lobes insert a "pause" between stimulus and response. In that pause, a number of crucial "executive" processes occur that greatly expand our response options. For example, we don't immediately have to respond with a mean comment when someone says something mean to us. Instead, we can *inhibit* the first response that comes to mind (a mean comment) and choose a response based on a goal such as not getting in trouble with the teacher.

As you can see, one of the most important roles of the frontal lobes is impulse control. This is very often impaired after TBI. It is important to note that control is ordinarily achieved, not by *eliminating* automatic responding, but by inhibiting or suppressing it. If this inhibitory process is damaged, automatic, stimulus-driven responding returns. Without impulse control, a child has fewer *choices* in behavior.

Working Memory

Where do our choices come from? How do we go about selecting an alternative behavior that may be more appropriate in a particular social situation, or more beneficial in the long run, than an impulsive response? The frontal lobes take care of this problem, too. Through their extensive connections with other brain regions, they create a mental "scratch-pad" called "working memory." In working memory, all stored and incoming information relevant to a particular situation can be called up into consciousness, represented, combined, and manipulated. As working memory interacts with impulse control, it becomes possible to *organize* our behavior, as described below.

Organization

As the child in the example above inhibits his impulse to respond to a mean comment with his own mean remark, his working memory brings up information to help him decide how to react. He remembers his mom's advice to ignore bullies and his teacher's recent instruction to complete work quietly or lose recess time. He remembers his plans to play ball with a friend at recess, and the anticipated enjoyment acts as a temporary reward. He chooses to remain silent, move away from the bully, and complete his work. Thanks to working memory, he was able to anticipate a future desired state and plan a series of actions needed to reach that goal. Because of impulse control, he was able to use this plan to direct his behavior instead of immediate needs and wants unrelated to his goal.

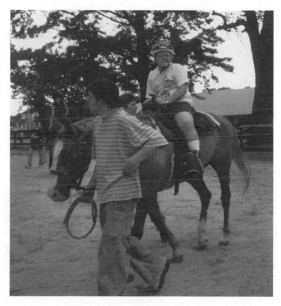

When behavior is consistently governed by plans and goals, it becomes *organized* and purposeful, rather than fragmented and "scatterbrained." Another way of looking at it is to say that our thinking and behavior become controlled by internalized language, rather than by impulse. Because our goal is kept alive in working memory, we can constantly compare our current status with where we want to be, and adjust our plan as circumstances change. That is, our overall direction stays organized, even in an unpredictable world. We can tolerate some unexpected "bumps in the road" and make mid-course corrections.

Executive Management of Attention

The frontal lobes, through "feedback loops" with the sensory input unit, have developed the ability to direct our attention to information in the environment that is important to future goals and to "filter out" non-relevant distractions. With age, this ability to control attention and behavior by future goals increases.

In the example above, the child whose behavior is controlled by the goal of playing ball at recess will be better able to focus on the teacher's voice and the work on his desk, and less distracted by the noise around him.

When your child has difficulties with executive function, his attention is easily captured by any passing sight or sound. He appears disorganized and distracted.

Acquiring Abstract Concepts and Rules

Because of our mental "scratch-pad," we can consider multiple aspects of a situation, even if we experienced them separately over time, and draw out common features. In so doing, we develop concepts, generalizations, and rules. For example, after repeated experiences in a variety of situations, people in the U.S. learn the rule of "stay to the right" and can apply that rule in traffic, on a busy sidewalk, or on a high school stairway. In contrast, a teenager with an executive function deficit might learn to use his memory book effectively in the rehabilitation setting, but be completely unable to carry over that skill to his school. Likewise, he may have difficulty applying a math operation learned in one context to a word problem using a different situation.

Once we have internalized rules and concepts, they can control our behavior, instead of immediate internal impulses or external "triggers." This helps free us from concrete thinking, and we can appreciate symbolism, humor, innuendo, sarcasm, and other forms of abstract thought and indirect communication. Children with executive function dysfunction, on the other hand, tend to think in very concrete, literal terms. I am reminded of a teenager with TBI who was working diligently on a reading comprehension exercise while in rehab. When asked, "What happens at the end of the story?" she replied, "I stop reading."

Frustration Tolerance

Ordinarily, as a child grows older, he is able to wait for a reward because he can mentally represent that reward in working memory. In other words, when working memory is working well, the *anticipation* of the desired goal becomes an effective stand-in for the real thing. The child who can keep an anticipated reward in working memory is able to accept a brief delay when Mom says, "Just a minute" or the teacher says, "It's not your turn yet." To the child with an executive dysfunction, the situation seems quite hopeless and intolerable if demands are not met *immediately*.

Flexibility, Creativity, and Initiation

As we hold bits of information in working memory, we are able to mentally combine them in new ways, to generate new solutions in unfamiliar situations. We can mentally try out new ideas and consider their long-term consequences. Thus, we can be flexible and creative. We can come up with activities to fill unstructured time by creating possibilities through working memory, without needing an external stimulus or prompt to get started.

In contrast, children with TBI may become dependent on others to structure his free time. He may become quite "clingy" and complain of being bored, or he may simply appear disinterested and apathetic. This lack of initiative is sometimes interpreted as emotional depression.

Children with TBI may also become easily "stuck" on one approach or solution and be unable to come up with alternatives. They may repeat the same unsuccessful response over and over, or be unable to get restarted after encountering an obstacle. This mental inflexibility often interferes with a child's ability to independently complete academic work.

Insight, Empathy, and Responsibility

Through working memory, we are able to mentally replay our own actions and then observe them objectively, as an outsider "looking in." In so doing, we gain insight and the ability to judge the appropriateness of a particular course of action. As an observer of ourselves, we are able to take the perspective of another. We lose some of our self-centeredness and gain empathy. We develop a sense of ourselves as independently acting entities, responsible for our own behavior.

Children with TBI, on the other hand, may have great difficulty evaluating their own behavior and appreciating the effects of that behavior on others. Parents sometimes report that their child seems "selfish" or "uncaring." He is not intentionally acting that way, however, and will generally respond well if you give him calm, nonjudgmental feedback.

Help for Children with Executive Function Problems

Many of the suggestions provided earlier for higher-level attention and memory problems are equally appropriate for executive function problems. Other strategies for encouraging impulse control include:

- *Teach your child to use "self-talk,"* such as "STOP, LOOK, and LISTEN" for the younger child, or "Calm down—keep it small" for teenagers.
- *Break complex, lengthy tasks down into individual steps.* For example, "Clean your room" may overwhelm your child, but he may happily comply when told, "Put all the clothes on the floor in this hamper and tell me when you're finished." Then give step 2, etc.
- *Encourage him to make notes and lists.* Incorporate use of a daily, weekly, and monthly planner book into everyday routine. Model this behavior yourself, and it may help *you* get organized!
- *If your child has difficulty getting started, provide two choices.* For example, ask, "Do you want to color a picture or help me bake brownies right now?" Or, provide very concrete, specific directions for beginning a task.
- *Model goal-setting and problem-solving by "thinking out loud"* with your child as you make everyday decisions and deal with unexpected events.
- *Encourage self-monitoring* by asking your child to predict how he will do on a task, then comparing prediction with reality. Be positive about his successes, but trouble-shoot when his prediction doesn't match results.
- *Tactfully check on your child frequently* if he is doing independent work, to be sure that he is still "on track."
- For the older adolescent, *consider a job coach* or organization skills tutor.
- *Supervise social interactions,* and, for the younger child, *provide structured activities* with one or two friends at a time.

Long-Term Effects on Executive Function

These are very complex and important cognitive processes! They will not all suddenly disappear after TBI. Children with TBI may have problems with executive functioning ranging from quite mild and subtle, such as distractibility under highly stimulating conditions, to very severe, such as dangerous impulsivity or almost complete inability to initiate any activity without external prompting.

Some problems your child experiences early in recovery may get better. On the other hand, new problems may emerge with age as higher levels of abstract thinking and impulse control are expected. Problems with impulse control and working memory have such a big effect on social/emotional behavior and are such a pressing concern for many parents that they are discussed more thoroughly in Chapters 7 and 8. Since executive function problems also have a significant effect on academic achievement, additional suggestions for compensating for these difficulties are offered in Chapter 9.

▌ The Neuropsychological Evaluation

This chapter has emphasized the complexity of cognitive issues after TBI and the importance of obtaining accurate information about your child's needs and abilities. The person who is most likely to provide this piece of the puzzle is a *neuropsychologist*. A neuropsychologist is a psychologist who has completed specialized training beyond the Ph.D. level in the cognitive and behavioral problems that result from changes in normal brain function. These changes may be due to injury, illness, a developmental (inborn) disorder, or other neurological event. The *pediatric* neuropsychologist has further specialized in the problems of *children* with brain disorders, and how those problems will affect development.

If your child is placed in a rehabilitation program, either as an inpatient or on a day-hospital basis, he will probably be seen regularly by a neuropsychologist as part of the multidisciplinary evaluation and treatment team. The neuropsychologist in the rehab setting will help develop an initial treatment plan, will monitor changes in cognitive status and confer frequently with others on the rehab team; provide information and support to your family; and communicate with school staff before and after discharge, as needed. The role of the neuropsychologist is to help parents, teachers, and others understand:

- how the injury has affected learning, information processing, and behavior;
- what interventions are appropriate at different stages of recovery;
- what services and accommodations may be needed to support learning upon return to school; and

■ what improvements, problems, and changes to watch for as the processes of recovery and development continue.

If your child will not be receiving rehabilitation care after he is discharged from the hospital, ask hospital staff if there is a neuropsychologist at the hospital who could complete an evaluation prior to discharge. If this is not possible, the task of completing appropriate evaluations may fall to the school. In working with school staff to plan your child's transition back to school, it is advisable to specifically request a neuropsychological evalution for your child. In most cases, this goes beyond the scope of generally available school-based psychological evaluations. Names of neuropsychologists may be obtained from medical schools in your area, state professional psychology organizations, state chapters of the National Brain Injury Association, and the Brain Injury Association's *Directory of Brain Injury Rehabilitation Services.*

After the neuropsychologist sees your child, he or she will provide a written report of findings, based on information from:

■ a developmental history obtained from careful interview with you, the parents;

■ an educational history from school records;

■ a review of the medical records of the injury and subsequent course of recovery;

■ observations of your child in different settings;

■ consultation with other therapists;

■ formal testing of major cognitive domains: These will vary depending upon your child's status and stage of recovery, but may include general intelligence, memory, attention, visual-perceptual and visual-motor abilities, and executive functions. The important areas of academic function and language abilities will also be assessed, if this information is not available from specialists in these areas.

Make sure that the school special education team receives a copy of the neuropsychologist's report. Be sure to keep a copy in your permanent files. At the end of each school year, request that your child's teachers for the upcoming year review the report and meet with current teachers, so they will be familiar with your child's strengths and needs. Remember, the neuropsychologist is another member of your "circle of support." Don't hesitate to contact him or her if you have questions or concerns, whether early in the recovery process or well down the road!

■■ A Closing Note

The goal of this chapter has been to present the full array of changes in thinking and learning that may occur after moderate or severe TBI. Being familiar with these terms and symptoms will better prepare you to understand the connection between your child's injury and current needs. You will be able to communicate effectively with the professionals who work with your child, and you will be a confident advocate in school programming decisions. We have tried to be thorough. Does this mean that you should expect to see *all* of these difficulties, and to the degree of severity described? Absolutely not! Remember, every brain injury is unique.

What about the question of changes over time? In the past, the rule of thumb was that all recovery that is going to occur takes place within the first year or so after injury. This is no longer considered valid. Yes, the *rate* of recovery is most rapid during that period, but most rehabilitation specialists would agree that improvements in function can continue to emerge indefinitely into the future. Schools are increasingly aware of the unique needs of children with TBI, and many are developing exciting new programs to meet those needs. Most are willing to work creatively with parents and other professionals in the best interests of the child. Community agencies are beginning to respond to the longer-term needs of young adults, with innovative programs such as job coaches and group homes, which will allow most individuals with TBI to eventually live independently or semi-independently and to do satisfying, productive work.

Brain injury is a life-changing event for all involved, but you do not have to navigate this new territory alone! Along the way, you will connect with other families who will offer support, encouragement, and invaluable information. You will work with many dedicated, relentlessly optimistic pediatric specialists! And you will gain some very satisfying insights about your own inner strengths. You will burst with pride at times, at the strength you will see in your child. As one father said, "I say to my son whenever he faces a challenge: 'Remember, you got through your TBI – you can handle anything!' And he says to me, 'You too, Dad!'" And it's true.

❚❚ Parent Statements

Sometimes the things he blurts out are so honest and up-front that we just have to laugh.

❧❀❧

It's so hard to be patient when he forgets the simplest things, or insists we haven't told him something we went over a hundred times. I get angry and then I feel guilty.

❧❀❧

It has been helpful for us to try to focus on the progress she has made since the accident, and not on how things were before the accident.

❧❀❧

It still hurts when people who know about the accident say things like, "You shouldn't let him talk to you like that," or, "If he were my child, he'd never get away with that." They just have no idea how much every normal thought and action depends on a normal, uninjured brain.

❧❀❧

Most of the time now, he's doing great. I guess we've all learned to make adjustments. It's only when he gets really tired or things get too busy and complicated that I can see that the problems—mostly attention and memory—are still there.

❧❀❧

I always feel so anxious for her every time the school has to do an assessment. I hate the idea that she may not "perform" as well as she can on the day that they're doing the IQ testing, and get really anxious about finding out the results.

❧❀❧

It's very important to me to find out the results of any intelligence testing before the IEP meeting, so I have time to absorb the results and deal with my feelings about them in private.

❧❀❧

It's very hard for me to bring myself to discipline him for anything. I never know if it's his fault or the accident's fault. How much should I expect? The professionals can't really answer that for every situation.

❧❀❧

One of the most helpful things I ever heard from a therapist was to have faith in my own judgment and my own instincts. The fact is, there aren't any magic solutions. You have to do what works best for your child and your whole family.

HOW TBI
AFFECTS SPEECH
AND LANGUAGE

Lisa Schoenbrodt, Ed.D., CCC-SLP

At the rehabilitation unit, Mrs. Smith expressed concern that Johnny was unable to talk or communicate his needs. In response, the speech-language pathologist at the hospital developed a communication board for Johnny consisting of a few pictures of family members and his favorite foods. Johnny was not always able to use the board and frequently became irritated and pushed the board away. However, as time passed and his overall condition began to improve, he became better at using the board to communicate his needs. Eventually, he was able to use his voice again. His voice was somewhat hoarse at first, but improved on its own without any formal therapy.

Daily speech-language therapy was recommended during his rehabilitation stay. Therapy sessions were short, and focused first on his overall orientation to his surroundings and on communication needed to function in this environment. As Johnny continued to improve, the length of therapy was increased and goals changed to focus on language skills needed to return to school.

Johnny was discharged to a day hospital, where he continued to receive daily speech-language therapy. Goals focused on helping him develop methods for retrieving words and on improving his memory. Johnny found it helpful to think of categories of words, such as foods, or to visualize the word he was trying to retrieve. Despite this success, Johnny continued to have trouble in social situations. He rarely initiated a conversation, and once he began, he continually jumped from topic to topic without any warning. In addition, his word retrieval difficulties were more noticeable during conversations, as he frequently circumlocuted, or talked around a word instead of just saying it.

As the time neared for Johnny to return to school, the speech-language pathologist (SLP) at the day hospital contacted the SLP at Johnny's school. Together they discussed Johnny's progress, goals for transition back to school, and how much speech-language therapy Johnny would need upon his return to the school. The school SLP was somewhat knowledgeable about TBI, as she had recently attended a course and planned to attend the inservice to be provided by the rehabilitation staff. While the school SLP was eager to help with the transition, she was not sure how much speech-language therapy Johnny should receive each week. She decided to wait until Johnny returned to school to re-evaluate his needs.

At an educational meeting held at the school, everyone agreed that Johnny should receive direct speech-language therapy services. That is, the SLP would work with Johnny directly, rather than consulting with teachers about his difficulties. The SLP was to see Johnny on a weekly basis, both in the classroom and in a small group or individually, when needed. She would continue to work on communication needs for the classroom, such as vocabulary and word retrieval, and would also work on social skills in less structured settings, such as the playground, recess, etc. She would be in daily contact with Johnny's teachers and re-evaluate his progress monthly.

Now, after six months, Johnny's overall communication skills have improved. His parents were very helpful in coming in at the beginning of the school year to meet with everyone involved in their son's program. However, Johnny continues to have some problems with social skills. This area will need to be monitored, particularly upon transition to middle school. An in-depth speech-language evaluation will be conducted to aid in the development of goals for the transition to middle school.

▪▪ The Effects of TBI on Communication Skills

Children who have an acquired brain injury can have many problems with communication—with giving and receiving information. They may have problems with both major components of communication: speech and language. Or they may just have problems with language. These difficulties may be only temporary and improve over time, or they may be permanent. Unfortunately, communication problems often persist for years, largely depending on the severity of the TBI.

The type of speech and language difficulties your child has depends upon how her head moved during the injury. A "straight-line" trauma such as hitting a windshield may cause less damage than a trauma that causes extreme force from side to side. The side-to-side action can result in a *coup contrecoup injury,* where the brain strikes the front of the skull and then rebounds, hitting the back of the skull. This type of injury results in more widespread damage, including bruising of the brain tissue. In addition, more damage can result due to post-traumatic swelling and bleeding that may occur in the brain. In general, the more widespread or diffuse the damage is, the more significant the speech and language problem will be.

Speech Problems

Speech is the process of producing sounds and combining the sounds into words and sentences for communication. Effective speech involves coordinating the structures involved in respiration (breathing), phonation (voice production), and articulation (sound production). A brain injury may cause difficulties in any of these areas. Overall, however, speech problems are less common than language problems in children with TBI (see below).

Children with TBI may experience *dysarthric* or *dysfluent* speech in the initial phases of recovery. Dysarthric speech is slow and labored, sometimes with imprecise articulation. Dysfluent speech is otherwise known as stuttering. It is characterized by repetitions of sounds, syllables, words, or phrases, which impair the overall flow of speech. Both conditions may make it difficult for a child to make herself understood. Following a TBI, these conditions may eventually subside without any treatment, or they may persist.

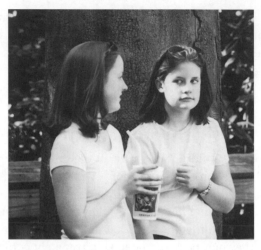

Other speech problems that can result from a brain injury include:

- **Respiration (breathing) difficulties:** Improper respiration can affect voice quality, making it sound very labored, excessively breathy, and out of sync.
- **Speech sound production difficulties:** These include dysarthria, as well as *apraxia* or *dyspraxia*. In apraxia, a child is unable to plan and make the movements needed to produce sounds or words. In dyspraxia, the child has difficulty with these movements.
- **Vocal problems:** Problems with resonance, or how the air vibrates within the throat and head, can result in a child's voice sounding either too nasal or too hollow. Problems with voice quality can result in a hoarse, breathy, or other atypical voice quality.

Language Problems

Language is any set of arbitrary symbols that people use to communicate with one another. These symbols can take the form of spoken words, written symbols, or gestures. For example, English, Spanish, French, and Chinese are languages that can be spoken and written, Braille is an exclusively written language, and American Sign Language is a language made up of gestures.

To communicate with others, a child must develop two types of language skills:

1. *receptive language,* or the ability to understand the language that others are using;

2. *expressive language,* or the ability to use language to express herself to others.

A child with a language disorder may have impairments in either receptive or expressive language or both.

Language problems are more common than speech problems in children with TBI, affecting many children. These problems can range from mild to severe and may be temporary or permanent.

One reason that children with TBI may have language problems is that language abilities are closely linked to cognitive functions. In particular, language abilities are related to *executive functions* of the brain:

- attention,
- memory,
- conceptual organization (being able to categorize information so that concepts can be stored in the brain and used when needed),
- speed of processing (how fast the child can respond to information she hears),
- analysis and synthesis of environmental cues and conversation (for example, being able to focus in on what is important in a noisy environment, or reading facial expressions and cues to get the message that a listener doesn't understand you).

When executive functions are disrupted by brain injury, language may also be impaired. This results in difficulties in:

- learning new vocabulary,
- thinking of the right word,
- following multi-step directions,
- understanding idioms, metaphors, and figurative language, and
- solving problems.

In addition, children may have difficulties with conversational speech following a TBI. Their conversations may be:

- *tangential,* meaning that they talk around the topic and switch topics frequently, leaving fragments or *tangents* of unfinished conversation;
- *irrelevant,* meaning that they add information that is not necessary or relevant to the conversation; or

■ *confabulatory,* or made up, meaning that they make up information about situations or people that are not real or true.

Although conversational skills generally improve, there may be lingering language problems. In particular, problems with *pragmatic language,* or the social use of language, may continue to be quite impaired. Conversational skills are a subset of pragmatic skills. Other pragmatic skills include the ability to make friends and the ability to express wants and needs. These problems with pragmatics may cause significant problems in communication with family and peers.

:: Who Can Help with Speech and Language Problems?

For help in regaining speech and language abilities, your child will need to work closely with a speech-language pathologist, a professional with expertise in evaluating and treating communication problems.

Your child should receive her speech-language therapy from a certified speech-language pathologist (SLP). The title speech-language pathologist means that the professional holds a master's degree from an accredited school in the area of Speech Pathology or Speech/Language Pathology. To obtain the degree, he or she must have completed appropriate coursework, as well as an extensive internship. To become certified, he or she must have earned the Certificate of Clinical Competence (CCC) from the American Speech Language Hearing Association (ASHA). In order to receive the CCC from ASHA, the SLP must complete a clinical fellowship program and pass a national exam in speech-language pathology. The SLP must also hold a license from the state in which he or she is practicing.

The area of speech-language pathology has grown tremendously in the past fifty years. For this reason, many SLPs specialize in either children or adults. In addition, many narrow their specialization to people with particular conditions, such as children with TBI, children with developmental delays, children with feeding problems, etc. If at all possible, look for a SLP who specializes in TBI. If none are available, your second choice should be a SLP who specializes in children.

In seeking speech-language therapy for your child, you may encounter professionals who provide therapy but do not have the level of education or meet the certification standards approved by the ASHA.

For instance, if your child is receiving speech-language services in a public school, the school may only require that the SLP have a master's degree, but not certification by ASHA. At a minimum, you should be sure that the professional holds at least a master's degree in speech pathology and specializes in children.

Particularly in schools, you may encounter specialists called speech pathology assistants. IDEA (Individuals with Disabilities Education Act) requires states to provide guidelines for the use of speech pathology assistants. The assistants, however, are not considered qualified by ASHA standards to perform assessment or treatment without the supervision of a licensed professional. As a parent, it is important for you to realize the difference between the two positions when you are seeking services for your child. If speech-language pathology services are recommended, you have the right to expect a qualified SLP will provide services. SLP assistants can play a useful role in providing additional practice or intervention under the guidance of a certified SLP. Assistants should not, however, be conducting assessments and should not provide treatment plans.

∷ The First Step in Beginning Speech-Language Therapy

In the early days following a TBI, the SLP may briefly assess your child to determine whether she is oriented to time (hour, day, date), place (where she is), and person (who is in the room, who she is, who you are, etc.). As time goes on, the SLP may use some informal tests to see whether your child remembers concepts she had mastered before the injury, such as numbers, words, and letters.

Once your child's condition is stabilized, she will be given a comprehensive, in-depth evaluation (assessment) in all areas of functioning: psychological, educational, speech-language, motor skills, behavioral. This evaluation will identify your child's profile of strengths and weaknesses and provide information for important decisions about therapies and her education. If your child is being considered for special education, the results of the evaluation will determine whether she qualifies. If she does, her test results will be considered in deciding where she should go to school, what services (speech-language therapy, occupational therapy, physical therapy) she should receive, and what classroom modifications may be needed. If your child is already receiving special education, or if you are seeking private therapy for her, the evaluation results will help in setting appropriate goals for the future.

If your child was not evaluated before reentering school, you should contact your child's school and ask that your child be tested. You will be contacted by a representative from the school admissions, review, and dismissal team who will set a date for you to meet with representatives from the school. More information on this process is covered in Chapter 9.

■■ Speech-Language Assessment

Your child's speech and language assessment should consist of both formal (standardized) tests and informal tests.

The results of these tests will identify the areas where your child needs support or remedial work. They also provide a way of comparing your child's performance before and after TBI. This, in turn, helps pinpoint areas that should be targets for short-term and long-term intervention. The assessment results will also determine whether your child's school must provide speech-language therapy services free of charge. Different school systems have different standards for determining who qualifies for speech-language therapy. Usually, however, if your child's test scores show that she has lost significant ground compared to her pre-TBI abilities, she will qualify for services. The amount of therapy to be provided would be determined by the school assessment team with the guidance of the SLP. See Chapter 9 for more information about eligibility issues.

Formal Assessment

During the formal portion of your child's speech-language assessment, she will be given a number of standardized tests. These are tests that are based on norms, which have been established through testing many individuals. A certified speech-language pathologist administers the tests on a one-to-one basis, generally in a quiet environment with a minimum of distractions. The results of these tests will be expressed in a variety of ways, including:

- **Standard scores**—numerical scores that are evaluated as being below average, low average, average, high average, etc., depending upon the degree to which the score differs from the mean (average) score. Tests using standard scores are constructed so that a score of 100 is exactly average.

- *Percentile rank*—a converted score that expresses a child's score relative to her group in percentile points. If a child receives a percentile rank of 60, for example, it means that 60 percent of the individuals who took the test had a score that was the same or lower, and 40 percent had a score that was higher.
- *Age equivalent scores*—a converted score that expresses the child's score in terms of chronological age equivalency. For example, a child who is chronologically nine years, two months, might receive an age equivalency score of six years, five months, meaning that she scored as well as the average child aged six years, five months.

The overall purposes of formal testing are: 1) to compare your child's performance after her brain injury to her performance before the injury; and 2) to determine areas of strength and weakness. The speech language pathologist will choose assessments covering a variety of areas, including:

- language (speaking, reading, listening, and writing);
- speech (articulation, fluency, rate of speech, voice quality);
- word finding difficulties (*anomia*), and
- pragmatics (conversational skills, social skills).

The following general characteristics also should be observed during your child's evaluation:

- Level of attention;
- Tolerance to stress (time constraints, noise, frustration);
- Degree of cueing and prompting necessary: If your child does not say the word "house," for example, can she retrieve the word if a prompt such as "you live in a ____" is given, or does a phonemic cue need to be given, such as "we live in a **h**____"?
- Use of compensatory strategies: Is your child already using some strategies to help her compensate for weaknesses? For example, perhaps during the testing session she was observed to think out loud in trying to identify steps to solving a problem. This "think aloud" strategy

should be noted as one that she is already using and may
be used in other situations.

- Processing time: whether your child needs a longer time
  to comprehend what is asked before giving an answer;
- Delayed response or slowed performance;
- Anxiety;
- Fear of failure;
- Fatigue.

The SLP may need to modify the way she tests your child to
accommodate for any of the above problems. For example, if your
child fatigues easily, assessments might be broken into several testing
sessions. Likewise, if your child has visual field deficits because of
TBI, printed material may need to be enlarged, or presented to the
nonaffected side.

Additional modifications may include:

- changing the modality or sensory channel of the test
  items (for example, if the item is to be presented
  auditorally, also present the item visually),
- allowing the test item to be presented several times
  before your child responds,
- allowing cues and prompts to be given to aid, for
  example, with word retrieval (for instance, the item to
  be named is a bird, and the SLP provides a phonemic or
  sound cue like "b" to cue your child into the beginning
  sound of the word).

There is one important point to remember whenever your child
is having a formal assessment. The examiner (in this case, the SLP)
must follow to the letter all instructions and time constraints outlined
in the standardized test. Adhering to the rules is necessary to ensure
that the results are reliable and valid, and to get an idea of how your
child performs under stress. However, valuable information regarding
your child's performance may be misinterpreted or missed altogether
if some modifications cannot be made. For example, if a test item is
supposed to be answered within twenty seconds, a modification might
be for the SLP to mark the item as incorrect if your child does not
respond within the time constraints, but then allow her a longer period of time to answer. It may be that your child simply needs additional time to process the information and give a correct response.
Without the modification, the SLP might conclude that your child does

not have the knowledge to complete the test, when in reality she just needs more processing time.

Informal Assessment

In addition to formal testing, an in-depth speech language assessment should also include an informal or *naturalistic* assessment. Naturalistic assessments are carried out in a child's natural environment and are not standardized. These assessments can provide important information about your child's language functioning that may not be apparent with standardized tests. Informal assessment can take many forms, including observation of performance through interviews, questionnaires, behavioral observations, narrative language samples, and assessment of the language demands of your child's classroom curriculum.

Interviews and Questionnaires. Through interviews and questionnaires, the SLP can obtain more in-depth information from you and your child's teachers about communication problems that may be occurring at home or in the classroom. Examples of questions that should be asked include:

- How do communication problems affect your child's ability to indicate her wants?
- How well is she able to hold an appropriate conversation with family members or peers?
- Is your child able to express the need for clarification or repetition of class assignments?

Behavioral Observations. Your child should also be observed by the SLP and her classroom teachers in a variety of settings and contexts, such as the gymnasium, cafeteria, playground, and classroom. For example, an observation in the cafeteria yields information regarding your child's ability to process information in a noisy environment, the ability to communicate under time constraints (in the lunch line), the ability to communicate effectively in conversation, word finding difficulties, and so on. Such invaluable information is not provided by a standardized assessment.

Curriculum Based Language Assessment. Curriculum based language assessment (CBLA) is another form of informal assessment. CBLA assesses:

- the types of language skills and strategies your child has for processing the language of the curriculum or her classroom content areas (math, social studies, science, etc.);

- the resources your child is using to handle the class curriculum;
- additional strategies or needs your child has to process classroom information more efficiently, and;
- any modifications that may be made in the curriculum or its presentation to make it more accessible to your child.

In the curriculum based language assessment process, your child's schoolwork should be reviewed with the understanding that this is only the end product and does not give insight into the process your child uses to complete the work. For example, in reviewing your child's science quiz, a pattern of errors may be obvious. However, this pattern of errors does not give insight into why your child was having difficulty or how she was solving the problem.

Your child should be observed by the SLP in different classroom environments at various times of the day. The purpose of the observations is to record the language and communication demands of the curriculum that may be problematic to your child. For instance, the SLP may observe that the teacher frequently gives directions orally to the class but does not write them down. If your child has difficulty processing language, she may never be able to write the information down, let alone comprehend what was said. Goals for intervention would then include working on methods to teach your child how to focus on important information that is said instead of being concerned with *everything* that is said. The SLP may teach your child to listen for key words like "turn to page ..." or "your assignment is ...." In addition, the SLP would talk to the teacher and your child about modifications that may be needed. For example, in this instance, the teacher could help your child by writing the directions on the board or tape recording them so your child could listen to them as many times as needed.

Observations of your child's current knowledge, skills, and strategies when completing tasks should be documented. The diagnostic information obtained from the CBLA can identify the language demands of the curriculum and how well your child handles those demands. The CBLA is the best way of gathering functional information that is useful in developing instructional goals that are meaningful to your child.

Narrative Language Samples. Another form of naturalistic assessment is *narrative assessment*—evaluating a child's ability to tell or retell a story. These types of evaluations are important because being able to produce and understand narratives is vital both to academic success (reading and writing) and to participation in conversations.

Several methods can be used to obtain narrative samples:

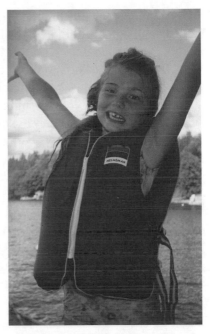

1. Having your child relate a personal experience;

2. Having your child create a fictional story from pictures or from a given story stem (for example, "One night in a dark and scary forest…");

3. Having your child retell a story after hearing the story presented orally or after viewing a filmstrip or videotape, and;

4. Having your child relate a narrative about routine events in her daily life (for example, getting ready for school).

In general, it is more difficult for children to create a novel story than to retell a story or tell about an everyday event. For this reason, it is important that as many narrative samples as possible be obtained in each of the above four areas.

Once the narrative samples are obtained, the SLP will analyze them for story components. For example, is there a beginning to the story, an introduction of the characters, a theme or plot, and a closing or resolution? The samples will also be analyzed for cohesiveness. That is, does the story make sense and flow easily from one thought to the next? In addition, the SLP will evaluate the number of words produced and the variety of words that are used.

The information collected through each of these types of informal evaluations yields a great deal of information about your child's communication needs at school and in less formal settings (on the playground, in the lunchroom, with peers, etc.). This information is critical to obtain in addition to the information collected through standardized assessments.

In fact, the information obtained from a standardized assessment may be deceiving. Your child may obtain "average" scores on the assessments because "old learning" is operating. Still, she may not be able to function appropriately at home or at school. On the other hand, your child may have below average scores on many assessments, but be able to function adequately in daily life activities.

Continuing brain development also can make it difficult to predict success from test scores. This is because brain function may or may not continue to improve, and there is no telling how quickly this will occur. Variability in performance is a hallmark of TBI and must be interpreted cautiously, as a child's performance can vary from day to day. All these factors make it essential to obtain a clear picture of your child's communication abilities through a combination of both formal and informal evaluations.

:: Speech-Language Intervention

Direct or Consultative Services?

The amount and type of speech-language therapy your child needs will depend upon the extent of the brain injury, as well as the setting where services will be provided. A child with a milder brain injury may not require speech-language pathology services on a long-term basis. She may need intensive services immediately following the injury, but as she progresses, may only need consultative services. A child with a moderate to severe injury may require more direct speech-language therapy and over a longer period of time.

Consultative Services. All children who have communication problems following a brain injury should receive consultative speech-language services. That is, a SLP should be provided to monitor any changes in your child's communication that occur in any setting, including at home, at school, and in therapy. The SLP also keeps track of communication strengths and weaknesses that would be important in developing or revising your child's speech-language program. The SLP should keep parents, teachers, and other service providers informed about how your child communicates in different environments.

In providing consultative services, the SLP does not work directly with your child. Instead, he or she suggests ways that parents and teachers can help your child improve her communication. Consultative services should be provided in addition to direct speech language services, if warranted, for as long as your child demonstrates difficulties with academics.

Direct Services. When a child receives direct speech-language intervention, she works with a certified SLP *at least* once a week. The actual amount of time that your child would be seen depends again on the severity of injury and the setting where therapy is provided. The following section describes areas that your child might work on when receiving direct services.

Intervention Goals

The goals of speech-language intervention for your child will depend on a number of factors, including:

- her chronological age,
- the developmental age or stage at which she is functioning,
- the extent of the damage from the TBI,
- how well your child functions in various settings, including home, school, and community, and
- how much family support is available (how much time your family has to work on communication with your child and how supportive you are of her efforts).

No matter what your child's characteristics are, however, intervention should focus upon helping your child to be functional in various environments. Rather than teaching or reteaching skills through drills, it is more helpful to teach them in a meaningful way that will help your child transfer skills from one setting to another.

Goals for Children with Motor Speech Disorders

As explained earlier in the chapter, TBI can result in motor speech disorders—disorders that cause difficulties planning movements of the articulators (tongue, lips, and jaw) for speech production. Problems can include difficulties with respiration, speech sound production, slow labored speech (dysarthria), and vocal problems (including resonance and quality of voice—hoarse, breathy, etc.). For children with motor speech disorders, the following types of therapy may be needed:

Oral Motor Therapy. Oral motor therapy may be recommended to facilitate speech sound production. This type of therapy involves exercises to strengthen the tongue, lips, and jaw. The SLP may use mirrors, tongue depressors, and pictures to help your child learn where to place her tongue, lips, and jaw for speech production.

Phonation Exercises. If the loudness or intensity level of your child's speech is too low, then phonation exercises may be recommended. These are basically breath control exercises. For example, to help your child speak more loudly, the SLP might have her speak into a tape recorder. She would watch the recorder's VU meter, which measures increases in volume, and try to get the VU needle to move by speaking more loudly.

Articulation Therapy. Articulation therapy may be recommended to help your child produce more precise sounds. Materials used for therapy should include vocabulary from school, from your child's job setting, or from home, including words related to your child's hobbies or special interests.

The SLP may help your child produce particular sounds by giving her direct cues. For instance, to produce the "f" sound, she might say, "Put your upper teeth on your lower lip and blow." She might also use a mirror so your child can see how she is producing the sound, or use activities to increase awareness of where the tongue or articulators should be to produce a sound. For example, to help your child produce the "l" sound, the SLP may put peanut butter on the ridge behind your child's teeth.

Goals for Children with Language Disorders

Besides having motor speech disorders, children with TBI may also have language disorders. In fact, language disorders are more common than speech disorders. Some children with TBI have both a motor speech disorder and a language disorder, in which case they would benefit from speech-language intervention in both areas. For children with language disorders, speech-language therapy may focus on one or more of the following areas:

Vocabulary. Vocabulary development is crucial for both comprehension and speaking. Your child needs to develop vocabulary that is meaningful in a variety of settings—home, school, work, hobbies, extracurricular activities, and social activities. She needs to learn not only the formal vocabulary used in these settings, but also commonly used slang expressions. At all costs, word lists that are unrelated to your child's needs should be avoided. Vocabulary that she cannot make practical use of in many situations will only frustrate her.

One useful way to help improve your child's vocabulary is to work on understanding categories. For example, the SLP may ask your child to name as many animals as possible. To develop this concept, the SLP may cue your child by saying, "Let's think of all the farm animals first" (then zoo animals, pets, etc.). The SLP may also work on visualization techniques, by saying, for instance, "Can you remember going to the zoo? Take a walk in your mind and remember what you saw." Learning visualization techniques and how to categorize will help your child link old information to new ideas.

Another good technique to help your child expand ideas is to use word webs. The SLP might start by writing a vocabulary word, such as "school," on a paper or chalkboard and then circling it. Then your child would list all the words related to the circled word that she could think of, with lines drawn from these words to the central word. For example, "school" might make her think of the words "homework," "classes" "lunch," "teachers," "classroom." These words can then be branched out even further to develop more vocabulary and concepts. For example, "social studies," "algebra," and "biology" might be linked to the word "classes."

Pragmatic Skills. Conversational and social skills are best taught in settings with peers. In the beginning, a good place for your child to learn or relearn skills may be in a quiet therapy room with the SLP helping her make conversation with her peers. However, in order for your child to transfer these skills successfully to more natural environments, therapy needs to move out of the therapy room to the cafeteria, playground, restaurant, or job setting. By monitoring your child's communication development in a variety of settings, the SLP can help your child evaluate where communication breakdowns occur, and then design ways to fix the problem. Your child needs to develop these problem-solving cognitive skills so that she has the ability to think about language and how to communicate effectively.

One reason for communication breakdowns is that children with TBI sometimes have a tendency to *circumlocute,* or talk around a topic, without getting to the point. The SLP may work with your child in developing a cue to help her get back on topic. For example, the SLP might put her finger on her chin to signal your child that she is off topic. This cue may be enough for your child to stop and think about what she is saying and get back on topic. This cueing system should then be taught to peers, teachers, and family members to help your child communicate more effectively in conversation. Likewise, if your child has difficulty choosing topics of conversation that are of interest to family members and peers, the SLP can help your child learn to identify appropriate topics.

Organizational Skills. The SLP should teach your child organizational skills to facilitate language learning. Examples of such skills include:

- *classification* (techniques given earlier in vocabulary section);
- *categorization*—the ability to understand that things belong to a category (e.g., animals include pets, farm animals, jungle animals, etc.). A typical activity would be to have your child name as many animals as she can in one minute;
- *association*—the ability to establish connections between two or more related symbols or concepts, such as hat/head and puppy/dog; and
- *sequencing*—the ability to connect a series of things or events (e.g., your child is given picture cards of a common activity like putting on shoes, and asked to sequence the cards and tell about them in the correct order).

Humor. Your child may need help in understanding and using humor appropriately. If she cannot understand humor, she won't "get" jokes and will have trouble fitting in with peers. She may also fail to realize when someone is being sarcastic. Understanding and using humor involves abstract language and is a higher level skill. The use of cartoons, comic strips, and books of jokes and riddles can be helpful.

The types of communication difficulties and possible interventions outlined in this section should not be regarded as an all-inclusive list. Because it is difficult to generalize about the communication problems and outcomes of children with TBI as a group, the guidelines may not be specific to your child. In fact, the suggestions may be only the "tip of the iceberg" for some. This underscores the need for your child's individual strengths and needs to be evaluated at the start of speech-language therapy and for her progress in communication skills to be monitored in all settings.

■■ Where to Go to Receive SLP Services

In the Hospital or Rehabilitation Center

If your child requires speech-language therapy services while in the hospital or rehabilitation center, those services will be provided upon your physician's recommendation. In most instances, your HMO or insurance will pay for it.

While your child is in the hospital or rehab center, the SLP will be working on goals that are functional for your child, at whatever stage of recovery she may be. For example, the SLP may help your child be oriented to the day of the week, month of the year, where she is, etc. If your child is at a more advanced level of recovery, the SLP may work on concepts such as naming opposites and synonyms. The therapist will evaluate how quickly your child is able to process this information, if she is able to retrieve it at all. The SLP should also try to get copies of schoolbooks and materials your child was using, both to reinforce old learning skills and to evaluate your child's ability to learn new information.

How long your child stays in the hospital or rehab center and her overall physical condition will dictate the intensity of therapy in this setting. At a minimum, however, the SLP in the hospital should thoroughly evaluate your child's speech and language skills before she returns to school. It would also be helpful for the hospital SLP to directly collaborate with the school SLP to help with the transition. As a parent, you should request that this type of collaboration occur.

At School

Most children who sustain a brain injury return to school, whether it is the school they were attending before the accident, or a more specialized school. As Chapter 9 explains, your child can receive a variety of types of therapy and special educational help at school. This includes both consultative and direct speech-language services. If your child qualifies for assistance under the Individuals with Disabilities Education Act, these services will be provided without charge to your family.

During the transition from the hospital or rehabilitation setting to the school setting, the SLP at your child's school should be notified. This way she can help identify areas for intervention. This type of

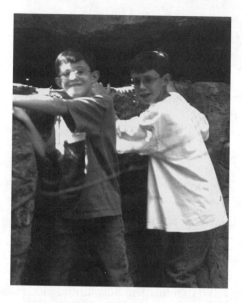

collaboration before your child returns to school may help prevent the territorial issues and miscommunications between hospital and school SLPs that sometimes occur. For example, when your child is first returning to school, the hospital or rehab center SLP may recommend that your child receive intense services many days of the week. The recommendation may be for only the first month of school so further evaluation can take place or because the SLP at the hospital believes a lot of growth will occur quickly if more intense services are provided in the beginning. The school, however, may feel that they do not have the capability to provide this amount of therapy, when, in fact, this may be a short-term recommendation that has long-term benefits. A collaborative meeting before your child goes back to school may alleviate friction between the hospital and the school and allow for a "meeting of the minds."

Even if your child has received a complete speech-language evaluation at the hospital/rehabilitation center, the school SLP should informally evaluate your child in the classroom setting. Some areas of intervention identified in the hospital setting may need to be modified to the academic setting, where there are more demands, more people, etc. For instance, at school your child may need to work on retrieving vocabulary words related to the classroom, whereas in the hospital, she may have worked just on strategies for word retrieval in general.

If your child receives consultative services at school, the SLP will contact your child's teachers and other service providers to find out how she is communicating in class. The SLP should also be available to provide further training or resources to your child's teachers.

If your child receives direct services, the school SLP will see her as often as is recommended by the school assessment team. Her speech-language therapy might be provided as pull-out therapy. That is, your child will leave the classroom and see the SLP either individually or in a small group. Or, she may remain in the classroom, where the SLP may co-teach with a teacher and introduce concepts and strategies to a larger group of students, including your child. Often, a combination of both approaches is used. It is important that you monitor how and when your child is receiving services and which type of intervention or combination of interventions is best for your child. In addition, the school SLP should continually monitor your child for any changes that may be needed in your child's program.

▪▪ Your Child's Case Manager

Whether in the hospital, rehab setting, or school, the speech-language pathologist may act as your child's *case manager,* or *service coordinator.* This professional makes sure that your child is receiving all the appropriate services and that the various professionals working with your child communicate with one another when necessary.

Speech-language pathologists are often uniquely qualified to serve as case managers for children with TBI. They have training in neurological functioning and in how a TBI can affect a child's educational performance. Frequently, they have had specific coursework or continuing education related to this area. This foundation allows the SLP to act as case manager even if specific speech-language therapy goals have not been recommended for your child.

As your child's case manager, the SLP will be responsible for providing information to your child's teachers about the injury and the impact it can have on your child's functioning at school. The SLP should also provide information about how your child's current level of performance compares to her performance before the injury ("premorbid history"). In addition, the therapist should help teachers understand the differences between children with TBI and children with other types of disabilities. In particular, teachers need to understand how TBI affects a child differently than learning disabilities do, as there are similarities but also important differences.

The other important responsibility of the SLP as case manager is to be in frequent contact with your child and your family. The SLP should act as a resource to your family, providing you with relevant information about your child's transition back into school. In addition, the SLP should monitor your child's overall well-being in various school settings, including the classroom (academic performance), the cafeteria/recess (social integration), and after-school/extracurricular activities. The SLP should share her observations with you and with other people involved with your child at school on a monthly basis.

▪▪ How to Locate a Speech-Language Pathologist for Your Child

As explained above, if your child qualifies to receive speech-language therapy at school under IDEA, this therapy will be provided by the school system at no extra cost to you. Even if the school does not have a speech-language pathologist for some reason, the school system is still obligated to provide speech-language therapy services for the recommended number of times at no cost to you.

When your child receives speech-language therapy through the school, you do not have to locate a speech-language pathologist to provide the services. Your child will see the SLP who is assigned to the school.

Some families are completely satisfied with the speech-language therapy their child receives through the school. Other families, however, seek a private speech-language pathologist for their child. Common reasons for arranging for private therapy are that the parents think their child would benefit from additional therapy or from more one-to-one therapy in an office setting. Parents might also pursue private therapy if their child attends a private school by choice. Although the child can still receive speech-language therapy through the public school, the child will probably need to travel to that school to receive services. It may not be convenient for parents to take their child to the public school and back again to her school.

If you decide to seek private services, there are some considerations to bear in mind. Most importantly, you should make sure that the therapist you are interviewing is certified by the American Speech Language Hearing Association (holds the CCC—certificate of clinical competence) and is licensed in the state in which he or she is practicing. It is crucial that you ask about the professional's experience and knowledge in the area of acquired brain injury. You should ask questions such as:

1. How many *children* with TBI has the SLP evaluated and treated? Many SLPs advertise experience with brain injuries, but their experience may be specific to adults. They assume that that knowledge is sufficient for children, but it is not.
2. Will he or she be available to work with the school SLP (if your child is also receiving services in the school) to develop a meaningful program that will carry over between the two settings?
3. If your child is not in a public school, will the SLP be able to provide services at her school and consult teachers regarding curriculum, assignments, etc.?
4. Does the SLP conduct therapy that facilitates social skills such as conversational skills, friendship-making skills, etc.?
5. What specific courses, workshops, or training has the therapist had in TBI, and how recently?
6. How and how often will the therapist monitor progress and change the intervention program, and how will you be informed (through weekly conversations, progress reports, phone conversation, etc.)?

If your family's health insurance is provided through an HMO, the HMO will have a list of SLPs that your child is "allowed" to go to. It is possible that none of the approved therapists will be experienced in working with children with TBI. If so, it is imperative that you explain to the insurance consultant the necessity of having a SLP who has training and experience in providing services for children with TBI. The SLP at the hospital can help write a letter that explains why this is important.

To locate a SLP with the right experience and training, you can begin by checking your local telephone directory. You may also contact the American Speech Language and Hearing Association in Rockville, MD, as listed in the Resource Guide at the back of this book. They can provide either a listing of individuals in your area or the name and phone number of the local speech and hearing association in your state that would have a listing of therapists who provide private services.

Private services can also be provided on an outpatient basis at local hospitals and rehabilitation centers. Even in these facilities, it is still critical that you make sure that the SLP is experienced in *pediatric*

TBI. The issues faced by children and their families are vastly different from those faced by adults. The communication needs for children and adults are also very different following a brain injury.

■■ Enhancing Communication Skills Is Not Just the SLP's Job

Although the SLP plays an important role in helping your child improve her communication skills, the SLP does not play the only role. For your child to make as much progress as quickly as possible, parents, peers, and others who regularly interact with her need to be involved in helping her communicate.

Speech-language pathologists Roberta DePompei and Jean Blosser have identified a series of strategies that can be used to enhance communication skills in children with TBI. They advise that it is important not to use or teach all of the strategies at one time. Instead, the strategies should be matched to each individual child's needs. The strategies developed by DePompei and Blosser are outlined below:

1. *Monitor the quality of your child's conversations.* Think about whether you (or another speaker) need to reduce and simplify the length, rate of speech, and complexity of your speech in order for your child to understand the message.

2. *Provide instructions and directions.* Directions may need to be repeated more than once and not just given verbally. The speaker may need to use pictures or point in combination with speaking so your child comprehends.

3. *Explain new concepts and vocabulary.* Because new learning is so difficult for children with TBI, only introduce a limited amount of new vocabulary at one time. In addition, new vocabulary should be used over and over in a variety of contexts until your child masters the concept.

4. *Monitor selection of words, expressions, and comments.* As explained earlier, children with TBI have difficulty comprehending abstract language, such as idioms (e.g., "your eyes are bigger than your stomach" or "it's raining cats and dogs"), and humor. Sarcasm is also difficult for

children with TBI to grasp. If these types of language are used, the meaning needs to be explained. Do not use this type of language when it is critical that your child understands the information being given to her.

5. *Organize and sequence information.* Children with TBI have difficulty with informal conversations because they sometimes lack organizational skills. Conversational partners should be aware of signals from your child that she is confused and be ready to step in and help her understand by using terms such as first, next, etc. This will also help your child learn to structure her conversations.

6. *Announce and clarify the topic of conversation.* For example, when preparing to switch topics, say, "Now let's talk about the *Rugrats* movie."

7. *Permit adequate response time.* Conversations and classroom discussions generally move at a rapid rate. Controlling the pace will help your child comprehend. You may need to make peers, teachers, and extended family members aware of the need to slow down and allow your child time to process the information.

8. *Teach your child to be aware of other's responses.* Because children with TBI are often unaware of others' reactions, breakdowns in communication frequently occur. You can teach your child to watch other people and identify facial expressions that may signal confusion, loss of interest, etc. Then teach your child how to repair the situation so she will not be embarrassed.

9. *Reinforce communication attempts.* Anyone who is working with your child should be made aware of what can be realistically expected in the way of communication and should reinforce attempts to communicate in a positive manner. For example, tell her that she is making excellent use of her strategies to help her communicate thoughts and ideas. Conversational partners should let your child know whether her communication is accurate, and if not, how it can be improved, but in a positive way.

10. *Encourage communication through any means.* Although most children with TBI are eventually able to communicate effectively with speech, some can benefit from using

other systems of communication for a short while, or even indefinitely. For example, some might use an *alternative communication system* to provide another means to communicate if they cannot use speech. Examples include sign language or a communication board with pictures or words that your child can point to. For others, the best choice might be an augmentative communication device to augment or add to the speech they already have. For example, there are electronic or computerized devices that can generate spoken words or sentences. Augmentative or alternative communication devices should be introduced as early as possible so that your child has a way to communicate and does not become frustrated. If this system is one that will continue to be used, encourage its use in all settings.

11. *Arrange the physical environment to encourage communication.* Look for barriers in the environment that may impede communication, and be ready to make modifications in the environment. For example, rearrange the physical location of desks and chairs to encourage, rather than discourage, communication.

12. *Help your child improve her memory skills.* For instance, gradually expect your child to remember longer instructions and to answer questions about what she did at school.

▪▪ Conclusion

Communication is essential in all aspects of life. Your child's communication needs should be identified and monitored continuously throughout the journey from acute care to rehabilitation to reentry or entry into school, and possibly to a work setting. Goals for successful communication should also be monitored and frequently reworked to match your child's unique needs in her environment. Plans for intervention should take into consideration your child's overall functioning in all areas, including cognitive skills, motor skills, and behavior. The ultimate goal should be to enable your child to function effectively at home, school, and in the community.

It is vital that you be actively involved in your child's speech and language program. Ultimately, the skills that your child learns from her speech-language pathologist can only be enhanced if you help her practice and apply those skills. The earlier you are involved, the faster your child will learn to use many of these skills in other settings and situations. If you ever feel that your child's communication needs are not being met in speech-language therapy, speak up! By advocating for your child now, you increase the chances that she will be able to advocate for herself in the future.

∎ Parent Statements

When Kevin first came out of his coma, his speech was very soft and slurred. Most of what he said made sense, although his short-term memory was very poor.

❧

Julie didn't talk much in the hospital, and seemed very tired. Her eyes were very expressive, though.

❧

At first, Kevin spoke with little expression in his voice or on his face. He had always used his eyebrows a lot when he talked and had been a fairly animated person. After about three weeks, he began moving his eyebrows again when he talked. His laugh returned a few days later, but it wasn't the same laugh he'd always had. Even now, three years after his accident, his laugh is still different.

❧

Sophia has a hard time getting her thoughts together and expressing herself clearly. She tends to ramble and takes a very long time to get her point across. Often she talks for awhile without ever really answering a given problem. She doesn't seem to be aware that this is a problem.

❧

Our son's speech has improved a great deal in the three years since his car accident. But he still is not as concise as he once was.

❧

The school speech-language pathologist was our main source of information following Jamie's incident. She was helpful in relaying *information to his teachers, and then helping us with Jamie's needs at home and at school.*

⋙❀⋘

The SLP at the rehabilitation center worked together with my wife and me to develop a system to cue Rebecca when she was not talking on the topic of conversation. This cueing helped Rebecca a lot to be able to communicate again and feel comfortable in social situations.

⋙❀⋘

The SLP in the hospital prepared us for some of the continuous communication problems that Zachary would have when he returned to school. We were grateful to have that information so we could look ahead.

How TBI Affects Behavior

Cindy L. Tucker, Ph.D.

*J*ohnny and his parents, Ann and Tom, arrived a few minutes late for their first appointment in Rehabilitation Follow-Up Clinic. Keeping Johnny on-task and getting him out of the door every morning was becoming more and more challenging. It had been exactly four months since Johnny's accident. Thinking back on that day, it was hard to believe how much progress he had made in such a brief time. He had progressed from lying comatose in the intensive care unit to looking as if nothing had ever happened to him except for a slight limp. However, during that same period, changes to Johnny's personality and behavior had also begun to surface, as various rehab staff members had warned might happen.

Because Johnny had always been an active child who often needed to have rules repeated, Ann and Tom initially did not believe that their son had any problem behaviors. When the rehab staff described his behavior as "impulsive," they saw it as a natural response to being cooped up in the hospital and frustrated with the demands of his rehab therapies. When staff members expressed concerns, they replied that Johnny always had been strong willed and prone to act without thinking. To them, he really didn't seem all that different. Johnny's grandparents agreed, stating, "He's all boy. There's nothing wrong with him. He just needs to get back home with his family."

All the rules, points, and prizes being used by the hospital staff to encourage Johnny to cooperate with his therapies seemed unnecessary. Tom worried that his son would begin to expect prizes for everything once home. Ann sometimes couldn't believe her ears when the staff talked about various disciplinary and management techniques. "How could they be suggesting discipline for a child who was on a ventilator in the ICU only a few weeks ago? I still can't believe he is physically okay. I couldn't care less how he behaves." Ann and Tom did agree to follow most of the recommendations for making their home safe for Johnny's return (such as restricting his access to knives, medications, and cleaning supplies), but wanted to wait and see how he adjusted to being home before going forward with a formal behavior program.

Now, just seven weeks after Johnny's discharge from the day hospital program and return to school, Ann and Tom were beginning to wonder if their hopes had been realistic. Initially relieved just to have Johnny home with them again, they now worried that the honeymoon had ended. Things weren't getting better and life was definitely not returning to normal.

Johnny had challenged their parenting skills from the beginning. As an infant, he had been much more demanding than his sister, Susan. As he grew, he had become increasingly disorganized and distractible, and seemed to need constant reminders to complete even routine tasks. Just before the accident, they had met with the school to discuss similar problems observed with completing homework. Since his injury, all of these problems seemed significantly worse. Just getting ready for bed or dressed for the day was a major project, and everything took twice as long as before. Yet, for now, Ann was just grateful to have Johnny alive and home with her. She couldn't muster the emotional energy to focus on how he was behaving and how that might affect his future adjustment. She just wanted to hold him and keep him safe.

Johnny's father, Tom, found himself growing more and more frustrated with Johnny. "I'll bet he has asked me 100 times today if he can go out and ride his bike. I've told him over and over that he can't, but he doesn't seem to understand why. It's as if he doesn't realize how seriously he was injured, not to mention that his balance is off now. I can't let him out of my sight. Yesterday I caught him trying to pull his wrecked bike down from the hooks in the garage, right after I had told him 'no.' It's like that with all of the restrictions the doctors have placed on his activity. He wants to rollerblade and skateboard and play baseball with his friends, and he becomes so belligerent when I won't let him. I don't know how we will keep him busy this summer without his usual activities."

Tom also was concerned that Johnny acted so immaturely. He talked loudly and was overly familiar with strangers. Tom had noticed people looking at Johnny and whispering comments. Tom was angry at people he felt were being insensitive, but he had to admit that he was embarrassed by Johnny's behavior, and, as a result, felt guilty as well. The way Johnny behaved made him look impaired, and Tom struggled with his feelings about this. He wondered if they would ever be able to go places as a family again. He wondered if his son would ever be himself again. He wondered if he had the skills necessary to parent a child with Johnny's problems.

In Follow-Up Clinic, Ann and Tom were pleased to learn that Johnny's medical status was stable and that he would not need to return to clinic again for another six months. When asked how they were doing at home, they both automatically responded that things were fine, but after more questioning by the psychologist, they shared some of their concerns and difficulties in dealing with Johnny. They also confessed to being worried that Johnny's problems would affect his brother and sister. They were exhausted and somewhat overwhelmed. They acknowledged that they had not always seen eye-to-eye on parenting style in the past and that this was further complicating their efforts to manage Johnny. Although they still hoped that some of Johnny's troubling behaviors would resolve, they agreed to meet with the psychologist in the meantime to develop strategies for managing Johnny's behavioral problems. An appointment was scheduled for the next week and they were asked to list their top three concerns in preparation for that session. This would help in setting treatment priorities for the *most disruptive behaviors first. Johnny and his siblings would be seen at this initial session as well so that the needs of all family members could be assessed.*

At their one-year visit to Follow-Up Clinic, both Ann and Tom reported significant improvement in many areas. More importantly, they reported that they had learned several strategies that now could be applied to new problems as they emerged. They expressed increased confidence in their parenting skills and no longer focused primarily on when Johnny would be back to normal. They stated that they were "taking things a day at a time," and working hard to keep things at home structured and consistent. They felt that this had been beneficial to Susan and Billy as well. They were able to share both positive and negative feelings about the accident and its impact on the family.

Although Ann and Tom were feeling less guilt and blame, they expressed regret that they had so little time to spend with Johnny's brother and sister. Growing awareness of the persistent changes in Johnny contributed to ongoing feelings of grief and loss. They were most concerned about Johnny's lack of insight into his problems with relationships and the loss of most of his old friends. Unable to understand why old friends no longer wanted to play with him and lacking the skills needed to acquire new friends, he sometimes seemed lonely and sad. The psychologist agreed to begin meeting individually with Johnny to assess and assist his adjustment to his injury, and to refer him to a therapy group to work on social skills.

■■ Introduction

If your child or adolescent has recently experienced a traumatic brain injury, you may be wondering if you need to read this chapter. You may be feeling overwhelmed with more immediate problems, such as physical disabilities, communication difficulties, and learning problems, and with obtaining the services needed to treat these conditions. Or, considering that your child has recently survived a life-threatening injury, you believe that whether or not he follows rules or behaves appropriately in public is a trivial concern. Grateful that your child is alive, you may feel that it is inappropriate to complain about anything. "After all he has been through," you may think, "it's no wonder he is a little hard to manage now." Extended family members and friends may support this opinion.

The fact is, when a child is left with no observable signs of a TBI, parents and others tend to assume that the child is "back to normal" in all areas of functioning. Even when a child is left with many visible and profound physical differences, parents often have a need to see their child as being the same, at least in terms of his personality and general manner of interacting with others. For parents, this is a normal way of coping with the many losses they may face.

Parents may need to view their child's adjustment and behavior problems as temporary, or as unrelated to the effects of the brain injury. Perhaps, they think, the behavioral problems just reflect their child's frustration with a demanding rehabilitation program and physical limitations or challenges. To think that some of these changes might be more or less permanent can be overwhelming for some parents. Having nearly lost your child's life to a serious injury, it may be unthinkable that parts of your child's personality or basic self could have been lost as well. Feelings of grief, fatigue, and, in many cases, guilt, can strain a parent's ability to cope with the changes that may accompany a child's brain injury. In addition, some parents may be concerned that focusing attention on their child's behavior problems could reflect poorly in some way upon their parenting skills.

As difficult as it can be to face, adjustment and behavioral problems *can* have a variety of short- and long-term effects on your child's functioning. For example, some children with TBI have disruptive behavior that interferes with their ability to pick up new knowledge and skills in the classroom. Coping with changes related to TBI can also lead to poor self-esteem and emotional problems such as depression, anxiety, and anger outbursts. In addition, a brain injury can lead to long-term difficulties with impulsivity, judgment, and safety awareness. Children with TBI who ignore medical restrictions on contact sports and other recreational activities are also at increased risk of sustaining a second TBI.

If you or others involved in your child's care are concerned about his behavior or adjustment, it may be helpful to learn how TBI affects these areas of functioning. This chapter examines the relationship between injury to the brain and behavior, focusing on some adjustment and behavioral problems that are commonly associated with TBI. It also offers some general strategies for managing adjustment and behavioral disturbances.

▪▪ Will My Child Develop an Adjustment or Behavioral Problem after TBI?

It is relatively common for children to have behavioral or adjustment problems after TBI. Research has shown that up to one-half of children develop a new emotional or behavioral disorder in the first year after suffering a moderate or severe TBI. In another study, 30 to 35 percent of children with acquired brain damage were found to have an emotional or behavioral disorder. This is five to six times the rate for children with no chronic illness or brain injury.

A variety of factors may determine whether or not your child develops an adjustment or behavioral problem after TBI. Some of the factors that increase your child's risk cannot be altered. For example, children with more severe brain injuries, boys, and younger children are more likely to develop behavioral, adjustment, or emotional problems than children with less severe brain injuries, girls, and children who experience a TBI at an older age. Similarly, children who had behavioral or adjustment problems before their TBI tend to be at higher risk of developing new emotional or behavioral disorders after their injuries. Also at greater risk are children who have physical disabilities, lowered intellectual abilities, or seizures as a result of traumatic brain injury. Finally, adjustment or behavioral problems are more common among children whose parents have had prior problems with parenting and discipline.

Some risk factors that you and your child may be able to control include:

- how you cope with your child's injury,
- additional stresses on your family,

- your child's response to the injury and its effects (especially related to poor self-awareness, frustration tolerance, and anger management), and
- how any behavioral disturbances that occur during emergence from coma are managed.

Therapy for your child or family to address these issues can sometimes prevent or decrease behavioral and adjustment disturbances.

Learning as much as possible about your child's particular brain injury is a good first step in preparing for potential problems. Ask your child's physicians and therapists about the location and severity of your child's injury. Some skill losses and behavioral problems are related to injury of certain brain structures, while other behavioral problems are more unpredictable. Especially in the early days after a TBI, professionals may adopt a "wait and see" approach to predicting your child's level of injury and prospects for recovery. Just as every brain injury is unique, so too is every recovery. Hoping for the best and preparing for the worst, in terms of behavioral management skills, may be a practical approach. This is particularly true if your child leaves the hospital after a relatively short stay.

Many of the behavioral problems that occur soon after TBI will likely lessen, or perhaps disappear over time. However, it is difficult to predict which problems will go away and how long that may take. It is also possible that new behavioral and adjustment problems may emerge over the years as your child develops and meets with new challenges and higher demands.

For parents, the best advice is to learn the skills necessary for managing behavioral problems as soon as possible after their child's injury. This provides several benefits:

1. It increases your confidence in your ability to care for your child at home soon after a serious injury. This is particularly true if your child has other injuries requiring specialized care.
2. Being prepared for common behavior problems allows you to address such problems prior to, or as, they occur. This reduces the likelihood that behavior will worsen, you and your child will have stressful interactions, or possibly, that unsafe practices will place your child at risk of further injuries.

3. Managing disruptive behaviors appropriately can help prevent secondary behavioral problems that result from mismanaging and giving too much negative attention to undesirable behaviors.

4. When you are able to identify and address adjustment problems such as depression and anxiety, you can get help for your child in a timely manner.

▪▪ The Beginnings of Behavioral Disturbances Following TBI

What Kinds of Behavioral Problems Occur as a Child Emerges from Coma?

Children emerging from coma usually follow a typical pattern of recovery. The *Rancho Los Amigos Cognitive Scale* is one method used by rehabilitation professionals to assess a child's degree of recovery from brain injury. The levels of cognitive functioning in this scale provide us with a loose roadmap of the stages through which someone must pass as he emerges from injury-related coma. (See the Appendix.)

Although the Rancho Los Amigos Scale can give you an idea of your child's level of functioning, it does not predict how quickly he will recover or how long he will remain at any one level of functioning. Your child's level of functioning may fluctuate among different levels for a period of time. In addition, his recovery may stall at any functional level along the way. Although most children continue to progress up to the higher levels of recovery, the time frame varies widely.

Level I. Initially, a child in a coma does not respond in any way to his environment. Medical concerns are the biggest issue during this period.

Level II. Over time, the child may respond to visual, auditory, and tactile (touch) stimulation with actions that are mostly reflexive and involve large areas of the body.

Level III. As further recovery occurs, the child may begin to respond more specifically to stimulation in his environment. For instance, he may turn away from or blink at a bright light, may look toward the source of a sound, or may pull his arm away from cold or painful stimuli. A child at this level of functioning may seem as if he is attempting to follow simple directions, such as "Squeeze my hand" or

"Look at Mommy," but these efforts are inconsistent and imprecise. Sleep and wake cycles remain altered and the child seems drowsy much of the time.

Level IV. Further recovery typically leads to a level of functioning that includes a great deal of confusion, nonpurposeful (and somewhat random) physical activity, and agitation. Children at this level generally are unable to acquire new learning and remain disoriented. It is at Level IV that parents often begin to have concerns about their child's behavior. Children at this level often behave in a very disinhibited manner that can be quite distressing to their parents. They may:

- exhibit bizarre behaviors, use inappropriate language, behave provocatively, wander about, speak too loudly, or engage in unsafe acts;
- exhibit repetitive behaviors such as rocking, rubbing, picking, pacing, or other forms of self-stimulation;
- have emotions that are highly *labile* (full of mood swings), unpredictable, and that often do not match events in the environment or the content of their speech;
- have difficulty responding well to reason or verbal reprimands;
- have an extremely short attention span;
- show a low tolerance for frustration and discomfort.

Faced with the unfamiliar setting and demands of a rehabilitation program, their confusion and disorientation may lead to anxiety, resistance, and noncompliance. They may become combative or physically aggressive toward anyone who attempts to intervene, including parents.

Parents who are unprepared for such uncharacteristic behavior may become uncomfortable and apologetic, and try to control their child's behavior. Instead of viewing these behaviors as an expected part of their child's recovery, they feel embarrassed and ashamed. They may feel that such behavior reflects poorly on them as parents or on their family's home life. Parents should be reassured that brain injury professionals understand how these kinds of behaviors are related to a child's level of cognitive functioning. In fact, they view such behavior as a sign that the child's brain is continuing to emerge from a comatose state. It is because the child is becoming increasingly aware of his environment (but is not yet able to make sense of everything going on around him and control his responses) that he becomes agitated.

The key is to manage these complex behaviors appropriately. If not, too much attention may be paid to the disruptive behaviors, thereby reinforcing and strengthening them. This can result in these behaviors continuing into other phases of recovery. Remember, there is no way to predict how long your child will remain at this level of functioning, and therefore, how long these behaviors may persist. This makes it important to start managing the behaviors as soon as they appear.

Managing Behavioral Problems during the Confused, Agitated Phase of Recovery

Much of the agitation and other behavior problems common at this point in recovery result from injury to the brain itself. As a result, they cannot be eliminated entirely. However, steps *can* be taken to prevent the underlying agitation from being exacerbated. The key is to avoid overstimulating and placing excessive demands on your child. In addition, you must take care to keep your child away from dangerous situations. This is because children with TBI often regain their motor (movement) abilities before other abilities such as orientation (that is, knowing who and where they are), memory, safety awareness, and judgment.

It may help to remember the time when your child first learned to crawl, cruise, climb, and take his first steps. He was able to move about better and better, but without any sense of danger. Telling him to be careful was of little use because he was not capable of doing so. Instead, you had to modify the environment to protect him from injuries and unsafe activities. Over time, with consistency and repetition, your child learned to avoid certain activities and areas of potential danger, but adult supervision was still required for some time. It can be much the same when your child is recovering from a traumatic brain injury. If you modify the environment and match demands with your child's current abilities, you can reduce the likelihood that your child's behavior problems will worsen, keep your child safe, and smooth the recovery period.

Rehabilitation professionals have developed a variety of strategies to use with agitated and confused children. In general, you need to keep your child's environment calm and quiet, avoid excessive stimulation from conversations, televisions, video games, and radios, and be careful what you discuss in your child's presence.

Some points to bear in mind when communicating with your child at this time include:

- Keep communication concise, concrete, and direct, using simple words and gestures.
- Keep subject matter appropriate to your child's developmental level and avoid excessively violent or emotionally upsetting topics.
- Only one person at a time should talk to your child, especially when giving directions or asking questions.
- Be prepared to repeat information frequently due to deficits in your child's attention and memory.

Some points to bear in mind when managing your child's behavior during this phase of recovery include:

- Give your child only a few selected and appropriate choices in nonessential activities. Too many choices can be overwhelming to children at this stage of recovery.
- Give your child frequent breaks, changes in activities as attention wanes, and rest periods to combat fatigue.
- Only ask your child to perform tasks that are essential to his safety, physical well-being, or current level of recovery.
- The goal at this stage of recovery should be to develop a pattern of compliance (doing as asked) by calmly praising or rewarding even very small efforts to follow directions.
- Do not attempt to force your child to comply with demands, which could easily escalate into combativeness, physical resistance, and aggression. Do not scold, lecture, or get into power struggles with him.
- Focus positive attention on desired behaviors and ignore those that are inappropriate, bizarre, or undesirable, unless it would be unsafe to do so. Instead, attempt to redirect your child's attention to a more appropriate activity and provide information to reorient him, such as "Today is Wednesday and you are at the hospital. It is time to go to Physical Therapy and see Janet. Then we can go back to your room."
- If your child becomes aggressive, try to move out of range or block acts of physical aggression. Use comments to redirect him instead of commenting on the aggres-

sion. For example, "Stephen, you need to sit here and keep your hands down so we can watch the video you have chosen."

■ Provide praise and rewards calmly, including a statement of the specific behavior you approve of. For example, "I like the way you kept your hands to yourself in the elevator just now."

Ideally, rehabilitation therapists should match their demands on your child to his level of tolerance. This should help keep agitation and disruptive behaviors at an easily manageable level. As recovery progresses and your child's tolerance increases, rehabilitation therapy demands should be gradually increased to keep pace with, and gently challenge, your child's recovery. Any time your child regresses to previous forms of disruptive behavior, the behavior needs to be assessed and addressed on an individual basis. When this happens, your child may require more specific behavioral interventions targeting the problem behaviors. (See Chapter 8.)

While your child is functioning at the confused, agitated level of recovery, members of the rehabilitation team should use the strategies mentioned in this section. Further, you and your family should receive guidance and training in the use of these methods. If you believe that your child could benefit from these strategies, but they are not being used or are being used inconsistently, discuss your concerns with a member of the rehabilitation team. Request that a plan for modifying your child's environment and reducing agitation be developed. Conversely, if you or members of your family are having difficulty consistently using the recommended strategies with your child, ask for assistance from the behavioral specialist or psychologist on the rehabilitation team.

How Does Behavior Change Following the Period of Confused Agitation?

Level V. As your child continues to recover following the period of confused agitation (Level IV), he becomes calmer. However, overstimulation still can lead to agitation. He remains frequently confused and highly distractible, and often behaves inappropriately. Your child's ability to learn new information is still impaired, and he often needs constant redirection to complete even the simplest task.

Level VI. At the next level of functioning, your child's behavior becomes more appropriate to environmental demands, but is still frequently confused and disoriented to place and time. He begins to follow simple directions under optimal conditions and can complete steps toward a goal with plenty of assistance and guidance. Your child's ability to learn new material is variable, inconsistent, and highly affected by his level of fatigue.

Level VII. The next higher level of functioning is met when your child is able to perform his daily routine activities in a familiar setting, at a level appropriate to his development, with minimal prompting and assistance. Children at this level of functioning seem to perform routine tasks in an automatic, or robotic, manner. Your child may show few, if any, signs of emotional expression, although he may try to use some vocal inflection in his speech. Your child is unable to set realistic goals for the future and has poor awareness of his difficulties, especially in the area of thinking and judgment.

Level VIII. When your child reaches the highest level of functioning, his behavior becomes purposeful and appropriate. He is no longer confused, disoriented, or disruptive, and has no trouble with new learning. His cognitive functioning is normal. Some children who have had a severe brain injury may never reach this level of functioning. And children who reach this level of functioning may regress to lower levels of functioning at times when they are fatigued, stressed, or in unfamiliar settings or situations.

∷ Why Are Behavioral Disturbances So Often Associated with Brain Injuries?

A large proportion of childhood head injuries result in damage to an area of the brain called the *frontal lobes*. (See Chapter 1.) The frontal lobes are extensively connected to many areas of the brain and are involved in the oversight of many brain functions, ranging from emotional expression to decision-making. As a result, injuries to this region can result in a wide range of behavioral changes, affecting many areas of day-to-day functioning.

It is difficult to foresee how damage to the frontal lobes may eventually affect behavior, especially if a child is young when he acquires a brain injury. This is because the frontal lobes do not ordinarily finish developing until early adulthood. As a child with TBI grows older and encounters increasing demands for independent functioning, the limitations caused by frontal lobe damage become more noticeable. At this point, a wide range of difficulties can emerge—not due to misbehavior or willfulness, but because the child's frontal lobes are not functioning properly.

Executive Functions. The primary job of the frontal lobes is to perform the brain's "executive functions." These executive functions include a lengthy list of complex activities that most of us typically take for granted in our daily lives:

- The frontal lobes are responsible for planning, initiating, and evaluating complex motor actions and all sorts of other goal-directed behaviors.
- They are involved in performing abstract thinking, planning, judging, evaluating, and decision-making activities.
- The frontal lobes are involved in regulating emotional expression, appropriate social interactions, and expressive language.
- They allow for flexibility in thinking and behaving that is important in problem-solving.
- The frontal lobes act as regulatory mechanisms for behavior. They start, stop, refrain from, or suppress certain behaviors and thoughts. They also allow us to step back, observe our own behavior and the impact we are having on others, and modify our behavior if it is not achieving the desired effect. Commonly called insight or self-awareness, this skill is crucial to appropriate social functioning.
- The concept of personality, or who one is, resides in the frontal lobes. Therefore, an injury to the frontal lobes can result in a loss of the person's self, or changes that can make the injured person seem unlike his former self. This loss can be distressing to family and friends, as well as to the injured person himself. For example, this is what one seventeen-year-old said about his old self twenty months after suffering a TBI, "I don't remember him, but I miss the old Rob."

These executive functions remain underdeveloped and immature in all young children. In essence, adults serve the functions of the frontal lobes for young children by providing structure, organization, predictability, and direction. As an uninjured child matures and enters early adolescence, his frontal lobes gradually take on these functions. The functions continue to refine and develop well into adulthood, allowing for greater independent functioning.

Understanding the far-reaching effects of frontal lobe damage is crucial in trying to cope with and manage your child's behavioral difficulties. Otherwise, you or others caring for your child can develop many misperceptions, including the belief that your child has control over his troubling behaviors, or that he is being lazy, uncooperative, or manipulative. Lecturing or punishing a child for these neurologically based problems in brain functioning is not only insensitive, but ineffective since it does not help the child learn skills to compensate for his loss. As a parent, you can serve a vital role as advocate by educating others about the nature and underlying cause of your child's problematic behaviors and deficits, and the need to teach him ways to minimize the effects of the brain damage.

■■ Behavioral and Adjustment Problems Associated with Frontal Lobe Injury

There are several ways to understand the behavioral problems associated with injury to the frontal lobes. Considering that the frontal lobes regulate a multitude of brain activities, some researchers have suggested that frontal lobe injuries can result in two related, global patterns of behavior.

The first pattern of behavior is characterized by a tendency for the child to become easily aroused or overstimulated. Behaviors associated with this pattern of overactivity include distractibility, irritability, agitation, hyperactivity, impulsivity, disinhibition, social inappropriateness, and aggression. The second pattern of behavior results in a tendency for the child to be underactive or less easily stimulated. Behaviors associated with this pattern include apathy, lack of motivation and initiation, shyness or social withdrawal, depression, and physical complaints such as stomachaches, fatigue, or general malaise. Depending on the nature of the injury, a child may exhibit either one or a mix of these behaviors. Furthermore, different patterns of behavior may be present under different circumstances or at different locations or times of the day.

Another approach to understanding the impact of frontal lobe injury on behavior is to look at frontal lobe functions and the kinds of difficulties that can result if those functions are impaired by TBI.

Attention Functions. The frontal lobes play an important role in directing attention to relevant stimuli and filtering out irrelevant stimuli in the environment. When injury to the frontal lobes disrupts this attention function, it can result in:

- distractibility,
- poor sustained attention,
- random behavior,
- preoccupation with irrelevant or trivial details,
- confusion when confronted with choices,
- difficulty dividing attention when necessary, and
- failure to recognize the significance of important events or stimuli in the environment.

Personality. The frontal lobes provide continuity to our behavior across time. This results in a sense of predictability and coherence to our behavior that can be thought of as "*personality*." Therefore, injury to the frontal lobes may result in:

- unpredictable and erratic behavior or impulsivity,
- lack of foresight,
- an inability to anticipate predictable outcomes,
- difficulty in setting goals (or even seeing the need for goal-setting), in planning and executing a sequence of behaviors needed to meet a goal, in deciding which actions would best achieve a given goal, and in acting in a manner consistent with stated goals.

Emotional and Interpersonal Behavior. The frontal lobes regulate *emotional and interpersonal behavior* so that we are able to meet our own needs without violating norms and rules of society or our personal values. Consequently, injury to the frontal lobes may result in:

- mood swings or rapid, extreme shifts in emotional expression,
- irritability and agitation,
- poor self-control,
- immaturity and silliness,
- overfamiliarity, and provocative or uninhibited sexual behavior,
- belligerence and opposition,

- apathy and indifference,
- lack of emotional expression,
- poor frustration tolerance,
- quick temper, and
- aggression.

"Overseer" Functions. Finally, the frontal lobes serve as a monitor, evaluator, and modifier of behavior based on internal and external feedback. Injury to the frontal lobes' "overseer" function may result in:

- an inability to benefit from experience, instead learning only from repeated encounters with the negative consequences of their actions,
- difficulty accepting or using feedback from others, and refusing feedback that contradicts one's own perceptions,
- rigidity and inflexibility in thinking and acting,
- poor insight into one's deficits and behavior,
- an inability to monitor oneself for inappropriate behavior, and to detect and correct mistakes in a timely fashion,
- and difficulty with *generalizing,* or applying learned information to novel situations. For example, your child may interact appropriately with others at home and school, but be unable to demonstrate that same skill with strangers or in less familiar or new places, such as a restaurant.

How Do These Behavioral Problems Affect Children with TBI?

When you review all the problems that can result from damage to the frontal lobes, it becomes clear that the frontal lobes are essential to efficient, safe, congenial daily functioning. The difficulties resulting from frontal lobe damage can have far-reaching effects on your child's day-to-day life. Areas of particular concern for many parents of children following TBI are:

- poor safety awareness and judgment,
- poor impulse control (or self-control) and uninhibited behavior,
- poor social skills and peer relations,
- poor emotional control or rapidly shifting emotional states,
- poor anger management and aggression,
- poor self-esteem and depression,

- apathy and a tendency toward being overly dependent on others for completing tasks,
- disorganization and memory problems, and
- lack of insight into, or denial of, disabilities and deficits.

In real life, these problematic behaviors tend to occur together rather than in isolation. This makes it crucial to put together a comprehensive plan to manage them. Strategies specifically designed to address these problem areas will be discussed in the next chapter after we explore some important elements of general behavior management here.

How Can Any Strategy Help Change Behavior Caused by a Brain Injury?

It is important to understand the neurologic basis for your child's adjustment and behavioral difficulties. It would be a mistake, however, to assume that nothing can be done to help your child and family with these problems. Behavior management strategies, individual and family psychotherapy, and environmental modifications and supports all can help reduce or eliminate a number of behavioral problems related to TBI.

Behavioral disturbances that occur as a child is emerging from coma often get much better over time if they are properly managed during the agitated phase. The key is to handle these behaviors in a calm, neutral manner, taking necessary safety precautions, while remaining patient.

When behavioral disturbances result directly from damage to the frontal lobes, some abilities may be regained if the child receives the right kind of support early in his recovery. Some abilities, however, may never be regained, but the child can learn strategies to compensate for his difficulties with executive function. For example, some children may have difficulty remembering to take their completed homework to school each morning. A reminder sign ("environmental prompt") could be taped to the mirror in the bathroom prompting the child to pack his backpack and place it by the door before going to bed the night before. A reminder might also be placed on his desk at school prompting him to turn in his homework before beginning new work.

Sometimes treatments cannot eliminate a particular behavior problem. In this case, environmental supports and modifications must be used consistently to help the child function as well as possible. An example would be a child with serious attention difficulties who becomes easily distracted and disruptive in settings with other children. In addition to other interventions, the child might need to be placed in a smaller, quieter classroom with fewer children, reduced demands, and more frequent breaks and activity changes. If the child's attention problems improve, the environmental supports can be systematically reduced to determine how much support he needs to continue his recovery.

Besides helping to manage behavior problems that are a direct result of a brain injury, these strategies and supports can help keep secondary behavioral and adjustment disturbances from developing. As discussed above, these secondary disturbances can develop when too much negative attention is given to the problem behaviors that developed soon after the brain injury or when excessive demands continue to be placed on the recovering child. For example, as a child emerges from coma, he often will use inappropriate language or behave in strikingly immature ways. If this behavior is ignored and the child is redirected to more appropriate conversation and activity, the behavior generally ceases as recovery progresses. On the other hand, if care providers or others comment on, punish, or laugh at the undesirable behavior, the child may repeat the behavior in the future in order to receive attention or to escape some demand. He may do so even after he is once again capable of more appropriate behavior and self-control.

Since no one can accurately predict which functions will return and which will remain impaired as your child recovers, it is crucial to maintain a consistent approach to adjustment and behavioral disturbances throughout the recovery period and beyond. This is the best way to avoid inadvertently reinforcing, and thereby increasing, problem behaviors.

▪▪ When Should I Seek Professional Assistance for My Child?

This chapter was written to help parents understand, assess, and manage their child's adjustment and behavioral problems following traumatic brain injury. However, the range of problems encountered by children with TBI is broad and unique to each child. In addition, extenuating circumstances may make problematic behaviors more dangerous for some children. For instance, you may be concerned about impulsive behavior in a toddler, but you can physically remove him from a dangerous situation. In contrast, impulsive behavior in an adolescent can be life-threatening if he takes keys to the family car and drives without permission.

Clearly, you must waste no time in seeking professional assistance for more serious adjustment and behavioral problems. If you are wondering whether you need professional assistance, always err on the side of caution. Seek professional assistance for your child or adolescent *immediately* if he:

- threatens to harm himself or others,
- causes injuries to his own body,
- abuses alcohol or other drugs,
- sets fires, or
- behaves aggressively or cruelly toward younger children or animals.

You also should obtain immediate professional assistance *for yourself* if you become so overwhelmed that you feel that you may harm or injure your child, and especially if you use physical discipline excessively or while you are angry. Professional help also is recommended if your child has problems with theft; destruction of his own or others' property; sexual acting out; overfamiliarity with strangers; and persistent depression, anxiety, or periods of excessive activity or excitability.

■■ Where Can I Find Professional Assistance?

Your child's rehabilitation team should be able to refer you to qualified mental health professionals in your area. Sometimes, these professionals are members of the rehabilitation team and can meet with you and your family at the treatment center. Other times, you may need to seek a local professional with experience in brain injury. Depending on your community, it may be difficult to find a mental health professional with experience in the complex issues confronting children with TBI and their families.

The ideal therapist should have training and clinical experience in clinical child psychology and neuropsychology, family therapy, parent training, and applied behavioral analysis. When medications are recommended, referral to and collaboration with a child psychiatrist is often advisable. Various types of mental health professionals meet some of these qualifications to greater or lesser degrees. Professionals who offer therapy to children and their families include psychologists (Ph.D. or Psy.D.), family therapists (Ph.D., M.A., or M.S.), clinical social workers (M.S.W.), and psychiatrists (M.D.). Practitioners from each discipline may approach your child's problems from a different perspective. When seeking professional help, try to match your most urgent or biggest problems with the skills, training, and general approach of the mental health professional.

Once you have the names of several prospective therapists, determine their experience during an investigative telephone call. During these calls you may want to ask any or all of the following questions:

1. After sharing a brief overview of your child's history and your concerns, ask the therapist if he works with children with such difficulties and his general approach to treatment. If he is not an appropriate therapist for your child, ask him to refer you to another professional for help.

2. Ask about the therapist's education, training, and experience in working with children following brain injury. Try to determine how recent and extensive his experience is.

3. Ask about the cost of the therapy, how many visits may be required, and over what period of time. Ask about payment options and the possibility of health insurance reimbursement (e.g., is the professional a preferred provider with your health plan?).

4. Ask how quickly you may be seen. Some agencies and private practices have waiting lists for services.

5. Ask who is expected to attend sessions. Some therapists will want to meet alone with your child, only with you, with you and your spouse, or with the entire household. Determine if these arrangements will be suitable to your family.

6. Ask if the therapist has evening or weekend hours, if that would be more convenient for your family.

7. Ask if the therapist is willing and able to coordinate his treatment plan with your child's school. Rarely do problems exist in isolation. Treatment approaches work best if they are used consistently by all of those responsible for the child in all settings.

If you do not find the ideal therapist in your area, you may need to educate an otherwise experienced local mental health professional about childhood brain injury. Most rehabilitation treatment centers have mental health professionals on staff to work with the children during the acute phase of recovery. These professionals can be a valuable resource in providing relevant literature, guidance, and consultation to a therapist in your community. Packets of reading materials, as well as information specific to your child and his injury, can be requested for the local professional. Sometimes, these professionals can provide educational programming and consultation to your child's school personnel. This is especially crucial if your school has never dealt with a child following TBI, or if your child is having significant behavioral problems at school.

Therapy for adjustment and behavioral problems may be difficult and awkward under the best of circumstances. Following your child's head injury, you may feel that this is too much for you to take on right now. But seeking treatment of your child's behavioral problems can result in much improved quality of life for you, your spouse, your child, and your other children. It can also prepare you and your child for the many challenges you will face in the future by providing you with the skills necessary for managing new problems that emerge as your child matures and reaches new developmental levels.

** General Strategies for Managing Adjustment and Behavioral Disturbances

How Should I Use These Strategies with My Child?

There is no such thing as "one size fits all" when it comes to developing effective behavior management strategies for children with TBI. You should therefore consider this discussion of strategies as a starting point rather than the definitive answer to your child's problems. The examples given are necessarily simple in order to best illustrate the proper use of the strategies. This is not meant to imply that children's behavior problems are simple, straightforward, and easy to resolve. Certainly, if there was an easy answer, you would already have found it. These are merely some suggestions to consider when attempting to improve how you manage your child's behavior.

All of the strategies described here have been demonstrated to be effective with many children with brain injury and their families. These approaches are based on sound principles of human learning and behavior, and take into account the types and degrees of cognitive deficits that are common in children following a TBI. The strategies share many features and are consistent with one another. This means they can be easily adapted into a comprehensive behavior management program for children who have multiple adjustment and behavioral problems.

You should strive to adapt interventions to your child's age and developmental level, his stage of recovery from TBI, and your parenting style and preferred approach to discipline. By following the steps described here, you should be able to pinpoint more clearly the specific behaviors that concern you, and develop an initial plan for managing them. However, you should seek professional assistance if:

1. You have difficulty implementing these initial steps.
2. Consistent use of your behavior management plan does not bring the desired results after several weeks.
3. Any of the severe behaviors described on page 224 occur.

Both parents should work together to develop and carry out the plan. Consistency among caregivers is vital to the success of a behavior plan. Rules, expectations, and acceptable behavior for your child should be determined jointly. For example, one parent should not reward a behavior that the other parent punishes. Likewise, both parents must agree on the kinds of rewards and punishments that will be used. If parents need to compromise, they should not discuss differences of opinion in their child's presence. If one parent is less committed or enthusiastic about using these strategies, try to get that parent to agree to a three-month trial period to evaluate their effectiveness. At the end of the agreed-upon period, the plan can be reevaluated and changes made if needed.

If others provide care for your child, such as older siblings, other relatives, daycare providers, or teachers, they need to carry out your child's behavior management plan as consistently as you and your child's other parent. If any care provider refuses or is unable to implement the behavior plan, you should reconsider whether you want them to care for your child. You can ensure, at least, that teachers will participate in your child's behavior plan by having it included in your child's Individualized Education Program (IEP). (See Chapter 9 for more information on IEPs.)

Remember that behavior management strategies will probably be help-ful for your child even if medications are prescribed to control certain behaviors. For example, a child who seems very impulsive, inatten-tive, and disorganized may benefit from certain types of stimulant medications. However, if his environment remains overly stimulating and unpredictable, he will not receive optimal benefits from the medi-cation and his symptoms may remain difficult to manage. If strategies are used to modify the child's environment and reward appropriate behavior, the medication's effects will be augmented, so that the dos-age may be reduced or even eliminated over time. Always discuss this two-pronged approach with the prescribing physician. Try to work with professionals who are open to using medications in combination with behavior management strategies, and be skeptical of those prom-ising miracle results from medications alone.

Finally, no matter where your child is in recovery, always re-member to jot down behavioral and adjustment concerns to take with you to your child's follow-up appointments at the rehabilitation clinic. Experienced staff members there should be able to recommend pro-fessionals who can help you develop interventions specifically designed to address your child's problems.

Getting Started

In order to change a behavior, you first must determine some basic features of the behavior. The best way to do this is to systemati-cally observe your child for a relatively brief time. Your goals are to:

1. Define the behavior of concern (i.e., *target behavior*) in specific terms.
2. Determine how often the target behavior is currently occurring.
3. Develop interventions for modifying the target behavior based on the information gathered.

Defining the Target Behavior. The target behavior is the spe-cific behavior that you want to change. For example, you may want to stop your child from hitting his baby brother, or you may want your child to put away his toys before bed. The behavior that you target needs to be observable, measurable, and described in specific terms. For instance, you could say that you want your child to "be nice" to his baby brother—which is a vague, nonspecific goal that cannot be measured. It would be better, however, to say that you want to reduce the number of times each day that your child uses his hand, arm, or any object to strike his baby brother—which is a clear, specific, and measurable goal. Similarly, you could try to get your child to be "neater" with his belongings (vague, nonspecific, not measurable), or you could seek to increase the number of times each week that he puts away his toys before bed within two minutes of being told to do so (clear, specific, and measurable). The target behavior must be observable in order to be measurable. For instance, you cannot track the number of times that your child *thinks* about hitting his brother, only the number of times that he actually hits or attempts to hit his brother when they both are in your presence.

Tracking the Target Behavior. Once the target behavior is defined in clear terms, you can begin to track occurrences of the behavior. You could simply count the number of times in a day (or during any defined period of time) that the target behavior occurs. You can keep track of this *frequency count* by making tick marks on a calendar or data sheet and tallying up the sum at the end of the day. This method works well for behaviors that have discrete occurrences, such as using a curse word, kicking the dog, or putting dirty dishes in the dishwasher.

Other behaviors are better assessed by recording the length of time a child engages in the target behavior. This could be accomplished by noting the time that your child begins doing the target behavior and the time that he stops doing the target behavior, and adding up the elapsed time. This *duration method* works well when attempting to increase or decrease the amount of time spent on the target behavior, such as trying to decrease the amount of time your child spends getting dressed every morning or increasing the amount of time he spends attending to reading assignments.

A third tracking method, the *ABC Method,* provides both a frequency count and detailed information about the behavior that is useful in developing effective interventions. Using this method, three pieces of information about each occurrence of the behavior are recorded on a data sheet such as the one in Figure 1. The letters ABC refer to **A**ntecedents, **B**ehavior, and **C**onsequences.

- *Antecedents* are the conditions (actions, locations, people, time of day, interactions, and emotions) that occur immediately prior to an occurrence of the target behavior. One or more of these conditions may be

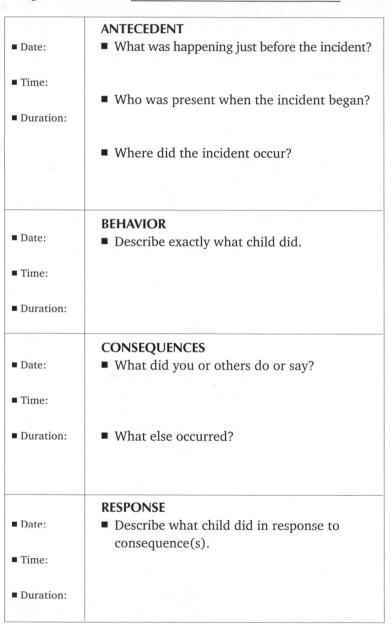

⁞⁞ Figure 1. ABC Data Sheet

Target behavior(s): _____

	ANTECEDENT
▪ Date:	▪ What was happening just before the incident?
▪ Time:	
	▪ Who was present when the incident began?
▪ Duration:	
	▪ Where did the incident occur?
	BEHAVIOR
▪ Date:	▪ Describe exactly what child did.
▪ Time:	
▪ Duration:	
	CONSEQUENCES
▪ Date:	▪ What did you or others do or say?
▪ Time:	
▪ Duration:	▪ What else occurred?
	RESPONSE
▪ Date:	▪ Describe what child did in response to consequence(s).
▪ Time:	
▪ Duration:	

serving as a trigger or signal to your child to start the target behavior. This information can be important in determining strategies that can be used to prevent the occurrence of certain behaviors. As an observer, you cannot accurately determine your child's specific thoughts and emotions just prior to a behavior, but you may notice that he tends to raise his voice and use inappropriate language more often when he is particularly tired or frustrated by a challenging task.

- The **behavior** is the action that has been targeted for change. On the form you would record characteristics of any occurrence of the behavior, such as to whom it was directed, how long it lasted, and its level of intensity.
- *Consequences* are the conditions that take place immediately following an occurrence of the target behavior. These conditions include both positive and negative events that come soon after a behavior and are believed to determine whether or not your child will repeat the same behavior in the future. Anything that is said to or about your child or the behavior, any action or attention directed toward your child, or any naturally occurring consequences, such as being scratched after pulling the cat's tail, may be important to note.

By noting consequences, you may find clues as to why the target behavior continues to occur, which can help in developing strategies for modifying the behavior. For instance, you may think that you are punishing your child when you scold him for throwing a temper tantrum (or having an angry outburst) every time you ask him to wash his hands for dinner. But by examining ABC data, you find that after you scold him, he comes to the dinner table with unwashed hands and is allowed to eat anyway. You have discovered that his temper tantrum allows him to both escape a demand and have access to something desirable (food). It is likely that he will continue to have tantrums when you ask him to wash his hands (or after any other requests), because in the past, that behavior has produced the desired results for him.

By becoming an astute observer of your child's behavior, you can pick up some very subtle indicators that can be valuable in developing successful behavior management strategies. As specific strategies are described below, types of information gleaned from ABC data that can influence strategy choice and implementation will be more fully discussed.

Once you have developed a plan for addressing your child's behavior and have implemented that plan, these assessment strategies continue to be useful. You should continue to track the rate and occurrence of the target behavior during implementation of the behavioral management strategies. This will enable you to determine the effect of your interventions on the behavior. If an intervention has not achieved the desired effect after a sufficient period of time, modifications to the plan should be made and evaluated as before. It is important to use this systematic approach when modifying a behavior plan. Otherwise, you may be tempted to make random changes or, worse yet, to abandon the plan altogether—for example, if your child briefly regresses due to fatigue, stress, or simply "a bad day." The observations you make during the ongoing assessment process will enable you to make effective modifications to the plan based on objective data rather than momentary frustration.

Preventing Predictable Behaviors from Occurring

As described in the previous section, you may find that there are certain predictable patterns or antecedents ("triggers") to your child's problematic behaviors. *Avoiding* disruptive or problematic behavior is always preferable to waiting for signs of a problem and then trying to manage it. Preventing problem behavior protects your child from unnecessary agitation, frustration, and disruption, which can leave him feeling out of control and distressed.

The best way to prevent problem behavior is to use *antecedent strategies*, or strategies designed to prevent the occurrence of an undesirable behavior. These strategies can reduce the time you spend trying to correct problems, increase the time you spend in positive interactions with your child, and increase the likelihood that your child will cooperate with you in the future. By increasing your child's sense of predictability and stability with you, you will reduce testing behaviors and avoidable power struggles. In addition, if you can effectively manage challenging behaviors through antecedent strategies, you will have greater confidence in your abilities to deal with future challenges and difficulties.

Successful use of antecedent strategies requires a thorough knowledge of your child and the situations or triggers that tend to lead to disruptive behavior. This knowledge comes from observations and ABC record-keeping, as described above. A good first step is to try to avoid situations that tend to trigger your child's disruptive behavior. This may mean not taking him to Chuck E. Cheese's Pizza for a friend's birthday party or limiting the amount of time there so the overly stimulating environment will not trigger disruptive behavior. It may mean limiting the length and scope of shopping trips and errands in order to avoid disruptive behavior brought on by fatigue and boredom. It does *not* mean allowing your child to escape an essential task that he does not want to do by having a temper tantrum or angry outburst. Instead, it requires that you think ahead about what helps and hinders your child's optimal performance, and then arrange the environment and situation appropriately whenever possible.

Children with TBI do best when the environment is highly predictable, organized, calm, and consistent across caregivers and settings. This is known as *increasing structure* in your child's environment. Your child should not be forced to use his limited executive function abilities to try to figure out what each adult is demanding of him in each setting each new day. Instead, this structure should be in place around him as much of the time and in as many places as possible, allowing him to focus on meeting the goals established for his optimal functioning.

Just as a child with a mobility or communication problem may rely upon a prosthetic or assistive device for walking or talking, the child with frontal lobe damage may require a well-coordinated system of external devices, memory aids, and environmental modifications to compensate for his executive functioning deficits. This means that you (and other relevant adults) must, in effect, take on the functions of the frontal lobes for your child. If you remember the lengthy list of functions and activities controlled by the frontal lobes under normal conditions, you can see what a daunting task this can be. Below are some suggestions that may help.

Establish a Daily Schedule. A daily schedule or routine can provide invaluable structure for your child. This daily schedule can be as general or as detailed as your child requires. It should include all tasks or demands that he must complete daily, such as morning and evening grooming, homework, medications, school attendance, and chores. Adults in the family should stick to established routines as closely as possible, even on weekends. For instance, mealtimes, waking, and bedtimes should be consistent from day to day with few exceptions. A predictable routine helps a child with TBI to stay more organized, and be less confused and more productive. It reduces time wasted in repeatedly reminding him what he needs to do throughout the day. The schedule should be kept in a prominent location and referred to as needed to keep your child on-task.

A sample daily schedule for a child with brain injury is shown in Figure 2. This particular example also provides a place for tracking target behaviors and providing feedback to the child about how he has performed his daily tasks.

Increase Structure and Predictability. A variety of other strategies can be used to increase structure and predictability for your child. For example, expectations and rules for your child should be clearly stated, specific, and achievable. Allow him to help set his own goals whenever possible, to a degree that is appropriate to his developmental level. Charts posting goals and progress toward them are useful for some children. Limits or rules also should be stated directly, specifically, and in a neutral manner. Better yet, general rules for the house or family, or for the classroom, should be posted in a prominent location to be referred to as needed by the parent or teacher. This is especially useful for rules regarding safety and socially appropriate behavior that may be hard for your child to recall.

Calendars, lists of rules or goals, daily schedules, alarm watches, timers, and the like are especially valuable if your child has any difficulty with memory, organization, or distractibility. These organizational tools are known as *prosthetic organizers* and they supplement the organizational role normally fulfilled by the uninjured frontal lobe. Such organizational devices should be built into all aspects of your child's daily functioning, along with prompts for their use. Goals in your child's IEP can be written to ensure these devices are used throughout the school day.

Avoid Overstimulation. It is easier to prevent overstimulation than to manage your child's disruptive behavior due to too much stimulation. This means that your child should have limited or no contact with topics that are highly emotional, violent, sexual, or otherwise overly stimulating. Do not assume that your child can understand that aggressive, rude, or promiscuous behavior seen in the media is socially unacceptable in the real world and should not be emulated. Serve as a filter for your child and be sure to discuss any

▪▪ FIGURE 2.   SAMPLE OF DAILY SCHEDULE

Jena's Daily Schedule

Date: _____   Day: _____

TIME	ACTIVITY	Refused	Delayed	Completed	COMMENTS
7:30 A.M.	Get out of bed, wash hands and face				
8:00	Eat breakfast and take medications				
8:30	Brush teeth and get dressed				
9.00	Do physical therapy exercises				
9:30	Reading time				
10:00	Free time				
10:30	Free time				
11:00	Free time				
11:30	Feed fish				
12 Noon	Eat lunch and take medications				
12:30 P.M.	Do physical therapy exercises				
1:00	Lie down for nap/rest				
1.30	Nap/rest				
2:00	Free time				
2:30	Free time				
3:00	Free time				
3:30	Playground				
4:00	Playground				
4:30	Free time—watch video if desired				
5:00	Do physical therapy exercises				
5:30	Eat dinner and take medications				
6:00	Clear table and help load dishwasher				
6:30	Free time				
7:00	Take bath, brush teeth, put on P.J.s				
7:30	Get out clothes for morning				
8:00	Read with Mom or Dad				
8:30	Get into bed, lights out				

Please indicate the occurrence (+) or nonoccurrence (-) of each target behavior.

upsetting material that he does encounter. Similarly, bear in mind that certain peers and social interactions may be overwhelming for a child who has difficulties making accurate social perceptions and interpretations. Peers may easily sway your child and lead him into socially unacceptable, immoral, or illegal behaviors and acts. Steer him instead toward activities, groups, and social activities that are highly structured and supervised, and that reinforce the values you want to guide his behavior.

Tailor Demands to Your Child's Emotional State. Parents need to be keen observers of their child's behavior and emotional state. Be prepared to modify demands or expectations if you see that your child is too fatigued, stressed, frustrated, or otherwise not at his best on a particular day. Your goal is to match the demands on your child with his realistic, present capabilities so as to optimize his chances for success. Success breeds success.

It is your job to help your child succeed as much and as often as possible. Again, this does not mean that you simply allow him to skip certain disliked tasks so that he will not become upset or act out. Nor does it mean that you abandon goals and expectations that are challenging for your child or that encourage his growth and development, or that you stop correcting or disciplining him. Instead, you should try to create situations that increase the probability of success for your child and avoid situations that set him up for failure. It is the difference between giving your child a chore to perform after he is well rested, fed, alert, calm, and attentive versus trying to have him perform the chore when he is fatigued, hungry, distracted, upset, or engaged in a highly preferred activity. If you plan ahead and have a good understanding of your child's capabilities and the factors that influence his behavior, you can optimize the chance that he will do as you request and exhibit more desirable behavior.

Redirect Your Child. Parents need to become experts at using a strategy known as *redirection*. Every parent of an infant has used this technique when diverting their baby's attention to a safe toy while removing an unsafe or breakable object from his reach. This strategy can be particularly effective with children with TBI, given the poor attention, high distractibility, and memory deficits that often accompany such injuries. It can be useful with many activities and behaviors, as well as with the persistent and unrelenting questions, demands, or other verbalizations that are common among children after TBI.

If you see that your child is headed for an undesirable behavior or activity, try to calmly divert or redirect his attention to a more appropriate activity. How you do this will depend on the age and developmental level of your child, the activity involved, and your own skill at redirecting. Even if your child is very young or impaired, you need to be somewhat subtle when using this strategy. Children can quickly discern that you are trying to keep them away from something, and that often prompts them to continue toward that activity if not properly redirected.

To use redirection effectively, you should understand the principle behind it. Redirection is intended to provide a smooth transition of the child's attention from one (inappropriate) activity to another (more appropriate) activity before or soon after the initial behavior has begun. It is not intended to punish a child for his behavior, nor to "trick" the child. Redirection should be used as a proactive strategy, to avoid or "short-circuit" disruptive or unsafe behavior. No mention or attention should be given to the initial or undesired activity. Only brief, calm, neutral directions should be given toward the new desired activity. If your child's attention is not easily diverted to the new activity, do not insist or plead. Stay calm and try again with another activity after a few minutes. Here are several examples of redirection:

Let's say that your young son recently has become insistent upon doing some restricted activity, such as climbing stairs unsupervised. Yesterday, you struggled all day with him over this. This afternoon, you see that he once again is headed for the stairs. You know that one of his favorite activities is to toss the ball with you. Without any mention of the stairs, you might say, "James, let's go outside and play ball until Sarah gets home from school," thereby diverting his attention to a more desirable, safer activity. Or, while out for dinner, your daughter becomes fidgety and loud while waiting for everyone to finish eating. Instead of attempting to talk her out of this behavior, you might say, "Kayla, let's go outside for a walk for a few minutes while everyone else finishes. Then we will come back and get ready to go home." In this example, not only have you short-circuited the disruptive behavior, you have provided an appropriate outlet for your child's need to move around and change activities.

Perhaps your adolescent is persistently taunting his younger sibling with a rude name or by telling an off-color joke. You might redirect him by saying, "David, tell me about that movie you were

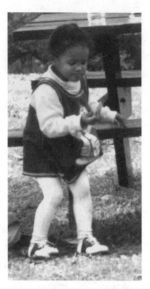

watching last night. It sounded really funny," knowing that David likes to tell others about movies he has seen. Once his attention is diverted to another topic, the undesirable behavior (taunting) ceases. It is replaced by a more acceptable behavior, without any risk of inadvertently reinforcing the undesirable behavior.

To be successful with redirection, you must stay a step ahead of your child. It can take significant energy and attention, but you must be prepared to guide him back to a more acceptable behavior whenever needed. Because children with TBI can be particularly persistent, you may need to use redirection frequently.

▪▪ How Do the Behavior Management Strategies Work?

This section presents specific strategies for increasing behaviors that you want your child to perform and decreasing behaviors that you don't want him to perform. An understanding of the principles underlying these strategies is necessary before we explore the use of these strategies.

The term *behavioral contingencies* refers to a principle of learning that states that behavior is determined by its consequences. These consequences determine whether or not the behavior will or will not occur again in the future, and at what rate, intensity, and duration. Consequences can be actions, statements, glances, gestures, rewards, punishments, and naturally occurring events that occur immediately or soon after the occurrence of an action or behavior. For example, when your child first learned to walk, you encouraged him for every tentative, wobbly step. He responded by taking more steps, and received more praise from you and self-satisfaction with his new skill. The positive consequences of pleasing you, pleasing himself, and increased freedom reinforced or promoted the behavior of taking steps. These consequences served as rewards for walking for your young child, and increased the likelihood that he would take more steps in the future.

A positive consequence also can result from the removal or avoidance of something the child finds *aversive* (unpleasant or painful). For instance, a child may learn that by throwing a temper tantrum, screaming loudly, or throwing something on the floor, he can get out of doing some task. If, as punishment, he gets sent to time-out (or the principal's office) for such behavior and does not have to complete the job he was trying to avoid, he learns that disruptive behavior is a successful way of avoiding an unpleasant task. The punishment actually serves as a reward or positive consequence for the child. In this case, disruptive behavior is likely to occur more often whenever the child wants to avoid doing something. This is what he has learned through the consequences following his behavior.

Consequences can be negative as well. For example, if a child is teased during his first days of school or has difficulty understanding the teacher's directions, he may be less likely to attend school in the future. He might refuse to go, complain of illness, or find some other means of avoiding the aversive consequences that were associated with his first school experience. These negative consequences served as "punishers" for attending school and decreased the likelihood that he would attend school in the future.

Naturally occurring consequences may serve as punishers for some behaviors. Being burned when touching a hot stove or breaking a toy after throwing it against the wall are examples of natural consequences that tend to reduce the likelihood of the behavior occurring again. The removal of a privilege or something else that is reinforcing to or valued by the child is another form of a negative consequence. If a child does not come in from playing at the agreed-upon time, he may not be allowed to play outside for several days. Being grounded, being sent to "time-out," and losing phone privileges are common examples of this form of a negative consequence and are designed to reduce the occurrence of that behavior in the future.

Consequences can also be events that become accidentally or inadvertently paired with a behavior. Superstitious beliefs are a good example of accidentally paired consequences. Let's say that a baseball player pitches a winning game after eating tuna for lunch. He may begin to eat tuna before every game, hoping to continue to pitch winning games. It is likely that he will continue with this lunchtime choice as long as his winning streak continues. However, if he eats tuna for lunch on a day when he is developing a stomach virus, and later becomes queasy and vomits, he may avoid tuna in the future, believing it to be the source of his upset stomach.

The point is, the actual relationship between a behavior and a consequence is not what is important, but what the individual *believes* the relationship between them to be. Perception is everything and must be considered when you are trying to develop appropriate consequences to modify your child's behavior.

Further, the meaning of a consequence to a child is highly individualized. A reward for one child may be of no interest to another. What one child might consider a punishment might be seen by another as a source of attention, and therefore affect his behavior differently. The value of a consequence can vary not only from child to child, but for any one child at different times and under different circumstances. Perhaps your child's favorite reward is chocolate ice cream. Using chocolate ice cream to reinforce or reward a desired behavior is likely to fail, however, if your child has just finished eating a large cone and is no longer hungry. In addition, it is probably not the healthiest practice to reward your child with a chocolate ice cream cone every time he follows a rule or completes a chore. If your child receives a chocolate ice cream cone every afternoon from his grandmother without regard to his behavior (*noncontingently*), it likely will not be a powerful reinforcer when you attempt to use it to reward him for completing a chore or following a rule.

Since choosing reinforcers is an important part of managing your child's behavior, you should spend the time to choose wisely in order to maximize the effect of your rewards.

Are Rewards for Following the Rules Really Necessary?

Some parents are uncomfortable with the idea of rewarding their child for "doing what he should do anyway." These feelings and beliefs must be considered before embarking on a behavior management program based on reinforcement. If one or both parents are against using reinforcement, it can undermine a program's effectiveness, potentially confusing the child and creating new behavioral problems. To help you sort out your feelings about using reinforcement, here are two thoughts:

Rewards Are a Part of Life. First, we all function within a system of reinforcement. Adults usually receive the reinforcement of a paycheck every two weeks as a reward for coming to work. In addition, praise and encouragement from a boss can increase motivation and work effort. Many people use desserts, sweets, or other snacks as rewards for completing unpleasant tasks. Vacations, weekends off, and breaks during the day are earned for timely completion of work projects. Compliments on a delicious meal reward the cook and increase the likelihood that he or she will prepare the meal again in the future. Rewards and consequences are common in everyone's daily life.

You may argue that adults also perform many tasks for which they are not directly rewarded or reinforced. For this form of motivation, known as *intrinsic motivation*, "a job well-done is its own reward" may be an apt description. This is the driving force for people with a strong work ethic. Many parents belief that this is the ideal under which their children should work, and fear that using rewards will undermine their efforts toward that end. This certainly is a laudable goal. However, after a traumatic brain injury, your child may have disruptive behaviors and severely impaired self-control mechanisms. At least in the short-term, you may need to use external rewards to eliminate undesirable behaviors and establish a new pattern of more desired behaviors. The use of a reinforcement system may be a necessary step on the path toward more appropriate functioning that is self motivated.

There Are All Kinds of Rewards. Rewards do not have to be edible, material, or cost lots of money to be effective. Social praise such as positive attention, smiles, hugs, gentle pats, nods, thumbs up, high fives, kisses, eye contact, and compliments are powerful reinforcers for most children. These rewards are free and should be used routinely. They teach your child what you want him to do by showing him what pleases you. They do not spoil your child or make him dependent upon external reinforcement, but serve instead as guideposts for your child to socially acceptable and desirable behavior. They can and should be a natural part of your relationship with your child; a loving way of expressing your pleasure with him.

Other reinforcers that can be used naturally are those commonly called privileges. Anything that is not essential to good health and safety can probably be defined as a privilege. Access to the phone, television, computer, video games, radio, CD player; special outings or time alone with a parent; bicycling, rollerblading, and other recreational activities; special foods and treats; visits to friends; eating out; and many other privileges can serve as rewards in a behavior management program, as long as you feel comfortable withholding them when your child's behavior warrants it.

Using social praise and privileges as your main rewards, with material rewards used intermittently to augment your basic system, will allow for a more natural approach to reinforcement. The gestures and privileges described here are likely to be given to your child anyway. By shifting the way that these reinforcers are delivered (that is, based on your child's behavior and not in spite of it), you can use them to modify your child's behaviors. As an aside, this is not meant to imply that you should show your child affection only when he behaves well. Children need unconditional love and acceptance from their parents. They need to know that they are loved no matter how they behave. But, in freely showing love to your child, be careful not to accidentally reward undesired behaviors by giving him attention only when he is disruptive or otherwise behaving poorly. Reinforcing negative behavior can lead to additional behavioral disruptions in the future.

▋▋ Choosing Reinforcers to Use with Your Child

Once you have decided to use reinforcement as part of your behavior management plan, you must determine the kinds of positive and negative consequences you will use with your child. The easiest way to choose positive consequences for your child is to observe what he enjoys doing. You can watch him in a store, with a toy catalog, or with other children's toys to determine the kinds of material rewards that might interest him. Listen to what he orders at restaurants or asks to eat at home to determine his favorite foods. Watch to see what he likes to do in his free time to determine the kinds of privileges that can be used as reinforcers. If he is old enough, you can ask him what he might like to earn.

Once you have a list of potential reinforcers, you can set up a system for earning them. Consider your ability to provide the reinforcers that you have chosen in a consistent and timely manner:

- Do you have time to provide the reinforcer?
- Can you afford to purchase the reinforcer if your child earns it often?
- Will your child become bored or satiated with the reinforcer?
- Are the reinforcers too big or too small for the behaviors required?

▪ Can you control your child's access to the reinforcers chosen for your plan?

For practical reasons, it generally is necessary to develop a system in which your child earns secondary reinforcers, also known as tokens, that can be accumulated and traded in for privileges or material rewards at a later time. The rate, frequency, and type of reinforcement arrangement need to be adapted to your child's developmental level and type of target behavior to be modified, among other considerations.

▪▪ Choosing Punishments for Your Child with TBI

You and your partner must decide upon the forms of negative consequences and punishment that you are willing to use with your child. You may come to the same decision that you reached as new parents before your child was injured. On the other hand, your child's injury may cause you to change your views on punishment, at least with this child.

There are two major issues to consider when discussing punishment approaches. The first involves the use of physical punishment, also known as corporal punishment, and it includes spanking, paddling, swatting, and other terms for striking a child, generally across his buttocks. (Other forms of striking children, especially with an object, are never recommended and may constitute child abuse.)

The decision to use corporal punishment is a highly personal, complex one. In my opinion, however, using physical punishment is inadvisable, at least with a child with TBI. First, the use of physical punishment serves as a model of behavior for a child, providing an example of how one should handle conflict and disagreement. Yet, striking another child is not acceptable behavior for a child. This contradictory message can be particularly confusing to a child following brain injury, because social rules can seem arbitrary to him under the best conditions. Clear rules and expectations, paired with models that are consistent with those rules, are most likely to help your child develop socially appropriate behavior.

Second, any time physical punishment is used, the potential for physical injury is present, especially if the parent is angry, frustrated, or fatigued. Further, I have observed that children with TBI often respond to physical punishment by becoming more disruptive and may become aggressive towards their parents, increasing the chance that someone will get hurt.

Third, physical punishment can only be used for a limited time. It cannot be used on a towering adolescent. When parents no longer have this strategy to fall back upon, they may be left with few effective management strategies.

Lastly, physical punishment often does not achieve the desired effect. In fact, it can create its own set of problems. The child may come to fear, resent, and be angry at the parent, and the parent-child relationship may be harmed. There are other effective ways for managing a child's behavior that do not carry these risks and potential negative outcomes, and I urge you to try them instead.

Whatever your decision, you must be aware of the danger of using any form of discipline, especially those involving physical management, when you are angry or feeling out of control. Having a child who has experienced a TBI, particularly one with behavior problems, is highly stressful and taxing. You have many demands on your time, energy, and attention. You may be in a state of chronic fatigue, never feeling at your best when dealing with your child. It is understandable that you may feel angry and overwhelmed from time to time. But if you attempt to discipline your child physically when in such a state, you may make the situation worse or injure your child.

All parents of children with TBI should have a plan to follow in case they feel they are at risk of harming their child. For example, you could prominently post the hotline number for Parents Anonymous, found in the emergency section of most local phone books. Your plan should also include a way for you to safely leave your child in a child-proofed place while you briefly retreat to another area of the house to calm down and regain your composure. Shut yourself in a room and turn on the radio if you need to block out sounds from your child. If possible, call on someone to come and give you a break from your child. For most parents, however, there is no one else at such moments. You must stay away from your child until you have calmed down enough that you will not cause him injury. If such an incident occurs, it is a strong indication for you to seek professional assistance for yourself and your child.

The second major issue to consider when making decisions about punishment involves withholding privileges. You must be comfortable with withholding a particular privilege if your child's behavior is unacceptable. If you are not consistently able to withhold a privilege such as access to the CD player, television, or the telephone, or if you cannot cancel a scheduled trip to a restaurant or other outing, then your plan will not be successful. Further, you must be present and able to keep your child from engaging in the privilege. If, for example, a behavior occurs when your child is at a friend's house, then you will likely not be able to withhold a privilege. Think ahead as you make decisions about both positive and negative consequences and make sure that you can follow through on all elements of the behavior management plan that you have developed.

▪▪ Strategies to Encourage Desired Behaviors

Make Good Use of Praise

As described earlier, social praise in all of its forms is a powerful method of increasing the likelihood that a desired behavior will be repeated. When your child exhibits a behavior that you like and would like to see in the future, let him know by smiling, winking, praising, hugging, or giving him some other form of positive attention. When using praise, clearly refer to the behavior you like. For example, if your child follows the rule to clean up after dinner, tell him, "Terry, I like the way you put your plate and glass in the dishwasher just now. That's very helpful of you." This is more effective in encouraging clean-up behavior than saying, "You're a good boy, Terry." At first, praise should be provided *immediately* after the behavior occurs each and every time you observe it. You must make a deliberate effort to watch for desirable behavior so that you can praise it promptly and specifically, especially as you are attempting to establish new behaviors.

Sometimes the behavior you are trying to encourage does not take place all at once. Perhaps you want to increase your child's ability to play independently and quietly for brief periods of time as you attend to his baby sister. You may be tempted to leave well enough alone when he is playing on his own, letting you get your other work done. Yet, this is exactly the time you should tell him that you like the way he is playing so calmly. If you wait until he stops playing independently to comment on his behavior, you will reinforce the wrong behavior and teach him that he needs to stop playing independently and perhaps become disruptive to gain your attention.

A better strategy would be to determine the optimal rate at which your child needs to receive positive attention in order to continue the behavior you desire. For a very young child, this rate may be as often as every minute or so. Slightly older children may be able to keep up the desired behavior with brief statements of praise every five to ten minutes. Older children and adolescents likely would find such attention annoying and intrusive, especially if peers or others were around. In these cases, you need to find a form of subtle social attention that you can provide your child frequently, but with little fanfare and notice from others.

Give Effective Commands

You can increase the likelihood that your child will comply with your requests by giving effective commands. *Compliance* means that your child does what you ask him to do with no more than a brief delay. Many parental requests are not followed, in part, because of the way they are given. Here are some suggestions for improving the way you give commands to your child:

1. Before giving any command, make sure that you are willing to follow through on having your child comply with the command. Don't give a command if it is optional, or if you don't have the time or energy to ensure that the command is followed.

2. Reduce the distractions in the room or area before you give a command.

3. Make sure that you have your child's attention prior to stating your command. You may need to have his eye contact, or you might have him repeat the command to you if his attention is in doubt.

4. Present commands as commands, not as questions, favors, pleas, or appeals. For example, don't say, "Amy, would you like to take your bath now?" Instead, say, "Amy, it's time to take your bath now; then you can have your snack."

5. Use simple, direct statements. Children don't want to listen to long explanations and reasons for why they need to comply. Simply state the command briefly and in a calm, neutral manner with an expectation of compliance.

6. Offer your child only realistic choices that are developmentally appropriate.
7. Don't offer your child an open-ended choice about a mandatory task. For example, don't say, "Stephen, when do you want to do your homework?" Instead say, "Stephen, you need to finish your homework now. Then, if there is time left before dinner, you can go out and play."
8. Give only one command at a time, especially with very young children or those who have trouble with memory or attention.

To increase the occurrence of a desired behavior, you first must determine whether your child is capable of performing that behavior. Children who do not have the skills to do something need different interventions than children who know what to do and how to do it, but still do not do it.

Let's look at a couple of training strategies first. If your child does not perform a behavior because he does not know how, you must find a way to train him to perform the behavior. You could simply tell him what he is to do. But for many children with TBI, simply giving directions may not be adequate for multi-step tasks. You could model the behavior for your child, demonstrating for him how to perform it. For some skills, it might be better to physically guide your child through the behavior or task while verbally describing the important elements of the task.

For more complex tasks, a strategy known as *task analysis* is useful. Through task analysis, the task is broken down into smaller, essential steps. The child then receives verbal (and other) instructions on performing each small step. Once he has mastered the first step, the next step is added. In a process known as *chaining*, each small skill is acquired step by step until the task is completed and the child has mastered the entire sequence of steps. Another, similar strategy is for you to guide your child through the steps of the task and gradually withdraw physical guidance and verbal prompts (*fading*) as he learns the new behavior.

Whenever your child is learning a new skill, the concept of *shaping* is useful to employ. With this strategy, you initially reinforce (through praise or other rewards) any effort that your child makes toward the ultimate goal. Let's say that you are trying to get your toddler to use a spoon to feed himself. At first you praise him for picking up the spoon and holding it, whether or not he uses it for eating. Later you praise him for touching his food with the spoon, then for picking up food on the spoon, until eventually you praise him only for neatly depositing food into his mouth from the spoon. These *successive approximations* toward the final goal must be reinforced promptly and generously in order to establish the new behavior and encourage your child to keep trying to do the skill correctly. The concept of shaping has many uses and can be applied to many behavior problems that are common following TBI.

Use Reinforcement Effectively

All of the strategies explained above can help your child learn a new, desired behavior. But once he has learned the new skill, how do you increase the likelihood that he will use it?

As described earlier, praise and other forms of positive reinforcement are powerful tools in increasing the occurrence of a desired behavior. In fact, if used correctly, positive reinforcement can be your most effective strategy for modifying your child's behavior.

Differential Reinforcement. In using positive reinforcement for the desired behavior, make sure that you withhold positive reinforcement for undesired behaviors. This technique is known as *differential reinforcement*. Ignoring mildly annoying behaviors and time out from positive reinforcement are two examples of the use of differential reinforcement.

The Premack Principle. Another simple strategy for using positive reinforcement is to have your child complete a less preferred activity (or less frequently performed behavior) before he is allowed to engage in a preferred activity (or more frequently performed behavior). Also known as the *Premack principle* or the *Grandma rule*, this common-sense approach can be used in many situations. Generally it is stated in an "If, then" format. Examples of typical uses include, "If you eat your vegetables, then you can have dessert," "If you clean your room, then you can go to the football game," "If you finish your homework, then you can go outside to play," and "If you feed the dog, then you can use the phone."

While it seems obvious, it is important that you do not reverse the order of this approach. Do not allow your child to do the preferred activity until he has successfully completed the less preferred activity or chore. If you stick to the rule and do not waver, refusals should be brief as your child learns that the only means of access to his preferred activity is to complete the less preferred activity.

Contingency Contracts. For older children and adolescents, parents can draw up a contract that spells out all of the events (contingencies) that will occur if the child performs certain behaviors. Known as a *contingency contract*, this list or document focuses on three important elements of the behavior management plan:

1. The contract must describe the target behavior in clear and specific terms.
2. The contract must make clear the goal or level at which the behavior is to be performed.
3. The contract must state exactly what the reward will be, how much will be given, and when.

For example, a simple contingency contract might state, "If Jason attends school every day for two weeks without being tardy, he will be allowed to go to McDonald's with a friend on the following Saturday." Children can be involved in the development of the contract so that the contract is seen as being fair to both parent and child. This helps increase the commitment of each to the contract. An example of a contingency contract and tracking sheet is shown in Figure 3 on the next page.

:: Strategies to Reduce "Undesirable" Behaviors

Teach Your Child a More Desirable Behavior

Whenever you seek to eliminate or reduce the occurrence of one behavior, you need to teach your child to replace it with a more desirable behavior. Just think about it. Your child may be exhibiting the undesirable behavior for a variety of reasons. For example: because it feels good, it is fun, it gets him something he wants (attention, a treat, etc.), it helps him to cope when he is frustrated (or tired or bored), or it gets him out of something he doesn't want to do. It is unlikely that he will simply stop the undesired behavior, forfeiting these benefits, and simply do nothing.

You must create a situation in which doing the more appropriate behavior is more rewarding than doing the inappropriate behavior. The more appropriate or desired behavior that you choose may be

:: Figure 3. Sample Contingency Contract and Tracking Sheet

WEEKLY GOALS:
1. If Megan earns 35 points, she may purchase a CD with Mom on Saturday morning
2. If Megan earns 28 points, she may go to the mall with a friend and Mom for 2 hours on Saturday morning
3. If Megan earns 21 points, she may choose a family activity on Saturday afternoon (select from the activity list)

Week of _____   *One point earned for each "Yes" circled
No points earned for each "No" circled*

Megan's Home Rules	SAT	SUN	MON	TUES	WED	THU	FRI
1. Megan will be where a parent or other adult (chosen by parent) can see or hear her at all times	Yes / No	Yes / No	Yes / No	Yes / No	Yes / No	Yes / No	Yes / No
2. Megan will leave the front yard ONLY with a parent or other adult (chosen by parent)	Yes / No	Yes / No	Yes / No	Yes / No	Yes / No	Yes / No	Yes / No
3. Megan will cook or operate household appliances ONLY with parent permission and supervision	Yes / No	Yes / No	Yes / No	Yes / No	Yes / No	Yes / No	Yes / No
4. Megan will keep her hands to herself and use appropriate language (no swearing) when angry	Yes / No	Yes / No	Yes / No	Yes / No	Yes / No	Yes / No	Yes / No
5. Megan will complete all homework and chores at the scheduled times before using the phone, listening to music, or watching television.	Yes / No	Yes / No	Yes / No	Yes / No	Yes / No	Yes / No	Yes / No

Daily Point Totals:
(total number of circled "Yes")   ____ + ____ + ____ + ____ + ____ + ____ + ____

Total Points for the Week = _____

any behavior besides the one you wish to eliminate. In the case of a child who hits others, the child might receive praise and positive consequences for doing anything as long as he isn't hitting another child. You could also choose to praise only those other behaviors that are incompatible with the undesired behavior. For example, the aggressive child described above might be praised for using his hands for an art project, or taking part in physical exercise.

When deciding on a substitute behavior to reinforce, parents often choose one that is more adaptable, socially acceptable, or functional. For instance, if the target behavior you want to decrease is grabbing toys from other children, a natural behavior to reinforce would be sharing toys.

Prevent Behaviors When You Can

Besides helping your child *replace* undesirable behaviors with more desirable ones, you should also use strategies designed to *prevent or avoid* undesirable behaviors whenever possible. These strategies, called *antecedent strategies*, were described on pages 232-38. Redirection can be a very valuable strategy in dealing with undesirable behaviors just before or as they are beginning to occur. Remember, it generally is easier to prevent a problem behavior from occurring than it is to manage it once it has begun.

Along the same line, limits and rules for appropriate behavior should be based realistically on your child's developmental abilities, clearly stated, and consistently enforced. Rules that are arbitrary, change from moment to moment, or are inconsistently enforced invite your child to act out in order to find out what the limits are. Don't make him guess what behavior is acceptable and what behavior is not. Be clear and direct, and make sure that other caregivers do the same. Serve as a role model for appropriate behavior for your child. If you don't want your child to swear when he is angry, do not swear yourself when you are angry. These preventive strategies require a parent to be organized, alert, and active. But they can be your best defense against being overwhelmed by a child who has no limits and who often engages in disruptive, dangerous, or other undesirable behaviors.

Ignore Mildly Annoying Behavior

Deciding which strategy to use for an undesirable behavior should be based, in part, on the kind or severity of the behavior. Once you have decided to address your child's disruptive behavior, it is tempting to try to modify all of his behaviors at once with equal zest and enthusiasm. This is not the most efficient strategy.

Some behaviors that are not unsafe for your child or others could be called mildly annoying behaviors. They include:

- whining,
- fussing,
- pouting,
- sulking,
- loud crying or screaming meant to upset the parent,
- complaining,
- demanding,
- and throwing mild temper tantrums.

For these behaviors, a strategy known as *planned* or *active ignoring* can be most effective when coupled with the differential reinforcement strategy described previously. Planned ignoring means that you briefly remove all reinforcement (attention, scolding, eye contact) when your child is engaged in a mildly annoying behavior. This prevents you from accidentally reinforcing a behavior that you want to eliminate. As soon as the undesirable behavior ends, you then reinforce your child with attention and social praise. Many parents find this strategy quite difficult to use since children tend to be experts at finding the behaviors that are most annoying and difficult for their parents to ignore. Here are some steps to follow when using this strategy:

1. When your child begins a mildly annoying, but safe, behavior, briefly remove all forms of attention from him. Turn your head away and avoid eye contact. Absolutely do not argue, scold, or talk to your child or mention his behavior. Do not show anger, annoyance, or frustration through your manner or gestures.

2. To divert your attention from the annoying behavior, try to become or act as if you are intensely absorbed and interested in some other activity. Look through a magazine or newspaper, tend to a plant, dust the furniture, wipe the counter, stare out of the window— anything but look at your child. (Of course, you will want to make sure that he has not begun to engage in an unsafe activity by glancing out of the corner of your eye periodically.)

3. Of critical importance: *Immediately* provide your child with attention and other forms of reinforcement as soon as the annoying behavior has ceased. You also may use redirection at this point, in order to move your child on to a more appropriate behavior or activity, praising him for engaging in behaviors besides the annoying ones.

4. It is important at this point to continue to refrain from commenting on your child's recently ended, annoying behavior. The episode is over; it's a new day, and no other action should be taken with regard to this episode.

When you first begin to use planned ignoring, there may be a brief, but significant increase in the frequency and/or intensity of the target behavior. Known as an *extinction burst*, this results from your child's expectation that the target behavior will be followed by the same reinforcer (for example, your attention or escape from some demand) he used to receive. He may redouble his efforts to gain the desired effect that he has typically received in the past. This may continue until he realizes that "things are different now" and he learns the new behaviors that will earn your praise and attention.

It can be disheartening for things to get worse before they get better. However, it helps to be prepared for this expected increase in undesirable behavior and to understand that generally it heralds an imminent improvement in your child's behavior.

Give Effective Reprimands

Many parents respond to their child's undesirable behavior by scolding, or by making a negative comment to the child about his behavior. Scolding for some parents typically turns into a lengthy lecture—one that the child soon learns to tune out. Some children scold or argue back, others mock or ignore their parent, still others become angry and throw a tantrum, while others appear to enjoy the attention that they are receiving or seeing their parent upset and frustrated. Make sure that scolding is not the only source of attention that your child receives from you.

Just like social attention and praise, reprimands are easy and quick to use. They take little effort and may be very effective for some children, for some behaviors, and in some situations, if implemented correctly. When giving a reprimand, make sure that you have your child's attention through eye contact and that distractions are reduced. Be brief, calm, serious, and firm. If you or others nearby actually find the behavior somewhat amusing or cute and you show this to your child, he will perceive the mixed message. The nonverbal message of approval likely will win out and he will be likely to repeat the behavior in the future.

Clearly state what behavior you do not like, labeling it and not your child. For instance, say, "Stacy, I don't like the way you took that toy from your sister. That was not good sharing," instead of, "Stacy, you are a bad girl for being so selfish." Then briefly tell your child what behavior you would rather see: "Stacy, you need to give the toy back to your sister." Scolding works best when the behavior is just starting.

Time Out

Many parents are familiar with the strategy known as *time out*. Although this strategy is quite commonly used, its purpose is often misunderstood, and it often is used incorrectly. The actual term for this strategy is *time out from positive reinforcement*, and it has little to do with a time-out room, corner, or chair. What is essential about time out is that the positive reinforcement that normally is present in your child's environment is suspended or removed for a specific time following the occurrence of certain behaviors.

Time out brings an immediate end to the target behavior and provides an opportunity for your child to calm down and get his behavior back under control. It is useful for a variety of problem behaviors, including aggression, sassing, spitting, engaging in dangerous activities, threatening, damaging toys or other property, and disobeying a direct command. It is not recommended for problems involving failing or forgetting to complete homework or chores, "attitude" problems, such as pouting, grumpiness, and irritability, or shyness and withdrawing from social interactions. That is because time out works best to stop a problem behavior, and not to get a child to initiate a desired behavior. Time out is intended to be boring for your child, but not frightening, painful, or shameful. Time out is useful for children from around age two to ten years.

Before using time out for the first time, you need to explain (and with younger children, practice) the time out procedure so that your child knows what to expect the next time that the behavior occurs. Initially, you should choose one or two target behaviors that you want to decrease, and use time out immediately and consistently after each occurrence of those behaviors. Usually, it is best not to threaten to use time out or give your child "just one more chance."

Ideally, time out should last one minute for each year that the child is old, and its duration should not vary with the severity of the behavior. A portable timer is useful for keeping track of time out. Place it where your child can hear it go off, but not manipulate it. You must be able to get your child into time out within a few seconds of the target behavior, and with very few words.

Find a location that is boring, safe, and free from any form of entertainment, such as television, radio, video games, toys, or other people. With some creativity, time out can be used in locations other than your home as long as these basic elements are employed. Young children should remain in the same room or area as you while being placed in a designated straight-backed chair or corner. Some older children (over five or six years) can be sent into a separate room for time out, but only if they are not a significant safety risk to themselves and the room is not filled with desirable toys or activities.

When putting your child in time out, express no anger, frustration, or other negative emotions. Remain calm, but firm, as you direct him to time out. Ignore everything he does in an attempt to avoid being placed into time out. During time out, give your child absolutely no attention—no scolding, no arguing, no talking at all. When the timer rings, your child should come to you and briefly review with you the reason that he was sent to time out. Once he has stated this, he is free to go on with his day. If he forgets or tells you the wrong answer, remind him briefly, have him repeat it to you, then allow him to return to play.

Toys or other objects can be placed in time out as well. For example, if two children are unable to share an item satisfactorily, the toy can be placed in time out so that neither child has access to it.

Most children do not like time out, but if time out is handled properly, they soon move on to more positive behavior after completing their time out period. If your child remains upset, do not attempt to alter his attitude directly. Simply allow him his feelings and use redirection and good listening skills.

Some children initially resist time out, but soon learn to accept it. If your child does not, there are a number of publications that deal with time out under these circumstances. You also may want to seek professional assistance. This is especially true if your child is aggressive and at risk of harming himself or other children and time out does not quickly eliminate or significantly reduce this problematic behavior.

Response Cost

Response cost is a strategy that can be used with children of all ages. It is, essentially, a fine or penalty for engaging in an undesirable behavior. A speeding or parking ticket is a common example of a response cost for adults. For children, the loss of a privilege, such as access to the television, telephone, outing, or other leisure activity, is a familiar consequence to a prohibited behavior. With children who have contingency contracts (see explanation above), engaging in the target behavior can result in the loss of tokens, points, or other secondary reinforcers that earn the child rewards at the end of the day, week, or other time period.

Response cost is most useful if the penalty is logically related to the negative behavior. For example, if your child rides his bike without his helmet, he is not allowed to ride his bike for a week. If he does not complete his homework, he is not allowed to play video games that evening. If he is late getting up and to school, he must go to bed thirty minutes earlier that night.

The danger with this strategy is the tendency for it to be overused. If you target too many behaviors at once, or give excessive penalties, your child may not receive any privileges or positive consequence for lengthy periods of time. When faced with such overwhelming odds, children often stop trying to modify their behavior. If they have no access to any privileges, they have nothing left to lose. If the standards are too high, they will have no hope of earning back privileges, and will give up.

Remember the power of positive consequences for appropriate (or approximations of appropriate) behavior. Your child must receive *some* positive consequences in order for these negative consequences (loss of privileges) to have an impact. It can be hard to allow your child access to a privilege if he has not behaved perfectly all day. Remember, however, that the behaviors you are trying to modify did not develop overnight, nor will they be eliminated quickly. Withhold privileges only for those behaviors that you have targeted and use active ignoring or another strategy for other ongoing problem behaviors. Once you have seen some success with the first targeted behaviors, you can target other behaviors that you wish to modify.

Ideally, your child's behavior plan or contingency contract will include ample opportunities for earning privileges and positive consequences, along with the conditions under which your child will lose tokens or privileges. When he does lose a privilege, remind him when he will have the opportunity to "try again" to earn back the privilege. Do not taunt, tease, or tempt him with the lost privilege during the period when it is being withheld, and do not let siblings do so either. The response cost itself should be sufficient. If your child seems always to be "on punishment," reexamine your target behavior and goals. They may be excessive for your child at this time. Advice from a professional may help you refine your behavior plan.

Overcorrection

Overcorrection is a strategy that may help if there is not a readily available logical consequence or loss of privilege to pair with the target behavior you wish to discourage. It is similar to response cost in that a penalty is imposed as a consequence of the target behavior. However, instead of receiving a fine or losing access to something, your child has to do something which, in some way, corrects the damage or harm done by the misbehavior or compels your child to practice a more socially acceptable activity.

Let's look at some familiar examples of overcorrection. Perhaps a child draws on the living room wall with crayons. As punishment, he may have to wash the wall several times to remove the crayon marks. (However, he is not forced to wash all the walls in the house or to paint the entire living room. This would be overly harsh and developmentally inappropriate.) Similarly, a child who wets his bed may be required to strip his bed in the morning, place the wet clothes and sheets in the washer, and make the bed with clean linens. These forms of overcorrection provide some *restitution* for the damage done by the child's behaviors.

There are also forms of overcorrection that do not provide any restitution, but provide the child with practice at more socially acceptable or appropriate behaviors (*positive practice*). For example, a child who copies from a classmate's paper during a quiz might have to write, "I will not cheat on tests," on the chalkboard 100 times. A child who swears may be required to brush his teeth a certain number of times after each episode, or a child who touches his genitals in public may have to perform a set of physical exercises with his hands and arms instead.

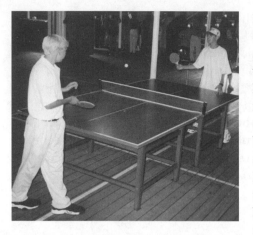

In order to be effective, the overcorrection penalty should be related in some way to the undesirable behavior, by using the same muscle group, or undoing damage resulting from the behavior. The punishment also must immediately follow the misbehavior. Lastly, the overcorrection act must be performed long enough that the child finds the punishment to be more unpleasant than the inappropriate behavior was enjoyable.

In selecting an overcorrection act, make sure your child is physically and cognitively able to do it, and that the number of repetitions is developmentally appropriate. Overcorrection has been found to be most useful with children who are late preschool aged and older.

There are several problems with the strategy of overcorrection to consider before attempting to use it as a part of your behavioral plan. First, it is hard to determine beforehand just how many repetitions of the overcorrection act will be sufficient to discourage your child from engaging in the target behavior again, but not be too harsh. More importantly, enforcing the overcorrection penalty may be quite taxing and time-consuming. If your child resists performing the overcorrection penalty, you need to physically guide him through the act for the prescribed number of times. Briefly providing gentle physical guidance to a young child to enforce putting away his toys is one thing, but physically forcing an older child to do a set of exercises or scrub the floor, or any other physical act, is likely to be risky (in terms of potential injury to parent or child), exhausting, and ultimately unsuccessful.

Take these points into consideration as you contemplate using this strategy, and if you do choose to use overcorrection, have a specific plan ready should your child physically resist performing the corrective act.

A Final Word about Reducing Negative Behavior

No matter what strategy you use to reduce your child's negative behavior, be sure that you can and will follow through on the intervention. Never use empty threats, lengthy lectures, or other power-less techniques. Children quickly learn when a parent does not intend to enforce a rule. When a parent frequently uses threats without ac-tion, a child learns that he can continue the disruptive behavior until his parent stands up, raises his voice to a certain volume, or threatens for the "final time." Do not fall into this trap. If you are too tired or distracted to follow through on your strategy, don't begin it at all. If the behavior is not unsafe for your child or others, you may just have to tolerate the behavior this time. Otherwise you will teach your child a lesson that will create more undesirable behaviors in the future.

∎∎ Conclusion

This chapter has examined the relationship between injury to the brain and behavior and has focused on some adjustment and be-havioral problems that are commonly associated with TBI. General strategies for managing adjustment and behavioral disturbances were presented. These strategies will serve as the foundation for more spe-cific recommendations to be discussed in Chapter 8 addressing prob-lems often seen in children following a traumatic brain injury.

∎∎ Parent Statements

It is so hard to see him being rejected by his so-called friends. Sure, they were right here when it first happened, but now that he is so difficult to be around, they've all gone on with their own lives. I guess I can understand that, but it leaves me feeling like I am the only friend he has and that gets in the way of my being his parent.

❦

She is really talkative now and says exactly what she is thinking, all of the time. It can really be embarrassing, and I am tired of trying to explain to people why she is like this. Sometimes I try, but usually I just smile and try to change the subject. Lindsay is so distractible that it usually works.

❦

I know those other boys put him up to it. But he's the one who gets caught setting fire to the guy's garbage can. Of course, his "friends" were half a mile away by then. Yet, he still wants to be with them and resents me for telling him "No." I don't think he really understands that they are laughing at him and just trying to get him into trouble. I don't know what he might do if they ask him to.

⋅⋇⋅

I have to watch her every minute. I fear what she might do if I left her alone. It is especially hard when we go some place. I can't always see all of the dangers that she can get into. People just don't understand when they think that I'm too overprotective. They don't realize how much she needs to be protected.

⋅⋇⋅

A year ago I felt like I might hurt him sometimes. He just made me so mad. I knew I needed some help. I still feel really angry with him sometimes, but it has helped having a psychologist to talk to. Knowing that she doesn't think I am a terrible mother and that she will listen when I am really upset has kept me from losing control with him.

⋅⋇⋅

Ever since he got into middle school, they just get in his face too much and it sets him up to get into trouble.

⋅⋇⋅

The county school system has a TBI specialist and she is great. She is trying to help with his behaviors, but her hands are tied somewhat because the school doesn't have the staff to provide him with the services he needs.

STRATEGIES FOR MANAGING YOUR CHILD'S BEHAVIOR

Cindy L. Tucker, Ph.D.

The behavior management principles and strategies discussed in the previous chapter form the foundation for any successful behavior management plan. For most behavioral problems, these general strategies and approaches are easily adaptable. However, parents of children with TBI frequently face certain behavioral concerns that may require some special strategies. The sections that follow examine some of these common concerns and describe some interventions that may be useful in managing them. If these problems persist or worsen, you should seek the services of a professional experienced in working with children with traumatic brain injury.

■■ Poor Judgment Resulting in Unsafe Behavior

Children with TBI have a higher risk of injuries due to their general lack of safety awareness, impulsivity, and poor judgment. These cognitive impairments may be short-lived or may persist long into recovery. Most children have at least some problems with safety awareness when they first leave the hospital.

It is vital that you plan for the safety of your child upon her return home. A partial list of precautions is shown in Figure 1. Other modifications needed will depend on your child's abilities, your home, and other settings where your child receives care or spends time. As you can see, it is recommended that all children who are impulsive

---

■■ Figure 1. Environmental Safety Strategies Following Your Child's Traumatic Brain Injury

1. Children and adolescents who display *impulsive behavior or impaired safety awareness* following TBI should NOT be left unattended at any time. Constant supervision by a responsible adult is necessary to assure the child's safety.

2. An older child or adolescent may have time for *privacy* in his or her room as long as he or she cannot leave the home unsupervised from the room and unsafe items have been removed from the room.

3. If there is *concern that the child or adolescent might attempt to leave the home* unsupervised, consider placing deadbolt locks on each external door. Deadbolt locks are most useful at night when supervising adults are sleeping. Supervising adults must have access to deadbolt keys at all times to allow for exit during an emergency. The child or adolescent must not be allowed access to these keys. Smoke and carbon dioxide detectors should be used in the home, especially under these circumstances.

4. *Medications* should be made inaccessible to the child or adolescent by keeping ALL medications, both prescriptions and over-the-counter (including vitamins and herbal supplements), inside a locked medicine chest or cabinet.

5. Access to *sharp and other potentially dangerous objects* (such as knives, matches, tools, razors) should be restricted. This may require reorganizing items typically kept in the kitchen, bathroom, gardening area, garage, and basement. Survey your home with an eye to potential dangers and place these objects inside of locked containers or cabinets.

6. Safety knobs should be placed on the *stove and oven* replacing the standard ones to prevent unsupervised use. Microwave use

and have poor safety awareness be supervised by a responsible adult *at all times* immediately upon discharge from the hospital. Some parents may need to keep their child within arm's reach, while for others, being in the same room is sufficient.

---

should be supervised. Use of a lock-out feature (if available) is recommended. Consider keeping a small microwave-safe container of water in the microwave when not in use in case of unauthorized use (consult manufacturer's manual to see if this is recommended).

7. Chemicals, cleaners, plant and lawn treatments, paint, inhalants, and other *hazardous substances* must be kept in locked cabinets, inaccessible to the child or adolescent.

8. *Keys to motor vehicles* must be inaccessible to the child at all times. This includes keys to automobiles, trucks, power mowers, boats, ATV's, jet skis, motorcycles, etc.

9. Examine the *child or adolescent's room* to determine potentials for injury. Remove any items which could pose a safety threat to the child if used without supervision or if used improperly. Examples include: electronic equipment, fish tanks, hobby materials and equipment, etc.

10. *Instruct all family members in these safety precautions.* Do not allow the child or adolescent to spend time in another home or location (including school) until similar precautions have been implemented there. The child or adolescent should always be supervised by an adult who has been trained in these safety precautions.

11. Should questions arise during a home visit or upon discharge, contact the Nursing Desk or Pediatric Psychology at your child's hospital. In an emergency situation (the child or adolescent is a danger to self or others, or has been injured in some way), CONTACT 911 IMMEDIATELY. Inform the emergency personnel that the child has had a traumatic brain injury, the name and dose of any medications the child is on, and the name of the child's physician.

Precautions for restricting your child's access to medications, chemicals, knives, cleaners, tools, garden supplies, and other toxic substances and unsafe items must be taken. Keys to motorized vehicles, including garden, farm, and recreational vehicles, must also be secured away from your child if there is even a remote chance that she might attempt to use them.

Safety rules can be printed and posted in several locations in your home. This way you can refer your child to these "standard" rules rather than continuously deal with questions or challenges about them. This is especially helpful for restrictions to physical activities imposed by medical personnel, such as contact sports and other activities with a potential for repeated brain injury. Safety precautions and physical activity restrictions can be integrated into a contingency contract to increase your child's compliance with these critical rules. (See Chapter 7 for information on contingency contracts.) A sample list of restricted physical activities is shown in Figure 2.

Most likely you will need to modify these precautions periodically as your child's safety awareness and judgment improve. As her impulsive, unsafe behavior decreases, you can provide her with limited, well-supervised access to a potential safety risk to determine her ability to exercise good safety awareness and judgment. For example, you might allow an older child or adolescent to help prepare foods that require chopping or slicing with a kitchen knife, or you might allow her to help heat water for cocoa. During such a planned trial, closely observe your child's ability to use devices safely. If, after repeated trials, she *consistently* demonstrates safe abilities, you can begin to modify some restrictions. If your child does not demonstrate adequate safety awareness, provide some brief, clear directions about how to perform the task safely, continue with the restrictions, and assess her skills again another time.

Remember that your child may demonstrate safe behavior when she is in a familiar setting such as home. However, she may have difficulty transferring this learning to a novel situation. Therefore, take care to assess her ability to function safely whenever potentially dangerous activities are attempted in new or less familiar settings.

For older adolescents who had driving privileges prior to suffering a traumatic brain injury, additional restrictions will be needed. See Chapter 10 for information about laws regarding driving privileges following a traumatic brain injury.

∷ FIGURE 2. PHYSICAL ACTIVITY GUIDELINES AFTER TRAUMATIC BRAIN INJURY

NOT ALLOWED	ALLOWED

Contact or high-risk sports, including:
  football
  soccer
  hockey
  basketball (competitive)
  baseball
  boxing
  wrestling
  lacrosse
  baseball
  ATV's
  jet skis
  motorized bikes
  trampoline
  balance beam / parallel bars
  diving
	swimming
	noncontact martial
	  arts
	bowling
	golf
	tennis
	badminton
	racquetball
	bicycling (with helmet)
	scooter (with helmet)
	tumbling
	weightlifting (as
	  appropriate for age)
	softball (with batting
	  helmet)
	most track and
	  field events
	dancing
	jogging

∷ Difficulty with Changes in Routine

Many children with TBI have difficulty easily shifting from one activity to another or tolerating changes in their daily routine. You may see these problems when you try to get your child to turn off the computer and eat dinner, or put on her coat to leave grandma's house. She may resist transitions even when she likes the new activity. Similarly, she may have difficulty when her daily routine is changed, such as when on vacation, or when meals are served later than usual. These difficulties are likely related to damage to the frontal lobes and executive functioning impairments, which make transitions (or shifting attention) and changing cognitive strategies (or ways of thinking) very difficult.

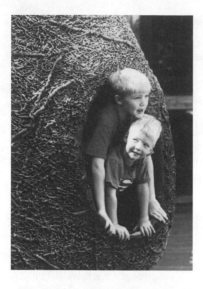

As described in the section on antecedent strategies in Chapter 7, daily schedules and other interventions for increasing structure in your child's day-to-day life are very helpful. Using a daily schedule, every morning you can review with your child the plans for the coming day, preparing her for any changes to her typical routine. While some changes cannot be avoided, it is important to stick as closely as possible to the remainder of your child's routine, especially to activities that give her a sense of security and stability, like meal and sleep routines.

For schedule changes that cannot be anticipated, you will need to make use of warning or transition periods. Warning periods are useful in managing transitions from one activity to another as well. A warning period consists of a verbal statement that one activity will be ending in a certain amount of time and another will begin. The statement is made in a calm, matter-of-fact manner with minimal conversation and explanation added. For instance, "Jason, in five minutes we will have to get our towel and pool toys, get dressed, and go home." About one minute before the end of the transition period, you would say, "Jason, you have one more minute before we have to get ready to go home." You would ignore requests, pleas, and demands to negotiate the length of the time period, and praise any signs of compliance with the transition. Long discussions and justifications of the activity change are not recommended, as they give your child the idea that the change is optional instead of required.

How much warning you give will depend on your child and the activity. For example, giving a four-year-old more than a three-minute warning may be too disruptive, and anything less than a fifteen-minute warning may be too brief for an adolescent. Your child may do fine with a very brief warning to end an activity before washing up for dinner, but may require a somewhat longer warning or transition period when it is time to leave the playground or a friend's house. Experience and careful observation of your child's reactions to warnings will lead you to the optimal amount of time for preparing her for transitions. Be sure to discuss this strategy with your child's educators so that they can use it to manage the many transitions that occur in a typical school day.

▪▪ Resistance to Therapy

Often, physical, occupational, or speech therapists provide parents with a list of exercises or activities that their child with TBI is to complete every day. When families try to carry out this therapy at home, it often results in power struggles, arguments, and neglected exercises. Given the numerous challenges and demands on a parent's day, this is not surprising. However, these rehabilitation exercises can be vital to your child's ongoing physical recovery. A number of strategies may help.

First, if the exercises seem to be boring, lengthy, painful, or otherwise unpleasant for your child, consult with her therapist. Specifically, ask whether the exercise routine can be shortened or streamlined, or if the required movements can be worked into a more naturalistic and fun activity, such as playing hopscotch or a game of catch. If your child complains of discomfort when performing the exercises, consult with the therapist or physician right away to make sure that a physical problem is not being aggravated by the exercises. If the exercises are determined to be safe and discomfort is to be expected, request assistance from the therapist or a psychologist trained in pain management strategies to help your child learn strategies for coping with the discomfort.

Other strategies that can help:

- Don't set yourself up for noncompliance by being inconsistent or unclear when you instruct your child to do her exercises. Make sure you know exactly what she is to do and how she is to do it by observing and consulting with the therapists. Obtain written instruction, diagrams, or photos if needed, and review them with your child.
- Do not leave the exercises until the end of the day, when fatigue and other demands are likely to interfere, and do not schedule the exercises at a time when you cannot supervise.

- Try "grandma's rule": have your child complete her exercises *before* you let her go outside to play, use the telephone, or do some other preferred activity.
- Have other family members engage in some physical activity while your child is doing exercises so she won't feel as if she is the only one with this additional chore.

⠿ Impulsive Behavior

Acting before thinking seems to be relatively common in children following a traumatic brain injury. This impulsivity can lead to involvement in dangerous activities, unsatisfying social interactions, and impaired opportunities for learning. Many publications address the issue of impulsivity in children with attention deficits or hyperactivity. Many of these strategies can be used with children with traumatic brain injury as well.

In addition, some strategies that work especially well for children with TBI include:

"Plan It, Do It, Review It" Strategy. In this strategy, your child is prompted by an adult (or given another type of cue or reminder) to plan out and verbally rehearse the steps she needs to complete. For example, let's say your child needs to complete a homework assignment, and typically rushes through the task, leaving the work unfinished or forgetting to take it to school the next day. You could start by asking her to list the steps involved in doing this task (*verbal rehearsal*). With some practice, she may respond that she needs to get together all of her materials, set up her materials at her desk, reread the instructions from the teacher, complete the assignment, check her work for completeness, have you check her work, place the completed assignment in her special folder, then put all of her materials in her book bag and place it by the door for morning.

If your child forgets a step, you may provide clues and prompts to remind her. For tasks that need to be performed routinely, it may help to prominently post a list (on her notebook, for instance) with key words or pictures illustrating the steps.

Once the steps have been rehearsed or stated, your child completes the task. Then you review her performance, noting what worked and what did not work, and making any necessary changes to the plan for next time.

Reviewing Rules about Behaviors and Consequences. A similar strategy can be used if your child often breaks rules, participates in activities that are off limits, or has trouble getting along with peers. You remind your child of the rule about the behavior and the consequences if she follows or breaks the rule. These contingencies are rehearsed and reviewed at an appropriate time before she typically engages in the problem behavior. For instance, just before your child goes into a friend's house to play, you ask her to recall the rule against, and the consequences for, grabbing toys from another child. You praise her for remembering and stating the rule and consequences or help her if she cannot remember. After her visit, you assess how she did with toy grabbing. If necessary, you develop plans for improving her behavior at the next visit, and praise her for her success. Both planning and reviewing are done in a simple, low-key, conversational manner, and should not become lengthy, critical lectures on proper behavior.

The goal of these activities is to promote your child's compliance, reduce her impulsivity, and provide opportunities for her to practice a "stop and think" strategy before acting. As with other antecedent strategies, you are attempting to provide the support necessary to ensure your child's success, not simply finding new ways to reprimand her.

Even though they may be able to state the rules and consequences of behaviors, many children with TBI continue to behave impulsively. Damage to the frontal lobes can seriously affect a child's ability to control certain actions or behaviors—sometimes for an extended time. Seek professional assistance if your child continues to demonstrate impulsive behavior that interferes with her safety, learning, or relationships.

▪▪ Difficulty Managing Anger

Following a child's traumatic brain injury, many parents report poor anger management, frequent and unpredictable angry outbursts, swearing and verbal threats, and destructive or aggressive behavior. These episodes can be quite violent and explosive, and may appear to be unrelated to any provocation in the environment. There are a number of reasons for these problems with anger management:

- Children with frontal lobe damage have a general decrease in the ability to control emotional responses to minor irritations or daily frustrations. This lack of emotional balance, coupled with an inability to control their responses to changing feelings, often leads the child to overreact to the day-to-day hassles and frustrations that everyone faces. Once set off, the child appears to have little awareness of, or control over, her behavior, and may shout, cry, swear, stomp, pound walls or tables, and throw nearby objects. Often the child can shift rapidly from this enraged state to one of amusement or nonchalance if something else engages her attention.

▪ Some children who have experienced a brain injury had difficulty with anger management before the injury. Damage to areas of the brain that inhibit impulses and modulate emotions may worsen these preexisting behavioral problems.

▪ For children with TBI, there are a multitude of new frustrations and challenges to face as a result of the residual effects of their injury, demands of rehabilitation, loss of friends, and other stresses that accompany brain injury. These stresses may overtax the child's ability to cope with the frustrations that all of us encounter every day.

▪ Children with TBI may come to learn that the "squeaky wheel gets the grease." Essentially, they learn that they can get desired or extra privileges or be excused from unpleasant tasks or rules by having an angry outburst. Behavior that initially may have occurred due to effects of damage to the brain may now be encouraged by responses from adults who do not have the skills needed to manage the child's behavior.

If your child's inability to manage her anger is placing her or anyone else in danger, you must seek professional assistance immediately. Although you may have empathy for your injured child and the many reasons for her disturbing behavior, allowing such outbursts to go untreated will not help. Your child cannot be allowed to intimidate her family or classmates, nor does she want to do so. Despite their poor insight and inability to control their behavior, children with TBI often are aware that their behavior is unacceptable and inappropriate after the fact, and many are quite sorry afterwards. If they do not receive help modifying their behavior, they are destined to repeat such acts again and again, and may lose self-esteem and feel more and more out of control.

Whether or not your child needs professional assistance, several anger management strategies can help:

Provide Positive Role Models. Most children today are inundated with images from TV, movies, video games, and music lyrics that glorify and promote disrespect, delinquency, aggression, and violence. Depending on your child's age and cognitive abilities, she may be able to differentiate between reality and fiction, and to resist acting in a way that reflects these violent influences. However, many children with TBI are very concrete, literal thinkers, and are strongly influenced by models in their environment. When they hear a movie crowd cheer an aggressive act performed by the hero, they believe that this is behavior worth imitating.

Likewise, your child with TBI will have difficulty understanding why she cannot hit her siblings or peers if her parents hit her as a form of discipline. She will tend to shout and swear when frustrated and angry if her most influential models, her parents, shout and swear when they are frustrated and angry. Many children, especially those with a brain injury, are not able to anticipate negative consequences to such actions if they do not observe them occurring to their aggressive models in either real life or the media.

It is crucial to surrounded your child with role models who exhibit positive and appropriate behavior. If you are creative and persistent, you can find many other experiences and activities that do not involve exposure to violent media images. Try to enlist the help of other parents who share your views and whose children can provide positive models for your child. If your child is to learn to manage her frustration and anger, she needs you to be a buffer between her and the harmful influences that pervade her world.

Reduce Unnecessary Frustrations. The antecedent strategies described in Chapter 7 are the best means of reducing unnecessary frustrations for your child. They can provide predictability and structure for your child, reducing the occurrence of situations that typically provoke impulsive and aggressive behavior.

Note that this recommendation refers to *unnecessary* frustration. There are many situations in the life of a child that bring frustration, disappointment, and irritation. You cannot protect your child from all sources of frustration, nor should you try to do so. Experience with unavoidable frustrations will provide your child with valuable opportunities for mastering skills for coping with and managing her emotional responses. However, too much frustration, or frustration that has no purpose, can overwhelm a child whose skills are already being taxed.

When you can anticipate that a particular experience will frustrate your child, try to use the experience to train her in responding appropriately. Review potential responses and the likely consequences of them with her. Discuss ways that she can remind herself to use responses that are more appropriate when actually confronting the frustrating situation. You may choose to provide her with an incentive for making an appropriate choice. Praise her for trying to prepare for frustration, as well as for any efforts made toward appropriate management of her anger in the actual situation.

Deal with Anger Appropriately. No matter what actions you take, some children will, at least occasionally, have trouble managing their anger. For young children whose behavior is aggressive, destructive, or otherwise out of control, the time-out strategy is recommended. Time out can quickly bring an end to the undesired behavior and provide your child with an opportunity to regain her composure. If your child is too old for a time out, consider taking away a valued privilege when she is aggressive or expresses anger inappropriately. All children may respond to the use of incentives or rewards for "aggression-free days" or other similar approaches. This strategy works best if you also provide your child with opportunities for learning alternate ways of responding to frustrating and anger-provoking situations. She cannot be expected to express anger appropriately if she does not have the skills necessary to do so.

Teach Anger Management Strategies. There are many approaches to training children and adolescents to better manage their anger. Some focus mainly on talking about feelings, while others concentrate on acquiring skills. All approaches stress modeling appropriate anger management by the therapist and others. During a series of sessions of either individual or group therapy, the child learns and practices a set of skills. The basic skills typically include some variation of the following list of abilities:

1. *The child learns to predict which situations trigger her angry outbursts or "push her buttons."* Learning to predict or anticipate these situations helps her either avoid them or be prepared to choose a more appropriate response when she "sees it coming."

2. *The child is trained to observe the internal signs and sensations that indicate that she is becoming angry before she actually has an angry outburst.* This eventually will enable her to plan her response before losing control, allowing her to make more appropriate choices or extricate herself from a problematic situation. Self-monitoring skills are taught and practiced in sessions using mock anger-provoking exercises and therapist feedback about observed signs of anger.

3. *The child learns several new responses to her anger, trying them out both in and out of sessions.* Once she has mastered several, she develops a list or menu of more appropriate responses to her anger and ways of prompting or reminding herself to use them. Generally, alternate responses should be incompatible with the expression of aggressive or destructive behavior. Possible alternate strategies include: relaxation exercises, the traditional "counting to 10," physical activity, getting out of the situation, and assertive communication skills.

4. *The child learns to complete some form of an anger log or record in order to assess her performance during angry episodes occurring between sessions.* Figure 3 shows an anger log used by an adolescent male after his traumatic brain injury. For this young man, going to his room to complete his log became a good way of gaining control over his angry impulses. Completing the log was helpful to him because he could use the "Notes" section as a journal to express his feelings and point of view about the situation that had provoked his anger. Review of these logs and his notes provided the information needed to troubleshoot and continue training him in anger management strategies in future sessions. The log also provided him with prompts for noticing signs of mounting anger and situations typically associated with his angry outbursts.

For many children with TBI, briefly leaving the situation to walk, pace, pound their pillow, yell in their room, or shoot a basketball may be the best of all possible alternate behaviors, or the only one that they can use once their anger has been aroused.

Unfortunately, even with skills training, children with TBI may still have inadequate impulse control when confronted with a real situation that provokes their anger. Parents may need to continue to serve as a back-up to their child's damaged frontal lobes, prompting

---

■■ Figure 3. Sample Anger Self-Monitoring Log

Date: _____   **Time:** _____

How Did You Know You Were Angry?

___ felt my face get hot   ___ heard my voice getting louder
___ noticed I was swearing   ___ felt my gut tighten up
___ noticed I had "shut down"   ___ other (specify)

Where Were You?

___ inside house   ___ in classroom
___ school cafeteria   ___ outside at home
___ school hallway   ___ friend's house
___ in car with: _____
___ other (specify): _____

What Triggered Your Anger?

___ I was nagged to do something ___ I was told I couldn't do
                                      something
___ I was rushed by someone   ___ I had to wait for someone or
                                      something
___ I was criticized   ___ someone messed with my
                                      things
___ I was frustrated   ___ I was tired
___ someone did something I didn't like (specify): _____
___ other (specify): _____

Who Were You Angry With?

___ Mom   ___ Dad
___ sister   ___ friend
___ teacher   ___ myself
___ other (specify): _____

her as needed to calm down, think through her alternatives, make a choice, and enact that choice.

It can help to make a contract with your child, outlining the prompts to be used to promote appropriate anger management. These

---

What Did You Do?

___ yelled	___ went to my room
___ cursed	___ told a lie
___ cursed quietly or silently	___ thought about something else
___ hit or tried to hurt someone	___ walked away
___ threw or hit something	___ damaged or destroyed something
___ listened to music	___ went for a walk or run
___ got an "attitude" with:	___ talked about what was bothering me
_____	
___ distracted myself with:	___ threatened to hurt someone or myself
_____	
___ cried	___ threatened to run away
___ made a joke	___ ignored them
___ took a deep breath	
___ other (specify): _____	

Additional Comments:

100   The angriest you can be—aggressive, destructive, out of control

75   Very angry—but not aggressive or destructive, threats to harm someone

50   Pretty angry—yelling, cursing, no threats

25   Kind of angry, annoyed, or irritated

0   No anger—not mad at all, no irritation or annoyance

How angry were you when your anger was at its worst or highest? ____

How angry were you when you first realized you were angry?____

How well do you think you handled your anger during this episode?

1	2	3	4	5
Poorly	Not so Great	Okay	Pretty well	Well

prompts can start at a more subtle level, like a small hand gesture, and become more direct if your child fails to respond to less obvious signals. An example of a direct prompt might be, "Tara, perhaps you would like to take a few minutes for a walk to cool down before we continue talking." As a parent, you may also benefit from training in frustration and anger management so that you can avoid inadvertently escalating your child's behavior during conflicts.

▪▪ Trouble Making and Keeping Friends

Soon after a child is injured, her friends tend to gather near, expressing concern and interest. They are eager to see her and play together once again. They also often have lots of questions about her injury and its effect on her appearance, speech, or behavior. If they witnessed or were involved in some other way in the incident causing the injury, they may experience signs of trauma, guilt, or fear and anxiety that make it difficult to interact comfortably with their friend. Typically, however, the greatest barrier to their ongoing relationship is the trouble that the child with TBI has with appropriate social interactions after her injury. Siblings as well as peers can be put off by the child's unusual behavior.

Some children with TBI are aware that they are being left out, laughed at, teased, or otherwise hurt by their old friends. They have little insight into the behaviors that have driven their friends away, however. Some children with TBI develop feelings of loss and sadness, while others respond with aggression and angry outbursts. Still others may not even be aware that they are the butt of jokes or that peers are avoiding them. They may think that others like them and therefore resist efforts to improve their social skills. These children are at risk for becoming involved in dangerous, delinquent, sexual, or otherwise harmful activities because they are naïve and easily misled by exploitative peers. Children with such significant impairments in social functioning may benefit from group therapy to learn more appropriate ways of interacting with others.

The types of social skill deficits that are seen after traumatic brain injury vary, depending on factors such as age, prior social skills, degree of injury, residual effects of the injury (such as speech impairments or physical disabilities), social environment, and quality of relationships. Problems may include:

- speaking too loudly or about inappropriate topics in public;
- difficulty respecting personal space, standing too close to others, and touching them or their clothing;
- touching or picking up items belonging to others, and then damaging or neglecting to return them;
- poor table manners;
- rudeness;
- making inappropriate comments about the appearance or behavior of others;
- conspicuous immaturity;
- lewdness;
- inappropriate styles of dress (inappropriate to the weather, activity, or location);
- a significant lack of regard for the feelings and needs of others, instead being demanding and insistent about having their own needs met;
- nose picking, scratching or touching private body parts, tending to private grooming tasks, or performing crude bodily functions in public;
- trouble engaging in a reciprocal or give-and-take conversation, tending instead to repeatedly turn the topic back to themselves or their interests.

Children with TBI may engage in these behaviors while seemingly unaware of their inappropriateness or how uncomfortable they are making others feel.

From this discussion of possible problems with social interactions, it should be clear that we are talking about more than simple etiquette *faux pas* or blunders. Children with TBI often seem totally unaware of the multitude of social rules that allow society to interact and function smoothly. Because they lack awareness of others' feelings, they think that the rules sound arbitrary, unnecessary, and overly complex. Efforts to convince them of the need for socially appropriate behavior are futile and do not result in significant behavioral change. Other approaches must therefore be used to help your child become more socially competent:

- Others who interact with your child need to understand that she may not be able to comprehend the purpose of social rules, but that she does not need to do so in order to conform to them.

- ■ Social rules and the consequences for following or not following them need to be stated clearly to your child.
- ■ Some children may benefit from the use of prompts and nonverbal cues from parents (or others) to modify their behavior in public. For example, your child may need you to tell her when she is speaking too loudly. You might indicate this to her by subtly placing your hand over your ear, or by pointing downward, or some other signal that you both agree on. If your child has particular difficulty accepting and using feedback from one parent, it may be best to have the other parent take the lead on this area of behavior change for a while.

Another way to provide your child with feedback about her social behavior is to use a social rules list where performance on each rule can be determined and recorded during specific periods of time throughout the day. See Figure 4 for an example of a rules lists that was used with a high school sophomore at school, where his social inappropriateness was particularly disruptive. A school aide accompanied this young man throughout the school day (due to his difficulties finding his classes) and was in charge of completing the tracking sheet and giving the student feedback about his performance each day.

When developing a social rules list for your child, target social rules that can be stated clearly, succinctly, and objectively, and are most likely to cause problems with others for your child. For instance, it is probably better to address your child's tendency to stand too close to and touch others than to insist that she never talk with food in her mouth. Similarly, it is preferable to eliminate overfamiliarity with strangers before tackling the more sophisticated skill of reciprocal conversation.

The chart may include rewards that your child will receive for following the rules (privileges, incentives, etc.), as well as targets for performance. The time periods for evaluation should optimize your child's opportunity to get back on track after infractions. Feedback should be given in a calm, neutral tone and be followed by a statement that she will have the chance to do better the next time.

Remember that your child does not need to agree with, or understand the need for, the rule you are working on. She simply must understand that this rule has been determined to be necessary for her and that

▪▪ FIGURE 4. SAMPLE SOCIAL RULES LIST

DATE: _____

DAILY GOAL:
Aaron must earn at least 36 points to walk home with his friends. If less than 36 points are earned, he will ride home on the bus or with a parent.

Aaron's School Rules	1st Period	2nd Period	3rd Period	4th Period	Lunch Period	5th Period	6th Period	7th Period
1. I will keep my hands to myself. I can give a handshake or "high five" when greeting a friend or someone I know.	Yes No	Yes No	Yes No	Yes No	Yes No	Yes No	Yes No	Yes No
2. I will ask and wait for permission before touching anything belonging to another person.	Yes No	Yes No	Yes No	Yes No	Yes No	Yes No	Yes No	Yes No
3. I will use appropriate language (no swearing, no insults, no rude jokes or comments) in class and in the hallway.	Yes No	Yes No	Yes No	Yes No	Yes No	Yes No	Yes No	Yes No
4. I will use my "inside voice" in class and in the hallway. I will make my voice quiet when reminded to do so.	Yes No	Yes No	Yes No	Yes No	Yes No	Yes No	Yes No	Yes No
5. I will raise my hand and wait until granted permission before speaking in class.	Yes No	Yes No	Yes No	Yes No	Yes No	Yes No	Yes No	Yes No
6. I will use an appropriate title (that is, "Ms.," "Mrs.," or "Mr.") when speaking to or talking about a teacher. I will not call a teacher by his or her first name.	Yes No	Yes No	Yes No	Yes No	Yes No	Yes No	Yes No	Yes No

Daily Point Totals:
(total number of circled "Yes")

____ + ____ + ____ + ____ + ____ + ____ + ____ + ____

Total Points for the Week= ____

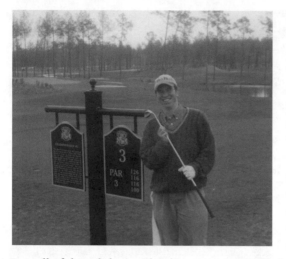

certain consequences will follow if she complies or doesn't comply with the rule. For example, you might explain a rule to a young adolescent with severe TBI like this: "Sarah, I understand that you disagree with me about this rule and that you think it is stupid. We will just have to agree to disagree about this. But, all of the adults involved in your care have determined that this rule is necessary for you to follow. In fact, everyone has to follow this rule when interacting with other people. Before your injury, you knew this and were able to follow the rule without thinking about it. Now, the part of your brain that allowed you to follow the rule has been damaged. Now you need others to remind you of the importance of the rule and to help you follow it when you talk to people. When you have learned how to follow this rule without reminders from us, we can stop using the chart."

If your child continues to have difficulty with social functioning, she may benefit from professional assistance—especially from group therapy specifically designed to provide social skills training to young people with brain injury. Ask staff at the rehabilitation facility for a referral. As a parent, you too may benefit from professional assistance. For example, you may need to learn strategies for coping with your self-consciousness when in public with a disinhibited child. You can also be empowered by learning strategies for modifying your child's social behavior.

It is critical that others in your child's environment be informed about your child's social skills difficulties and be given guidelines for dealing with them:

- Family and friends should be informed about the changes in your child's behavior and be given suggestions for responding that do not reinforce or worsen the behavior.
- Before your child reenters school, see whether rehabilitation staff can offer a program to your child's teachers

and classmates to provide information and an opportunity to ask questions.

- A peer helper may be assigned to help your child move from class to class or carry books and other materials. Given their unique position, these peer helpers need special guidance in how to respond to a youngster with a brain injury. Peer helpers can then serve as models to other children for responding to unexpected or unusual social behavior. An adult at the school should be available to the peer helper for managing problems and discussing concerns on a regular basis.
- Make sure that siblings receive special guidance in living with a child who has trouble conforming to society's conventions of behavior. Give brothers and sisters the opportunity to discuss their concerns privately with you. Giving them suggestions for addressing those concerns can help to alleviate some of the embarrassment, shame, and discomfort that they may be feeling.

■■ Lack of Insight into Strengths and Weaknesses

When under stress, many of us have trouble appreciating how our actions affect other people. When very upset, we seem only to be able to see things as they relate to us, our current situation, and our response to events and others. We cannot readily understand that others may be reacting or feeling differently than we are. In addition, we may not be able to see how our own behavior is affecting our situation, perhaps creating more problems than solutions.

Children with TBI frequently have these difficulties, even when they are not upset or under stress. It is not that they are just denying their deficits because they are stubborn or don't want to acknowledge them—they simply cannot accurately assess their abilities or see things from someone else's point of view. For example, here is how a sixteen-year-old girl who had a head injury two years ago assessed the changes in herself: "I know I can't think the same way anymore. It's like stuff is going on around me and I don't know what they're all talking about sometimes."

Your child's lack of awareness of her deficits cannot simply be "broken through," or challenged and changed any more than you could force a toddler to have insight and empathy for another's feelings. Because this lack of awareness arises from brain damage, it is not recommended that you try to force your child to acknowledge or admit her deficits through continual confrontation. This sort of approach tends to lead only to beliefs that are more entrenched and a resistant and defensive stance in future interactions.

This does not mean that you should withhold honest and direct feedback from your child. In fact, this type of feedback is crucial to helping her improve her functioning. However, doing so in an argumentative, confrontational, or emotional manner will only lead to resentment and conflict and will not give your child any useful information.

Instead, realize that your child's ability to accurately assess her strengths and weaknesses is impaired and may stay so for some time. Then go forward in setting limits when your child's judgment does not provide her with sufficient protection from injury or danger. For instance, if your child insists that she can ride her bike or use her rollerblades as before, you must restrict these activities to areas where there is less potential for serious injury, and require her to use helmets and other protective equipment, and provide supervision.

For some children, the natural consequences of their physical and other impairments provide the strongest feedback and route for behavior change. For example, a child with physical impairments who insists on trying out for a competitive athletic team will likely not make the cut for the varsity team, but may be offered a place on an intramural team. You can consult with physicians, coaches, physical therapists, and recreational therapists to provide your child with more realistic options for athletic or recreational endeavors.

Although many children with TBI freely acknowledge their more obvious physical deficits, they often deny any impairments in their ability to think, learn, and behave appropriately. Some notice that they have memory problems, and less often, trouble learning a new subject. This limited awareness can be useful in steering your child toward more appropriate classes at school. However, most children with TBI simply are not aware of their serious impairments in abstract thinking, social functioning, interpersonal relationships, and judgment and maturity.

Although it is challenging, it is very important to guide your child toward more realistic and achievable goals, while not underestimating her abilities. Sometimes, especially in adolescence, your child will accept suggestions about goals more readily if they come from someone besides you. Ask influential adults whom your child respects for this kind of assistance.

When your child insists on pursuing a goal that you believe she is physically, cognitively, or otherwise unable to achieve, you may choose to work with her on developing a plan toward the goal. This plan should be concrete and specific and include small, safe, observable steps toward your child's desired goal. Evaluate how your child does on these small steps and make further steps toward the goal contingent upon mastery of the smaller, intermediate steps.

Getting your child to "sign on" to such a plan can reduce conflict and keep you from having to restrict her efforts. This approach puts the responsibility of achieving the small steps into your child's hands. By sticking with this plan, she will either achieve the goal, fail to achieve the goal due to her failure to master the intermediate steps, or tire of the effort required if the goal is too difficult to achieve. Taking yourself out of the "spoiler" role can be important in reducing parent-child conflict.

▓ Depression

Children who have experienced a traumatic brain injury often are confronted with multiple losses, frustrations, and threats to their well-being. Such challenges may contribute to feelings of sadness or depression, especially as the child becomes more aware of the extent and permanence of her loss.

Children cope with sad feelings in a variety of ways. Some find that talking, writing, or drawing pictures about their feelings and fears helps them feel better. Others may use distraction, fantasy, or other cognitive (thinking) strategies to change the way they view the situation. If the stress is minor or brief, a child may quickly bounce back from low or blue feelings, using her own coping strategies. If the stress is prolonged or more serious in nature, the sad feelings may linger for a while, and the child may require parental or other adult intervention. Children who are truly depressed need professional guidance and treatment. In these cases, the depressed feelings may be the result of biochemical imbalances or, in the case of a child with traumatic brain injury, damage to a particular area of the brain involved in mood regulation.

If you are a parent, how do you determine if your child is sad or if she truly is depressed and in need of professional intervention? If you are concerned about your child, becoming familiar with the symptoms of depression is a good first step. Keep in mind that the symptoms of depression will vary depending on your child's age, temperament, family circumstances, and type and degree of impairment from her brain injury. Look for the following symptoms in your child if you suspect depression:

Emotions

- seems sad much of the time, with or without an obvious reason for the sadness;
- emotions change suddenly and unpredictably, is moody;
- may cry, become irritable, or lose temper easily;
- appears anxious, worried, or oversensitive and touchy;
- does not display a broad range of normal emotions, such as joy, pleasure, peacefulness;
- experiences excessive guilt, self-blame, or other signs of low self-esteem.

Thoughts

- is highly distractible;
- often has trouble concentrating;
- seems to focus on sad thoughts, memories, or worries much of the time;
- has disturbing or troubling thoughts that won't go away or that she can't ignore (called *intrusive thoughts,* because they are unwanted, yet persistent);
- may make statements such as "life is not worth living," or that suggest she is considering suicide (indicates a need for immediate professional evaluation and treatment).

Eating

- may lose appetite or refuse to eat; or
- seems to overeat to feel better or to soothe herself;
- has a significant weight loss or weight gain.

Sleeping

- doesn't want to go to bed or resists being alone at night;
- awakens more frequently during the night or unusually early in the morning without going back to sleep;

- develops nightmares, night terrors, bedwetting, or other sleep disturbances;
- seems particularly sleepy and not well-rested in the morning or at other times during the day;
- often wants to sleep during the day (in a child who had outgrown the need to nap).

Play and Recreation

- finds no happiness or satisfaction from activities that she once enjoyed;
- loses interest in activities, recreation, sports, play;
- becomes more sedentary, tends to just sit around, watching television or engaging in other solitary activities;
- seems to have no energy for play.

School

- tries to avoid attending school or completing homework;
- may develop school phobias (fear of being away from parent or home);
- loses interest in schoolwork, performance, or after-school activities;
- performance drops as child is unable to focus on learning due to fatigue, intrusive thoughts, or difficulty concentrating.

Relationships with Friends

- loses interest in friends, may avoid spending time with them;
- no longer seeks out friends or mutual activities;
- may get into petty arguments or disagreements with friends;
- becomes isolated and withdrawn.

Relationships with Family Members

- seems overly dependent on parents; or
- becomes withdrawn from and uncommunicative with parents;
- does not participate in family activities, or conversations;

- develops troubled relationships with parents, siblings, or other family members;
- spends a lot of time in her room, away from family.

Generally, parents know their child best and therefore often sense when something is wrong. When you review the list of symptoms, consider not only the number of symptoms your child has, but also the severity or persistence of those symptoms. A child may be sad, yet able to be redirected or distracted away from her sad thoughts for periods of time or still be able to enjoy a favorite activity or treat. If your child cannot do these things, her symptoms are more severe and more indicative of actual depression. Also, consider how her symptoms are affecting her functioning in these areas:

1. home and family life,
2. school grades and performance, and
3. relationships with friends and peers.

If your child's level of functioning in one or more of these areas is decreasing, her ability to cope may be failing. She will need you or another adult to intervene to help her find relief and to develop more effective coping strategies.

If you think your child may be depressed, she should be evaluated by a child psychiatrist for the need for medications known as antidepressants. These medications do not make children feel happy or mask the underlying problem. They do allow a child to focus on other thoughts and feelings besides those that are troubling, thereby increasing opportunities for enjoyment of her regular activities. Further, on medication, some children are better able to benefit from traditional "talking therapy" to learn ways of coping with the symptoms of depression.

It is important to stress that if your child indicates any thoughts of self-harm or suicide, or a lack of interest in living, you should seek professional evaluation and treatment immediately. If you think that your child is at risk of harming herself, take her to the nearest hospital emergency room and ask to have her evaluated by the psychiatrist (preferably, child psychiatrist) on call. Be sure to tell the psychiatrist about your child's traumatic brain injury and any medications she may be taking, as well as the current symptoms that have brought you for services. If your child is found to be at risk of harming herself, she will be admitted to the hospital for observation, further evaluation, and treatment, until she is no longer at risk for self-harm. In either case, a referral for ongoing treatment should be provided as a follow-up to this evaluation. Contact the psychologist, social worker, or psychiatrist associated with your child's rehabilitation center if you would like more recommendations for obtaining such services.

If your child's symptoms do not warrant professional assistance at this time, but you would like to help, here are a few ideas for promoting your child's emotional coping and improving her self-esteem:

- **Provide your child with adequate opportunities for emotional sharing and expression.** This means being available to her privately, calmly, and routinely in a non-judgmental way that invites her to discuss her feelings and concerns with you. She may choose not to share her feelings with you, but providing the opportunity to do so is still important.

- **Encourage your child to express her feelings by modeling how to do so.** When you experience sadness or disappointment, share these feelings with her as well as ways that you have learned to cope with your feelings. Be sure that you do not overwhelm or burden your child with your feelings.

- **Try using distraction and other strategies to help her to "escape" from her troubling thoughts and feelings for a while.** This may be particularly useful for children who are experiencing intrusive thoughts. Try to keep your child engaged in enjoyable, interactive, positive activities. Avoid letting her spend long hours alone or isolated in her room, if possible.

- **When planning activities for your child, focus on her strengths and abilities.** Provide her with opportunities where she can be successful. Of course, you must acknowledge her losses and difficulties, but try not to dwell on them. Instead, highlight the abilities and skills that remain after her injury and encourage her to develop interests in areas that maximize those abilities.

If these strategies do not bring about some positive change in your child's symptoms in a short time, reconsider the need for professional evaluation and treatment. Depression can be a debilitating and agonizing disorder, but treatment is available and relief can be found.

Lastly, be aware of your own feelings about your child's injury and residual impairments. The impact on your life and future may be profound, and, like many parents, you may feel overwhelmed by your new situation. Many parents report that they never had time to grieve the loss of the child they once knew before they had to begin caring for and adjusting to the new child that awoke following the injury. Eventually, the loss and grief do catch up with you and you may realize that you are experiencing many of the symptoms of depression listed above.

It is crucial for your own and your family's sake that you seek treatment for your depressive symptoms. Everyone copes with the challenge of a child with traumatic brain injury in his or her own way. If you are no longer able to manage your feelings, and especially if you feel that you may be at risk of harming yourself, immediately seek professional evaluation and treatment as described above. You also may contact one of the mental health professionals at your child's rehabilitation center, your physician, or your local mental health referral hotline to obtain advice on locating appropriate services for yourself in your area.

:: Conclusion

Learning about the profound and wide-reaching effects that traumatic brain injury can have on your child's future development and overall functioning may leave you feeling overwhelmed and without hope. Or you may be feeling that these issues have little to do with your child and that the suggested strategies are unnecessary. Possibly you are feeling a bit of relief knowing that you are not alone in facing these challenges.

Remember that no one can predict how any child's recovery from traumatic brain injury will progress. No one can tell you which of your child's deficits will be short-lived and which ones might be permanent. No one can assure you that life will eventually return to normal for you and your family, or that it won't. Certainly, you can be sure that no child has all of the problems discussed here all of the time and without any possibility for improvement. In fact, some children experience few of these problems, or experience them only for a limited period of time.

So many factors interact to determine your child's outcome and many of these are out of your control (for example, the severity and

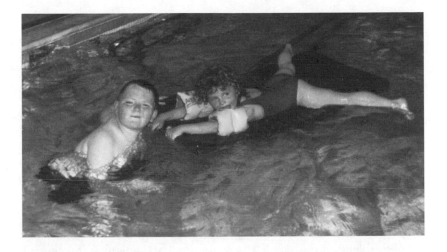

location of your child's brain injury). The goal of this chapter has been to provide you with ideas for strategies that might help your child by assisting you in changing some things that are *within* your control. As you have read, there are many ways to help your child, even when faced with serious, long-standing behavioral or emotional problems related to TBI. Furthermore, there are professionals with the experience and training to aid you in addressing your child's problems. Having to readjust your goals for your child's future, to rethink how you will parent her as she grows older, and to face the impact of this injury on each member of your family are daunting tasks. It can help to talk with others who have coped with TBI in a loved one, or to seek help from experienced and caring professionals.

You know your child, the members of your family, and yourself better than anyone else does. By honestly examining how all of you are doing now, you will know what you must do. Whether that means joining a support group, locating an experienced professional, implementing some of these strategies, or asking for help from your child's rehab team, the important thing to remember is that even if things can never return to normal, they *can* get better. You and your child deserve that opportunity.

■■ Parent Statements

I remember once our psychologist telling us, "If and when he realizes all that he has lost, he is going to be a very sad guy." Well, he is there now, and he really is sad. But he is hanging in. He is dating a girl who was head injured about ten years ago.

❦

I am having our second child in about two months. David is still so aggressive with other children. I need help controlling his hitting before this baby is born.

❦

He will suddenly burst in on me and tell me that he needs to be driven some place right away. He has no awareness that I may be in the middle of something, or that it is nearly time for dinner, or whatever. And when I tell him that he will have to wait, he goes off, calling me names, yelling, and swearing. It is so tense all of the time, just waiting for him to explode.

❦

He is so sad about the way his friends have abandoned him. I know that I need to set firm rules for him and be the parent, but it's hard.

❦

I am worried about the way she is around boys. She is overly friendly and doesn't seem to realize what they might think of her. She is so naive and vulnerable, but she won't listen to me and just gets angry if I try to talk with her about it.

❦

I just realized the other day that Bill and I never really got a chance to grieve over the loss of the child that we had known. There he was being kept alive by machines and we just had to keep our hopes up that everything would be okay. Then we had so much to learn to get ready to take him home. It still is like that; we just have to get through every day. But lately, I find myself thinking about my sweet, beautiful, little boy and realize that I will never see him again. That child is gone even though he is physically still here. I never got to bury the child who died, and I never got an opportunity to get to know the new child that occupies his body. All of a sudden one day, here he was and I was supposed to take care of him as if he had always been that way. I don't know how we did it.

❦

Things are so much better now that I know how to help him handle his frustration. I really enjoy being with him and I am so proud of the progress he has made. I remember right after his injury when we didn't know if he would live or die. And now just look at him!

❧❀❧

With special education support, she's earning A's and B's and doing great. She's developed into quite an artist as well.

The Educational Needs of Children with Traumatic Brain Injury

Joan Carney, M.A., and
Patricia Porter, M.S.

Prior to his accident, Johnny had been in a regular third grade class. Although his academic performance was average, his teacher had concerns about his distractibility. He had difficulty completing his work without a lot of reminders. In addition, Johnny had poor organizational skills and often had trouble locating assignments, homework, and school books. After the teacher raised these concerns at a parent conference, Tom and Ann Smith decided to discuss them with their pediatrician. The teacher agreed to make some adaptations to Johnny's program such as changing his seat to the front of the class and going over an assignment sheet with him each day. Thanks to these adaptations, Johnny made some improvement, but his teacher and his parents continued to have concerns.

While Johnny was an inpatient in the rehabilitation hospital, the hospital's educational specialist contacted his school. Until this point, the school staff had only heard about Johnny's head injury informally from his little brother Billy, and hadn't wanted to bother his parents at this stressful time. The educational specialist informed the school about Johnny's injury and gave them some idea of when to expect Johnny to return. She would be the contact person if the school ever wanted to check on Johnny's progress. These contacts allowed the school to anticipate when Johnny might return to school and what his needs might be at that time.

Once Johnny was medically stable enough for his family to care for him safely at home, he was discharged from the rehabilitation hospital. He still needed a great deal of rehabilitation therapy, so he began attending a day hospital rehabilitation program. Gradually, his ability to work on educational goals increased, while his need to work on rehabilitation goals decreased.

While Johnny was in the day hospital setting, the rehabilitation therapy team began collaborating with his community school. The school staff observed Johnny in the day hospital and the rehabilitation staff provided the school with inservice training regarding TBI and Johnny's particular needs.

Using information and recommendations from multidisciplinary evaluations completed by Johnny's rehabilitation therapists, the school's special education team held a meeting with Tom and Ann Smith. Here they discussed Johnny's needs and worked to plan an appropriate educational program for him. The team informed Johnny's parents that he qualified for educational services as a student with traumatic brain injury. Some of Johnny's needs identified by the team were: extra time to complete assignments; decreased written demands and/or assistance with the physical process of writing; small group instruction for reading comprehension; a structured environment to limit distractions; highly structured lessons to promote acquisition of new learning; someone to assist him with a variety of physical tasks; and physical, occupational, and speech-language therapy.

The team determined that Johnny's needs could be met through a combination of instruction in his regular third grade class and the special education classroom. His therapies would be provided within the classroom as much as possible in order to limit time away from class and to help him learn to use the skills in a natural environment.

Thanks to ongoing communication between the rehabilitation team and the school special education team, Johnny's return to school went smoothly. Like every child with a special education program, Johnny's educational program was reviewed and modified periodically. These adjustments and periodic reviews were needed more frequently during the first two years following his injury, to accommodate Johnny as his needs changed.

Ann and Tom Smith found it helpful to talk with Johnny's teachers at the beginning of each new school year to make sure they were aware of his current needs and of strategies that had been helpful in the past. This past year, prior to Johnny's transition to middle school, a full reevaluation was completed. His education team gave careful attention to planning Johnny's educational program, since the structure and demands in middle school differ drastically from those in elementary school.

∷ Introduction

Earlier chapters discussed many of the ways that a traumatic brain injury can affect a child's physiological, emotional, and cognitive functioning. Not surprisingly, many of these changes can have effects—ranging from mild to profound—on a child's ability to succeed at school.

Some problems may be obvious immediately. Others may surface later, as brain development is affected by the earlier traumatic brain injury. Even if your child has recovered medically and looks "normal," he may still have problems in learning and getting along with others that may not be apparent until he returns to school. Because we cannot see these problems, brain injury is sometimes referred to as a hidden disability.

If your child's TBI affects his academic achievement and school performance, he will be eligible for special services and/or a variety of adjustments in classroom or program requirements. Each public school in the United States has a process for providing your child with what he needs to benefit from his educational experience. This chapter, and the recommended readings, will help to acquaint you with your child's rights to an appropriate educational program and help to guide you through the process of obtaining one for your child.

∷ Why Is Special Assistance Needed?

Each child who has sustained a brain injury is unique. As discussed in previous chapters, many factors can affect your child's outcome, including: his abilities prior to the injury, the location and severity of his injury, his age at the time of injury, and the treatment that he receives after the injury.

Although each child with TBI is different, there are a number of common problems that can affect school performance. Other chapters discuss these changes in depth. Just a few will be mentioned here as examples.

Learning Differences

Generally, children do not forget the things they learned prior to sustaining a TBI. For example, a student who was reading on a third grade level prior to his brain injury may very well earn test scores at that same reading level when he returns to school. Despite this tendency to retain *over learned* (much practiced) skills such as math facts or the ability to read aloud, new learning may not continue at a normal rate. How well your child acquires new skills therefore needs to be monitored closely.

Another problem that often occurs following brain injury is that a child's rate of taking in and understanding information is slowed. This is sometimes called their information processing rate. When this happens, the student can still make progress in learning, but may need information presented in a simplified manner or may need more time to consider the information before making a response. In a traditional classroom setting without special assistance, this can be quite difficult and frustrating for the child.

Attention and concentration are other areas that are frequently affected by brain injury. Before your child returns to school, it is important to consider whether he can sustain attention as well as he could previously, or whether he is now more distractible or impulsive. Sometimes this is hard to assess in the hospital or at home before your child returns to school. Attention problems might, however, become very apparent when your child tries to return to his old school routine and has difficulty with the distractions in that environment.

Physical Differences

Sometimes physical problems resulting from TBI can also affect school functioning. Examples of motor problems that need to be addressed in school include: reduced balance and coordination, requiring a cane or a walker to walk, or reduced dexterity of one hand. These types of problems are more obvious than the learning problems and some very concrete plans can be made to assist your child in these areas. Even though they seem more obvious, it is still important to meet with the school and anticipate all

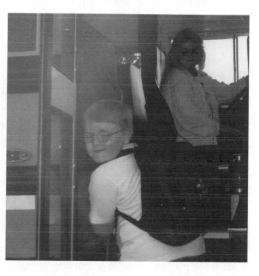

of the potential areas where your child might need assistance so that he remains safe in school and does not miss opportunities that other students are given.

Behavior Differences

Another important area to consider in planning a school program for a student with TBI is his behavior. Behaviors that a child had prior to his injury, such as calling out in class, are sometimes exacerbated or made more prominent. Other new behavior problems can emerge immediately or they might surface at a later point in the child's development.

Following brain injury, many children and adolescents develop problems controlling their impulses. A term sometimes used for this is *disinhibition*. When a child is disinhibited, he might, for example, say the first thing that comes to mind, not even realizing that he has offended someone or blurted out in class.

Disinhibited children can have trouble performing in school when they are required to make an appropriate, thoughtful response after considering several facts in a lesson. Disinhibition can also be a social problem for children. Friends often begin to make excuses not to spend time with disinhibited children, because interactions can be too uncomfortable.

If your child has any significant behavior problems, they will need to be managed at school so that your child can take advantage of all opportunities for learning and develop appropriate social relationships. See Chapters 7 and 8 for more information on disinhibition.

▪▪ Your Child's Rights to Special Educational Services

There are several federal laws that uphold your child's right to receive accommodations and/or modifications at school for any of the problems he might exhibit after brain injury. Three of the most important ones are:

1. Title V of the Rehabilitation Act of 1973 (commonly referred to as Section 504),
2. The Americans with Disabilities Act (ADA), and
3. The Individuals with Disabilities Education Act (IDEA).

These three laws work together to ensure that students with disabilities are not discriminated against, receive a free and appropriate public education, and have access to facilities. We will begin by discussing the Individuals with Disabilities Education Act, as it is the most comprehensive law relating specifically to the education of children with disabilities.

▪▪ Special Education

As it is defined in the Individuals with Disabilities Education Act (IDEA), special education means specially designed instruction, at no cost to the parents, to meet the needs of a child with a disability.

In addition to specially designed instruction, "related services" can also be provided if they are deemed educationally relevant. The term "related services" refers to transportation, therapies, and other services needed to enable a child to benefit from special education. Both this specially designed instruction and the related services will be discussed further in the pages that follow. In essence, though, special education is free, appropriate public education for all children with disabilities.

Furthermore, IDEA includes provisions to ensure the rights of students with disabilities and their parents. It does so by delineating specific requirements for local education agencies to follow in identifying, evaluating, and placing children in special education. It also includes procedures for families to follow if they have a dispute with the school about some aspect of their child's special education program.

Special education services can be provided completely within a general education class, or within very specialized school settings. Theoretically, there are an infinite number of possible variations in program design for a special education student because each child must be considered individually and have a program designed to meet his unique needs.

▪▪ Should You Consider Special Education?

Many families struggle with the decision of whether to access special education services. Soon after a child's brain injury, some families just do not realize the extent to which the injury has affected their child's school functioning. The truth may not sink in until the child meets with failure and frustration after returning to school.

Other families, or the children themselves, reject special education services because they have not accepted the fact that significant brain damage has been sustained. They still think of their child in terms of his skills and abilities before his injury. The family has probably seen ongoing recovery in many areas since the injury and they hope that all will return to normal and they can "put the incident behind them."

Still others families have had limited experience with special education services. They might think of special education only as special classes for children with mental retardation, when, in fact, a wide range of services is available.

Lastly, a common reaction from families is that they do not want the stigma or label of having a disability attached to their child.

Whatever situation you find yourself in, you undoubtedly want your child to experience success. Your child has sustained a brain injury and received specialized medical care. Now you also need to consider specialized care in the behavioral, cognitive, and/or learning areas. If your child has had a significant brain injury, he is probably eligible for special education services. As you will see when you continue your reading, you will have the right to refuse services if you do not feel they are right for your child. You will be a part of the team designing your child's school program, and this chapter will hopefully assist you in becoming an informed and active participant.

‼ Working with Your School System

If you and your child decide to investigate special education, many people will be involved in planning your child's educational program. They will come from a variety of disciplines, and have backgrounds in different areas. Along with you and your child, they will make up the *multidisciplinary team*. This team of people will be responsible for evaluating your child, reviewing evaluations, making placement decisions, planning an educational program, monitoring progress, and revising the educational plan, as needed.

Team discussions take place in scheduled meetings, which go by a variety of names depending on the terminology used in your school district. Some examples are Multidisciplinary Team Meeting (MDT), Admission, Review, and Dismissal (ARD) team meeting, Placement Advisory Committee (PAC), or School Services Team (SST) meeting. Ask your school what terminology they use to refer to their team meetings so that you will be familiar with it.

The core of most multidisciplinary teams usually consists of the following people:

- parents or guardians of the child;
- the child, when appropriate;
- school administrator (principal, assistant principal);
- school nurse;
- psychologist;
- guidance counselor;
- the child's classroom teacher;
- special education teacher;
- pupil personnel worker/social worker.

Depending on the needs of your child and the information needed by the team, other people may also be included on the multidisciplinary team. These might include any of the following:

- *speech-language pathologist*—a professional with expertise in diagnosing and treating communication difficulties, including problems with speech, language, or oral motor skills (such as chewing and swallowing)

- *physical therapist*—a professional who evaluates and treats gross motor skills needed for mobility (walking or wheelchair mobility)
- *occupational therapist*—a professional who focuses on improving skills necessary for independent functioning, such as writing, dressing, or feeding oneself
- *audiologist*—a professional who assesses and treats hearing loss
- *vision specialist*—a professional who assesses and treats visual difficulties as they affect school and educational activities
- *assistive technology specialist*—a professional with expertise in selecting, obtaining, and using technology at school
- *adaptive physical education teacher or motor teacher*—a physical education teacher with special training or knowledge in adapting activities for children with disabilities
- *transportation specialist*—a representative of the school system's transportation department with knowledge of accessibility of, and modifications to, transportation vehicles

One team member, usually an administrator or special educator, is identified as the team chairperson. This is the person who schedules the meetings, runs the meetings, and handles the paperwork. He is also the person to talk to when you want to request a team meeting.

Parents are also very important members of the multidisciplinary team. Because you are your child's first teacher and spend the most time with him, you are in a unique position to provide information and insights about your child to the other team members. You may also invite anyone else that you would like to join team meetings, such as a family member or friend, a health care professional, a rehabilitation professional, an independent evaluator, or an advocate.

You may find it helpful to keep a list of the team members involved with your child's program, along with their titles and phone numbers. See Figure 1 on the next page. In addition to this list, you should start a notebook to help you organize and keep track of the large number of papers that you will accumulate. Figure 2, on page 303, suggests organizational topics, but use any system that works for you.

▪▪ Figure 1. Parent Resource List of Multidisciplinary Team Members

POSITION	NAME	PHONE NUMBER
Team Chairperson:	_____	_____
School Administrator:	_____	_____
School Nurse:	_____	_____
Psychologist:	_____	_____
Guidance Counselor:	_____	_____
Classroom Teacher(s):	_____	_____
	_____	_____
	_____	_____
Special Education Teacher(s):	_____	_____
	_____	_____
	_____	_____
Classroom Assistant(s):	_____	_____
	_____	_____
	_____	_____
Pupil Personnel/Social Worker:	_____	_____
Speech/Language Pathologist:	_____	_____
Physical Therapist:	_____	_____
Occupational Therapist:	_____	_____
Others:	_____	_____
	_____	_____

▪▪ FIGURE 2. SECTION HEADINGS FOR ORGANIZATION OF PARENT NOTEBOOK

1. List of team members and their phone numbers
2. Telephone log
3. Copies of dated correspondence
4. I.E.P.s
5. Multidisciplinary team notes and summaries
6. School records (immunizations, standardized test results, etc.)
7. Multidisciplinary evaluation results and reports
8. Report cards and progress reports
9. Work samples
10. Teacher conference information
11. Medical information and reports
12. Procedural safeguards and special education law information
13. Miscellaneous (observations, notes)

▪▪ The Special Education Process

There are many steps involved in getting special education services for your child. After all that you have been through since your child's injury, these steps can often seem unimportant, drawn out, and ultimately frustrating. There *is* a purpose to these steps, however—to protect children's rights by preventing a rushed or premature placement in a special education setting.

Timelines and Timeliness

IDEA sets forth guidelines for the maximum amount of time that should be allowed to complete each step in the special education process. However, some states have stricter guidelines and permit less time for each step. This makes it important for you to obtain a copy of your state's timelines from your State Department of Education. As you can see from Figure 3 on page 305, the cumulative amount of time that passes, if all of the time limits are pushed to the maximum allowed by law, can be many months.

Time is especially important when your child has sustained a traumatic brain injury. It is critical that appropriate services be provided as soon as possible after your child returns to school. Schools are usually sensitive to this issue and typically do not use the maximum amount of time allowed. They will usually do their best to "speed things up" when requested to do so, and can often collapse two meetings into one in the interest of getting your child the services that he needs.

When talking to your school's team chairperson about scheduling, ask him or her if collapsing meetings and shortening the timelines would be possible so as to provide services as soon as possible. You may need to explain the importance of completing the process promptly and be persistent in asking to shorten the timelines whenever possible. However, you need to be aware that there are times when the school system's hands are tied due to issues that they may not be able to control, such as available evaluation times or a key team member's availability for a meeting.

Depending on the time of year that your child is injured, the school year calendar may also pose problems in obtaining educational services promptly. If your child's injury happens in the spring, there may not be enough time to complete the process and/or begin services for any significant period of time prior to summer break. You should be persistent in asking whether any services can be provided in the summer, such as summer school classes, home teaching, or speech-language, physical, or occupational therapy. If your child is injured during the summer months, it is often extremely difficult, and sometimes impossible, to even contact anyone within the school system who can assist you and answer your questions, much less arrange for evaluations and/or team meetings. It can be a very frustrating experience and often one that you cannot change.

Referral for Services

The first step in the process of obtaining services for your child is making a referral. This is usually accomplished fairly easily by contacting your school's multidisciplinary team chairperson or one of the school administrators. They should be informed as soon as possible that your child has sustained a traumatic brain injury and will need to be considered for appropriate services. This referral can be made by anyone involved with your child, including yourself, his classroom teacher, or his doctor. Depending on your school system, there may be

▪▪ Figure 3. Important Timelines

Stage	Time Allowed Between Stages
▪ Parent or other person requests evaluation ▪ Evaluation completed	90 calendar days
▪ Evaluation completed ▪ IEP written and approved by IEP team	30 calendar days
▪ IEP written and approved by IEP team ▪ IEP implemented	As soon as possible
▪ Annual Review	1 year
▪ Reevaluation	Every 3 years
Due Process Hearing Timelines ▪ Hearing request received by school system ▪ Hearing decision	45 calendar days
Timeline to appeal hearing decision to court:	80 calendar days

some forms that need to be completed and/or additional information needed to formalize the referral. Following the referral, a team meeting will be scheduled.

If your child is five or younger, the referral should be made to your school system's Child Find Office. If your child is aged six to twenty-one, the referral should be made to your neighborhood school. Contact information can be obtained from your local Board of Education.

Appropriate Educational Assessment

Once a referral has been made, the multidisciplinary team will hold a screening meeting to decide whether assessments are needed. Multidisciplinary assessments are needed to determine eligibility for special education services. There are two broad reasons for this. First, a student needs to be found to have one or more of the disabilities listed in IDEA in order to qualify for special education services. Second, the school system needs to determine whether or not a student's disability has an impact on his ability to learn. Information from assessments is also used in planning each student's individualized education program (see below).

Specific requirements vary from state to state and among local jurisdictions as to what type of assessments are required to document which disabilities. In some areas, only medical documentation and an educational evaluation are needed to determine that a child has a traumatic brain injury that qualifies him for special education services. Your state Department of Education will be able to provide you with the specifics for your area.

In general, information for your child's assessment may be gathered through standardized, printed tests, through observations, and from parents and other sources. The formal tests should be individually administered standardized tests. The assessment materials should be designed to identify specific areas of educational need, rather than just a single general intelligence quotient. If your child has impaired sensory, manual, or communication skills, the academic assessments used should accurately reflect his abilities and achievement levels, rather than his impairments. That is, tests may need to be adapted so that your child can show what he knows without being penalized for difficulty with speech or motor skills.

It is important that a multidisciplinary approach be used in evaluating your child, because each professional brings his or her own perspective to each child. For example, the psychologist may find that your child has difficulty with copying shapes, a problem that may be further explained by a fine motor problem identified by the occupational therapist.

At the end of your child's assessment, the team will decide:
1. whether your child fits the definition of a child with traumatic brain injury that appears in IDEA;
2. whether he has a disability other than, or in addition to, traumatic brain injury;
3. whether your child's disability, if any, has an educational impact on him.

If the answer to question 3 is "yes," he will be eligible to receive special education services.

Traumatic Brain Injury as a Designated Disability Category

Traumatic brain injury was not originally included in IDEA as a disability providing eligibility for special services. In 1990, however,

TBI was added to the list of conditions qualifying children and adolescents for special education. (See Figure 4.) This is how IDEA defines traumatic brain injury:

> *Traumatic brain injury is an injury to the brain caused by an external force, resulting in total or partial functional disability or psychosocial impairment or both, that adversely affects the child's educational performance. The term applies to open or closed head injuries resulting in impairments in one or more areas, such as: cognition, language, memory, attention, reasoning, abstract thinking, judgment, problem solving, sensory, perceptual and motor abilities, psycho social behavior, physical functions, information processing, and speech. The term does not apply to brain injuries that are congenital or degenerative, or brain injuries induced by birth trauma. [IDEA; Section 3.0.5 (b) (12).]*

As you can see, the current definition includes only brain injury acquired as the result of external trauma. Thus, children who acquire brain injury through an internal occurrence such as stroke, aneurysm, infection, or disease are sometimes not considered eligible under the current IDEA definition of TBI.

Even so, the implications of this eligibility category for students with brain injury are important. Previously, students with brain injury who were found eligible for special education services were classified inappropriately in such categories as "learning disability," "mental retardation," "serious emotional disturbance," or "other health impaired." Although students received services under these labels, classroom placement, related services, and supports were often inappropriate.

Now that there is a specific category for traumatic brain injury, placement decisions and services will hopefully evolve to meet the unique and complex needs of students with this disability. To date, several states have issued guidelines to schools on providing appropriate services to students with TBI. You should contact your State Department of Education to ask if written guidelines are available and whether they have been provided to your child's school.

Traumatic Brain Injury Compared to Other Disabilities

An important difference between traumatic brain injury and other disabilities is the age that the disability begins. When TBI occurs, it interrupts development, whereas many other disabilities listed in IDEA are believed to be present at birth, even if they are not diagnosed until later.

Although TBI can cause problems that resemble some of the other disabilities defined in IDEA, it is important to understand how TBI differs. This is because the approaches that are effective in helping children with these other disabilities in the classroom are not always the most effective ones for children with TBI.

Learning Disability. Some students with traumatic brain injury benefit from teaching methods, strategies, and accommodations used with students with a learning disability (LD). Yet children with TBI are fundamentally different from children with LD, depending on their age when injured.

By definition, students with learning disabilities have a discrepancy between their intellectual ability (usually measured by a test that gives an intelligence quotient, IQ) and their academic achievement. That is, they have an average or above average IQ, but their academic achievement is significantly below average in one or more areas.

A student with TBI usually has just the opposite profile of a student with LD, if he was old enough to have acquired some academics prior to his injury. When evaluated following their injury, students with TBI often show average academic achievement on standardized tests. This situation can probably be attributed to two factors:

1. They have learned academics through such a repetitive process that they can do skills such as reading words or solving math problems without much thought, even though the brain was injured.

2. The standardized tests used to measure academic achievement optimize the performance of students with TBI because they are so highly structured and paced. This structure and pacing accommodates for distractibility, impulsivity, and reduced rate of processing—which are common problems after brain injury.

In contrast, a child's IQ scores following a significant TBI are usually lower than before the injury. This is because many of the subtests in an IQ test involve timed responses and reacting to novel material or situations. Unlike achievement tests for reading or mathematics, they do not just evaluate what a child has previously learned.

The true test of academic performance for your child with TBI will be whether his new learning will proceed at a normal rate.

Mental Retardation. Some children who have sustained a severe TBI might have very poor thinking and learning abilities. Before the addition of TBI as a disability code, they might have been designated as having mental retardation. Children with mental retardation have both intellectual and functional skills well below average. A major difference, however, is that mental retardation is present at birth, and TBI is not.

Sometimes a student with TBI whose cognitive skills are significantly affected might be grouped with students with mental retardation because they have similar educational goals. However, it is important to remember what skills the child with TBI had attained prior to his injury. Some of his previously known skills may recover to a useful level, even if he does not fully regain his earlier skills. The student with TBI might also remember what he was like before the injury. In this case, it would be very important to ensure that educational materials and activities are age appropriate so they are not rejected as being too babyish.

Emotional Disturbance. Before IDEA included TBI as a disability, students with TBI who had severe behavior problems affecting their education were often classified as seriously emotionally disturbed (SED). This category is now called emotionally disturbed (ED). Unfortunately, this practice continues in some areas today, due to lack of awareness.

The programs designed for ED students generally include increased psychological support and psychotherapy. Students with TBI who have significant behavioral problems, however, usually have different needs. Their behaviors are more frequently a result of poor impulse control and are better managed with behavioral management strategies, structuring the environment and student's routine, and providing external cueing to control the behaviors. Because of this difference, students with TBI are usually not best served in programs designed for students with ED. It is true, however, that it is probably the most difficult to develop educational programs for students with TBI who have developed severe behavioral problems.

Other Health Impaired. Finally, the category called "other health impaired" (OHI) has often been used to grant eligibility for services for students with TBI. The OHI definition describes a student with a chronic or acute condition that causes reduced vitality, strength, or alertness that affects his educational performance. This category has become a sort of "catch all" category for many disabilities that may be too uncommon to warrant a definition of their own.

The OHI category is still frequently used because of the constraints of the TBI definition mentioned earlier. Because the definition only includes children who have had traumatic brain injury from an external force, children with brain tumors, strokes, encephalitis, meningitis, and other diseases are technically excluded. Children with these types of brain injuries are still usually designated as "other health impaired." The OHI definition does qualify students for special education services, yet few school systems actually have educational programs dedicated to children with health impairments. Typically, students with health impairments are educated in programs among children with various disabilities or are included in regular classrooms.

Public vs. Private Assessments

Most children being considered for special education have a series of multidisciplinary evaluations completed by the school system at no cost to the family. You should know that your child also has the right to have evaluations done by an independent party, in place of, or in addition to, the school assessments. An independent educational evaluation is testing that is done by qualified professionals who are not employed by your child's school system.

You always have the right to obtain an independent educational evaluation from qualified professionals of your choice, at your own expense. The team must consider the information from independent evaluations when making any decisions about your child's program. You may also request that the school system pay for an independent evaluation for your child if you feel the evaluation requires expertise not available from your school system. Any independent evaluation that is paid for by the school system must meet their criteria for testing as stated in their assessment procedures. Sometimes a school system may balk at paying for an independent evaluation on the grounds that their evaluation was appropriate. If so, parents have the right to take the school to due process (see below) to try to force the school to pay for an independent evaluation.

Because TBI is relatively rare, it is highly recommended that you obtain a private evaluation done by rehabilitation professionals specializing in pediatric brain injury. The standard battery schools use to look for learning disabilities and mental retardation will not assess many of the areas that need to be investigated following traumatic brain injury. Some examples are memory, planning, organization, new learning, and judgment. Further, a regional specialty facility that provides rehabilitation for children and adolescents with TBI will have more experience with TBI than any one school or school system.

To avoid duplication of testing, it is important that the school and the rehabilitation professionals coordinate their services during this phase of eligibility. Your family should release hospital records to the school and provide a release of information for the rehabilitation center and the school to share information freely.

Generally, schools are happy to accept evaluations from private facilities if they are not required to pay for them. They may, however, still require that the school personnel observe your child and review the evaluation reports. This is to ensure that the reports are acceptable to the standards of the local jurisdiction and that they have no reason to believe that they are not valid.

One caveat about private assessments: The professionals who conduct a private assessment will be looking at *all* your child's areas of needs—not just his educational needs. They will make recommendations for therapies and services that could benefit your child at home and in the community, as well as at school. The school, however, will interpret the private evaluation only in light of educational need. This is because the school system is only required to provide services and accommodations needed to help a child succeed at school. Schools do not have to provide services to improve skills that are not needed to participate in the classroom. For example, a rehabilitation physical therapist may recommend ongoing physical therapy to maintain your child's strength and flexibility. The school team, however, may not believe your child needs this therapy to participate in school activities. In cases like this, you should seek to have private therapy paid through your medical insurance.

You can ask your school system for information about where an independent evaluation may be obtained.

Interpreting Your Child's Assessment

As mentioned above, it is important for the professionals assessing your child to evaluate the specific areas we know are often affected following TBI. There are also some specific things to consider when interpreting the scores yielded by the testing.

Comparing Your Child's Current Abilities with Previous Abilities. Standardized assessment scores compare your child to a "normative group." This means that when developing the test, the authors administered it to large numbers of children across the country to find out the average performance on those test questions. Normative comparisons are somewhat helpful for your child. However, a more useful comparison is to your child's own performance prior to his injury.

Consider the example of a student who was doing well in advanced placement classes or a program for the gifted and talented before he sustained a severe TBI. Following the TBI, this student may test in the average range when compared to normative scores. Yet, compared to how this student performed prior to his injury, he has lost cognitive/academic skills, and his injury has therefore had educational impact. This student is likely to need special education assistance to learn new study skills and strategies, so that he can acquire new learning. For a student who has always found it easy to learn, it is very frustrating to now have to devote a different degree and type of mental effort to learn new things. He needs to be formally taught these skills.

What the Scores Really Mean. When considering the scores yielded by academic achievement tests, we need to realize that these scores reflect the reading, math, or spelling level that your child currently possesses. If these scores are average, they do not necessarily mean that your child will go on to acquire new learning at an average rate. His progress needs to be monitored closely for the weeks, months, and years to come.

Also remember that standardized tests provide only a sampling of a student's academic skills. When your child actually has to, for example, read a chapter and answer comprehension questions in class, any number of other factors that were not present during the testing situation could interfere. Examples of these might be: 1) the chapter is so long that memory problems interfere; 2) the classroom environment is distracting; or 3) your child takes so long to process the information that he cannot complete the assignment in a reasonable period of time.

Impairments That Can Affect Test Performance. How your child's TBI affects all areas of functioning needs to be considered when interpreting assessment results. If the TBI has affected his attention, communication skills, and/or motor skills, for instance, this may affect his test performance and interpretation of results. For example, lack of motor coordination may result in trouble with tests that require constructional skills such as manipulating blocks or drawing. Poor speech might make it difficult to interpret your child's verbal responses. Visual impairment might make it harder for your child to use some testing formats. Any of these problems might be a reason to invalidate test scores. Still, the information obtained from presenting the tasks, even if modified, can be important in discovering your child's learning profile.

▪▪ Developing an Individualized Education Program (IEP)

Once the multidisciplinary team has determined that your child should receive special education or related services, the next step is to plan an educational program. The federal law (IDEA) stipulates that each child with a disability should have an Individualized Education Program, or IEP, designed especially to meet his unique needs. The IEP is a written plan or document that contains several components. If your child is under the age of three, the document is called an Individualized Family Service Plan (IFSP).

Designated Disability

In addition to containing standard identifying information such as name and birthdate, your child's IEP will list his designated disability. As discussed above, this will usually be "traumatic brain injury," indicated by the designated disability code of "13" on his IEP. However, depending on the specific effects of your child's injury, the multidisciplinary team may determine that he is "multihandicapped" (designated disability code "10"), since he may have multiple disabilities that will affect his education. For example, he might have traumatic brain injury and orthopedic impairment or visual impairment. And, as explained above, if your child's brain injury is due to an internal factor such as brain tumor or stroke, he will probably be identified as "other health impaired" (designated disability code of "08"). This is because it is expected that a variety of health-related issues, and not just the injury to the brain, will have a more long-term and global effect on his education. A complete listing of the designated disability codes is shown in Figure 4 on the next page.

The primary purpose of listing a designated disability on your child's IEP is to provide the federal government with a count of students with specific types of disabilities. It is also important information, however, for your child's teacher and all staff that work directly with him. If your child is identified as "multihandicapped,"

:: Figure 4. Designated Disability Codes

01   Mentally Retarded (Intellectually Limited)

02   Hard-of-Hearing

03   Deaf

04   Speech and Language Impaired

05   Visually Handicapped

06   Emotionally Disturbed

07   Orthopedically Impaired

08   Other Health Impaired

09   Specific Learning Disability

10   Multi-handicapped

11   Child in Need of Assessment

12   Deaf/Blind

13   Traumatic Brain Injury

14   Autism

ask the team to list all of the disability conditions on his IEP, so that anyone working with him and using his IEP will be able to easily identify that he has sustained a traumatic brain injury. As a rule, the decision to identify your child as having a traumatic brain injury vs. having multiple disabilities will not affect his overall educational program or placement.

Unlike with other disabilities, such as "learning disability," your child does not need to obtain certain test scores to be identified as having a "traumatic brain injury." Instead, identification of a student with TBI as an educational disability requires evidence of the injury's educational impact and medical documentation of the injury. A sample doctor's letter is shown in Figure 5.

Present Levels of Educational Performance

Your child's IEP will also contain a section that lists his present levels of educational performance. Most of this information will come from the results of his evaluations, with observations from team members that are more objective (e.g., sat still during tasks) added during the team discussion. The statement of present levels of educational performance should include a statement of how your child's disability affects his involvement in the general curriculum.

The present levels of educational performance provide a broad framework for developing a more specific educational plan for your child. Identifying your child's areas of strength is just as important as identifying his needs. Many parents indicate that they often feel that the discussions at multidisciplinary team meetings focus only on their child's difficulties. Discussing your child's strengths and reviewing them during the team meeting allows all team members to see that your child has a lot of positive qualities and skills. It is also helpful to your child's teacher, because she should use some of your child's strong areas or skills to help him compensate for his weaker areas.

Goals and Benchmarks

The largest portion of your child's IEP is usually the section containing the goals and benchmarks of his educational program. These will provide the framework for his daily instruction.

The goals are very general and broad in scope. They are a statement of the skills or abilities that your child is expected to achieve

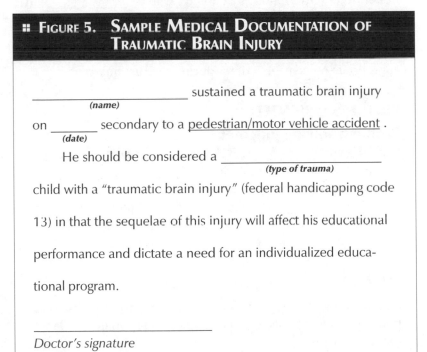

▪▪ FIGURE 5. **SAMPLE MEDICAL DOCUMENTATION OF TRAUMATIC BRAIN INJURY**

_____ sustained a traumatic brain injury
(name)

on _____ secondary to a pedestrian/motor vehicle accident .
(date)

He should be considered a _____
(type of trauma)

child with a "traumatic brain injury" (federal handicapping code

13) in that the sequelae of this injury will affect his educational

performance and dictate a need for an individualized educa-

tional program.

_____

Doctor's signature

over time. They are often referred to as long-term goals because they will most likely be appropriate for your child for a long period of time (i.e., one or two years or more).

Benchmarks—or short-term benchmarks—are more specific and intended to span a much shorter period of time, such as two months or a semester. The benchmarks are short-term objectives that your child needs to meet en route to achieving his long-term goals.

Some examples of long-term goals and benchmarks are presented in Figure 6.

■■ FIGURE 6. SAMPLE IEP GOALS AND BENCHMARKS FOR STUDENTS WITH TBI

CONTENT ORIENTED

Reading

annual goal: Given paragraph length passages, _____ will improve reading comprehension to the third grade level.

benchmark: Given multiple choice responses, _____ will identify the main idea of the passage 80% of the time over a two-week period.

benchmark: Having read a passage, _____ will predict an appropriate outcome 4/5 times during the first quarter.

PROCESS ORIENTED

Problem solving/judgment

annual goal: _____ will increase accuracy in evaluating a situation and choosing a solution.

benchmark: When shown pictures of safe and unsafe traffic conditions, _____ will choose a safe solution 75% of the time.

benchmark: When presented with a role play of a social dilemma, _____ will generate three possible solutions.

MEMORY

annual goal: _____ will increase ability to recall information over a short period of time to levels appropriate for classroom instruction.

Goals and benchmarks should be written in all areas of need that have been identified through your child's evaluations and discussion within the team meeting. This may include content-oriented goals from some or all of his academic areas, as well as process-oriented goals in areas such as memory, attention, visual processing, or auditory processing. It is important to remember that your child may not always have trouble with the content of the instruction, but rather with the learning process itself. This makes process-oriented goals a critical part of your child's IEP. In addition to these areas, goals and benchmarks may also

benchmark: _____ will restate oral directions upon request with 100% accuracy.

benchmark: _____ will recall four facts from a story read the previous day with 75% accuracy.

BEHAVIORALLY ORIENTED

annual goal: _____ will decrease incidents of classroom disruption.

benchmark: When presented with a choice of demands or expectations, _____ will choose and carry out one of them without verbal objections 50% of the time.

benchmark: _____ will ask permission before speaking out in class 75% of the time.

annual goal: _____ will decrease incidents of physical aggression.

benchmark: When agitated by physical assistance of caregivers, _____ will refrain from kicking for 80% of the episodes.

benchmark: When annoyed by a peer interaction, _____ will physically turn away from the situation 75% of the time without touching the peer.

need to be included on your child's IEP in the area of behavior. The need for behavioral goals and benchmarks may have been identified by you or hospital personnel or through observations made by school personnel during his evaluations.

You are an important member of the team and should be included in writing goals and benchmarks for your child's IEP. Although other team members often have prepared goals and benchmarks prior to the IEP meeting, they should be presented to you as a draft, not a final document. You should feel free to ask questions, make suggestions or changes, and offer any additional goals and benchmarks that you feel are appropriate for your child.

If your child is less than three years old, his IFSP will contain goals and benchmarks that address the needs of your family, as well as your child. For example, a family goal might be for the parents to learn to safely bathe their child.

Related Services

As defined in IDEA, related services consist of "developmental, corrective and other supportive services . . . as may be required to assist a child with disabilities to benefit from special education" (20 U.S.C. Chapter 33, Section 1401(17), 1991). These services may include any of the following:

- physical therapy
- occupational therapy
- speech/language therapy
- audiology
- psychological services
- school health services
- counseling services
- transportation services
- social work services
- medical services for diagnostic or evaluation purposes only
- parent counseling and training
- recreation therapy
- early identification and assessment of disabilities in children
- orientation and mobility

The federal regulations do not include an exhaustive list of related services. Some school systems have included other services that are not specifically mandated in the federal regulations, such as dance therapy or aquatic therapy.

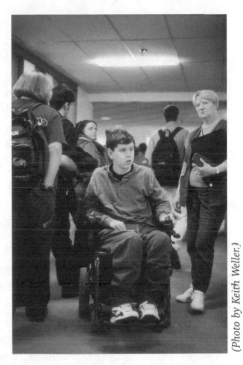

(Photo by Keith Weller.)

Keep in mind that a related service is any service that your child needs in order to benefit from his *educational* program, by helping him meet the goals and benchmarks on his IEP. It is important to note that school systems are only required to provide the amount of therapy that is needed for your child to participate successfully in his educational program. In the months immediately following your child's traumatic brain injury, he may require not only educationally based therapy in school, but additional medical therapy outside of school in order to facilitate his ongoing recovery.

If your child has been receiving intensive rehabilitation services since his injury, it may be difficult to understand and accept that he will not receive the same intensity of therapy at school. Once their child returns to school, many parents expect that all of his therapy needs will be met by the school and want the same intensity of therapy to continue. In reality, most children with TBI who return to school receive a combination of educationally based therapy at school and outpatient medical therapy that is paid for by their insurance providers. As time progresses, the amount of outpatient therapy, and sometimes educationally based therapy, usually decreases as your child's needs change.

The amount of time that your child is to receive each related service will be listed on his IEP (as hours per week). Sometimes a related service is provided at a "consult" level. This happens if your child does not need to work directly with a therapist (e.g., speech-language pathologist), but that therapist will work with his teachers as a consultant (e.g., regarding communication options within the classroom). Goals and benchmarks should be written for each related service listed on your child's IEP, with the possible exception of transportation.

Many times therapies are provided outside of the classroom using a "pull-out" model. This often results in a lot of time missed in the classroom, which may be difficult for a child with TBI to make up. Whenever possible, suggest that your child's therapy be provided within the classroom as part of his total educational program. Be aware, however, that one-on-one therapy is best for working on certain skills, such as walking or managing clothing after toileting.

Plan for Review of the IEP

Once an IEP has been developed and approved by your team, IDEA requires that the team monitor your child's progress to make sure the IEP truly is appropriate for him. There is a schedule of reviews that is outlined in the federal regulations. If your child was not receiving special education services before his injury, the law states that his IEP and educational program should be reviewed after 60 school days, since the services and program are new for your child. Once that review takes place, the next review is not legally mandated to occur until one year from the date of the IEP.

This review schedule is not usually appropriate for children with recent traumatic brain injuries. Children recovering from TBI can have frequent changes in functioning for at least one year following the injury. Consequently, it will be necessary to review your child's IEP and educational program more frequently than IDEA requires. Ideally, for the first year following his injury, your child's reviews should take place approximately every two to three months in order to determine whether his IEP, educational program, and related services continue to be appropriate to meet his needs. This review schedule should be discussed with the team before your child begins receiving special education services. It is important to know that you may request a team meeting to review your child's IEP and educational program at any time by contacting the team chairperson.

Program Accommodations and Modifications

The typical educational program at your child's school may need to be changed in various ways for your child to participate.

Changes that do not alter the content, expectations of the student, or level of the material are technically known as *accommoda-*

tions. For example, changes may be made in how your child communicates information—say, by giving oral, rather than written responses to a test. Or your child might be seated in a place where distractions are kept to a minimum.

Changes that alter what a student is expected to learn or demonstrate are known as *modifications.* An example might be requiring your child to learn ten of the weekly spelling words instead of twenty.

Many school systems write accommodations and modifications on the IEP, while others have a list on which they check the appropriate ones for your child. If other changes need to be made, they should be added to the checklist. These accommodations and modifications may be needed in many different areas depending on your child's needs. (Children with TBI can often receive accommodations even if they do not qualify for special education under IDEA. See "Educational Assistance for Students Who Are Not Eligible for IDEA," on page 342.)

Some common areas of accommodation for children with TBI are discussed below, with specific examples of accommodations given in Figure 7 on the next page.

Educational Accommodations and Modifications. In addition to having individualized goals and benchmarks on his IEP, your child may need some other changes in his educational program. One typical area for educational accommodations and modifications is testing. Examples include:

- increased or no time limits;
- having tests read to your child;
- multiple choice formats;
- dictating responses to the teacher.

Your child may also need to have the amount of classwork or homework decreased due to slowed processing, written language difficulties, or fatigue issues.

Physical Accommodations and Modifications. As a result of his TBI, your child may need some physical changes to his educational program. For example, he may become easily fatigued and may need a scheduled rest period.

If your child returns to school in a wheelchair, there are many physical accommodations that need to be made. He will require a handicapped accessible school building, inside and out. This will include:

- ramps into the building;

:: Figure 7. Samples of Program Accommodations & Modifications for Students with TBI

Educational
- peer notetaker
- taped lectures
- study guides
- structured outline provided by teacher
- extra set of books for home
- extra time to complete assignments
- decreased work load
- decreased written work requirements
- texts with key information highlighted
- homework assignment sheet

Testing
- increased time or untimed testing
- items read to student
- oral response allowed
- multiple choice format
- individually administered
- use of external prompts (e.g., charts, calculator)
- tests administered in shorter sessions over multiple days

Physical
- locker with a key, not a combination
- rest time provided
- preferential seating
- permission to move around the room as needed
- early dismissal to allow time to change classes
- extra set of books (one in classroom, one at home)
- peer buddy for assistance with materials

Accessible environment
- ramps
- elevator
- modified bathrooms
- door width

- evacuation plan
- furniture high enough to accommodate a wheelchair
- accessible general areas (e.g., gym, library, cafeteria, health room)
- water fountain
- public phone
- locker location

Emotional/Behavioral

- structured environment
- daily or weekly communication with the family (e.g., by phone, or traveling notebook)
- regular sessions with guidance counselor or school psychologist
- behavior management program (see Chapters 7 and 8)
- student contract for behavior
- permanent pass to guidance office or crisis intervention teacher
- teacher provides cues to redirect student before emotions get out of control (e.g., teacher walks by and touches corner of student's desk)
- student has a prearranged signal to indicate when emotional support is needed (e.g., student puts eraser on corner of desk)

Nonacademic

- peer buddy for getting around the building on time
- morning check-in period with teacher to review schedule, assignments, and preparedness
- end of day check-in period to review homework assignments and preparedness
- daily/weekly calendar
- materials checklist
- increased supervision
- provide necessary support for participation in appropriate extracurricular activities (e.g., holding activities in an accessible part of the building)

- an elevator (which your child should have free access to) in a multilevel building;
- doorways wide enough to accommodate his wheelchair;
- accessible bathrooms;
- a special fire plan to allow for immediate evacuation from upper levels of the building;
- accessible general areas (gym, cafeteria, auditorium); and
- classroom furniture high enough to accommodate his wheelchair.

It might also be advisable for the school to provide an extra set of textbooks so that your child does not have to transport them to and from school every day. A peer may need to be assigned to your child to help him with his books and other materials during the school day. The necessary physical accommodations should be written on your child's IEP so that there are no misunderstandings as to what is required for your child. If they are not written on the IEP, it can be more difficult to hold the school accountable if problems arise.

Emotional Accommodations and Modifications. Depending on the effects of your child's traumatic brain injury, he may need to have some accommodations or modifications included on his IEP to help him deal with new emotions and difficult situations. These may include:

- a permanent pass to the guidance office or crisis intervention teacher;
- a private signal between herself and the teacher to indicate that he is having trouble controlling himself;
- a regular weekly session scheduled with the school's guidance counselor or psychologist; or
- a structured behavior management program with a student contract, when appropriate.

Again, these should be specifically written into your child's IEP.

Nonacademic Considerations. There are many parts to the school day that may seem insignificant to most people, but may be a big challenge to a child with a traumatic brain injury. These should be addressed as carefully as the rest of his educational program. Some of the issues that should be considered are times when your child is in transition (e.g., changing classes, traveling to and from the bus) and times when the students are typically unsupervised (e.g., in the cafeteria, bathroom, or locker room, or on the bus). Your child may require additional structure, supervision, or assistance during these times.

Your child may have difficulty managing his locker due to memory or fine motor difficulties or trouble getting around the school because of orientation problems. It is not unusual for a child with TBI to show signs of distractibility or impulsivity following his injury. This affects his work within the classroom, as well as his behavior and ability to function appropriately throughout the school day. Acting impulsively without first thinking through the consequences may cause unsafe behavior, as well as social difficulties, which can lead to poor peer relations and low self esteem. It is very important that accommodations to address these nonacademic concerns be spelled out clearly on your child's IEP.

Signing the Individualized Education Program

At the end of the team meeting, you will be asked to sign your child's IEP. Before you do this, you need to ask what your signature means. In some school systems, signing the IEP means merely that you attended the meeting. In these school systems, another document needs to be signed to indicate your approval of the IEP. In other school systems, signing the IEP means that you agree with everything that is in it—the placement, the present levels of educational performance, the type and amount of related services, the goals and benchmarks in each area, and the accommodations and modifications.

If you are comfortable that the IEP shows a clear picture of your child and his needs, you should sign the IEP (or the document that your school system uses to signify parental approval). However, you should not feel pressured to sign the IEP right then and there. If you are uncertain, ask to take a copy of the IEP home and look it over for a few days. Tell the team when you will give them a decision about signing the IEP. If there are parts that you do not agree with, point them out to the team and discuss them further. If you still do not agree to certain parts after the discussion is over, you may choose to not sign the IEP. If you sign the IEP and then decide that you do not agree with it, you may revoke, or take back, your consent.

If your child has been newly identified as having a disability and this is his first IEP, no services will be provided for him until you sign it. You or the school system may request a hearing to work out any disagreements about the placement or IEP (see the section on "Procedural

Safeguards" for additional information about this). Until that happens, your child will not receive any special education or related services.

Another choice is to sign the IEP, but indicate in writing which sections you do not agree with and request a hearing to discuss your concerns. If you do this, your child will begin to receive special education and related services, but you will still be able to try to resolve the disagreements between yourself and the school system. If this is not your child's first IEP and you do not sign it, the school system can go ahead and implement it after giving you notice. You may still request a hearing to discuss your concerns and try to resolve your disagreement.

Extended School Year Services

Extended School Year services, or ESY, are an extension of special education and/or related services beyond the regular school year and are usually provided in the summer. These services may be considered part of a "free and appropriate public education," or FAPE, for eligible special education students. They are not automatic for every child receiving special education services and are not an enrichment program.

Your child is considered eligible for ESY services if it is likely that he will regress significantly in one or more "critical life skills" as a result of an extended school break, and not be able to recover those losses in a reasonable amount of time. A "critical life skill" is any skill on your child's IEP that the multidisciplinary team decides is critical to his overall educational progress. The team must discuss whether your child qualifies for ESY services every year. This usually takes place during the spring, which may also be the same time that your child's IEP and educational program are reviewed for the year.

In deciding if your child is eligible for ESY services, the team will look at different eligibility criteria. These usually include regression/recovery, degree of progress toward mastery of IEP goals, emerging skills/breakthrough opportunities, interfering behaviors, nature and/or severity of the disability, and special circumstances. The exact eligibility criteria may vary from school system to school system. If the team determines that any of these would prevent your child from benefiting from his educational program during the regular school year, then ESY services should be provided.

If the team decides that your child is eligible for ESY services, an ESY Individualized Education Plan (IEP) will be developed. It will contain:

- specific goals and benchmarks for ESY;
- the type, amount, and duration of the special education and/or related services, including transportation, that are needed to meet the IEP goals;
- the least restrictive environment in which the services can be provided;
- and the amount of time that your child will be with his nondisabled peers.

As a member of the team, it is important for you to express your opinions about the appropriateness of ESY services for your child. If you disagree with the final decision of the team, you can request a due process hearing to review that decision.

Placement Options

Every child with TBI has a different combination of needs when returning to school, as shown by the need for an *individualized* education plan. Few school systems have programs designed especially to meet the needs of children with traumatic brain injuries, and there are not many teachers who have experience with children with traumatic brain injuries or are familiar with the resulting difficulties. This may make finding an appropriate placement for your child a challenge. Children with traumatic brain injuries have received services in a wide range of placements. Options include:

- a regular classroom in which a special educator consults with the regular classroom teacher but does not work directly with your child;
- a regular classroom in which a special education teacher team teaches or co-teaches with the regular classroom teacher;
- a regular classroom with special education resource support in some areas (your child sometimes leaves the classroom to work in a smaller group with the special education teacher);
- a combination of a special education classroom in a regular school for some subjects and "inclusion" in regular classrooms for other academic subject areas or special area classes (art, gym, music);
- a special education classroom for the entire day in a regular school;

- a special education classroom for the entire day in a special education wing or school;
- a private special education day school;
- a residential special education school;
- homebound instruction.

Where your child is placed will depend on what the IEP team decides is the *least restrictive environment* for him. (See below.)

Least Restrictive Environment

IDEA clearly states that children with disabilities should receive their special education and related services in the *"least restrictive environment" (LRE)* possible. This means that your child should be placed in a program that will provide as much interaction as possible with his nondisabled peers, and still meet his needs. Before IDEA became a law, most children with disabilities were placed in separate special education schools, where their opportunities to interact with their nondisabled peers were nonexistent. We now know that both disabled and nondisabled children benefit from interactions with each other. Based on your child's needs, the team should discuss a variety of placements, beginning with the least restrictive and moving to more restrictive ones, as appropriate. (See the list of options above.)

While this approach is designed to protect children from being unnecessarily separated from their nondisabled peers, it is not always in the best interest of children with TBI. Brain injury is often considered a "hidden disability" because so many of the survivors look, and sometimes act, unchanged. Unless your child is returning to school in a wheelchair or with other obvious physical, motor, speech, or behavior difficulties, it is easy for the school to think that he has returned to "normal." Even if evaluation results indicate a variety of problems, the school system may think that your child "looks good" and place him in a program that does not provide enough support to meet his needs. This can quickly lead to frustration, low self-esteem, school difficulties, and increased behavior problems.

Even though your child will continue to recover and have fewer needs after he returns to school, it is better for him to initially receive services in a more intensive, or restrictive, environment than might first appear to be appropriate. This will provide him with a strong support system and will help smooth the transition back into a school setting. After your child has returned to school and is experiencing success, these intensive supports can be gradually taken away, resulting in a less restrictive environment. It is better to allow your child to succeed with additional help, than to wait to provide that help after he has failed. By then, it may be too late.

Scheduling Considerations

For a variety of reasons, the team may need to consider some changes in your child's schedule when he returns to school. It is common for a child with TBI to continue to fatigue even after he leaves the hospital and is ready to return to school. He may be able to attend school for only part of the day because of his fatigue. Which part of the day is best will depend on when your child is fresher and more alert.

Attending Part Time vs. Full Time. If your child attends school for part of the day, the team should consider whether he should also receive home teaching services provided by the school system for a few afternoons or evenings a week. This might allow your child to keep up with his schoolwork, as well as give him time to rest at home when he needs it the most. It may be that your child may be able to attend school for a full day if a rest period is provided at some point. The specific timing of this period and a location (usually the nurse's office) for resting can be worked out with your child's school.

Your child may not be ready to return to school for academics, but may be ready to interact with his peers and reestablish his social relationships. In this case, he may be able to attend school only during the times when the class has activities such as gym, music, and art or during lunchtime.

Home Teaching Services. Depending on his stamina and endurance, your child may need to begin with home teaching services before he is ready to return to a school setting. It is important to find out your school system's guidelines related to home teaching services. Your child will usually need to be out of school a minimum number of weeks in order to receive home teaching services. Your school principal should be able to provide you with this information or direct you to the head of the home teaching services for your school system.

Home teaching services can be very beneficial for a child with TBI because the scheduling is usually very flexible and is arranged at times that are convenient for both you and the teacher. Often you can arrange for the teacher to come when your child is best able to benefit

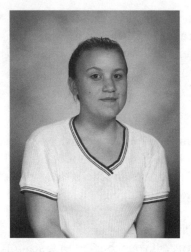

from the instruction. However, the maximum number of hours that can be provided each week is usually not enough to keep your child "caught up" with his class.

If your child has health problems related to his TBI that may keep him out of school for one or more days at a time throughout the school year, a plan should be made with your school system for him to receive home teaching services on those days. This will help him keep up with his schoolwork in spite of periodic, unavoidable absences. Many school systems already have a program like this in place and may refer to it as something similar to "CHIP," which stands for "chronic health impaired program."

Scheduling Adjustments at School. While your child is in school, he may need some additional scheduling adjustments to help him succeed. He may need to have a "check-in" with the special education teacher, assistant, or other personnel in order to be sure that he has his previous night's homework, his textbooks and supplies, and knows his schedule for the day. It may also be helpful to have a "check-out" with the same person to be certain that he has written down and understands his homework assignments and has the necessary books and supplies. In addition, your child may need a supervised study hall period to give him time to complete classwork and homework assignments.

If your child is having balance or distractibility problems or is showing poor judgment or safety awareness, moving through the crowded halls of a school will be a concern. He should be allowed to leave his classes a few minutes early so that he can move to his next location when the halls are not as crowded as during normal transition times. It may also be helpful to have a peer "buddy" accompany him to the next class.

Precautions Related to P.E. and Sports. Most doctors recommend that a child with a traumatic brain injury not take part in regular physical education classes or certain contact sports for at least one year following their injury. Their concern is to keep the child out of situations where he might suffer another blow to the head. The school system should provide your child with an adaptive physical education program that is safe for him to take part in. Adaptive physical education programs vary widely and can be based on recommendations from a doctor, physical therapist, or a physical education teacher trained in adapting physical education activities for children with disabilities.

It is also necessary to discuss the types of equipment that your child may use and the games that he may play during recess. School systems often require a doctor's note or order indicating that your child will need an adaptive physical education program. A sample doctor's letter is shown in Figure 8 on the next page.

All of the scheduling considerations mentioned in this section are reasonable to expect of your school system. The key is finding the ones that meet your child's individual needs and allow him to be successful in the school environment. Your child may need something different from what is suggested here. Be creative and work with your school to find the schedule that works best for your child.

Use of Support Personnel

In addition to your child's teacher, there are many school staff, or support personnel, who may be involved with him as part of his educational program. These support personnel will play an important part in your child's overall success when he returns to school.

Instructional Assistants. Instructional assistants are the most commonly used type of support personnel within the school system. Most special education classrooms have an instructional assistant in addition to the classroom teacher. Inclusion classes—regular classes that have special education students in them—often have instructional assistants assigned to them, too. Your school may use other titles for this role such as classroom aide.

As the title indicates, the role of the instructional assistant is to help the teacher carry out her instructional program. In many jurisdictions, the instructional assistant is not required to have an educational degree or specific training. The classroom teacher provides specific directions as to how he would like the assistant to help throughout the school day. Instructional assistants may:

- work with a small group of students to reinforce a new skill or practice a previously presented concept;

▪▪ FIGURE 8. SAMPLE LETTER OF PHYSICAL ACTIVITY GUIDELINES POSTBRAIN INJURY

The information below should be used as a guideline in developing an appropriate adaptive physical educational program for

_____.
(student name)

During at least the first year, we recommend no contact sports or other high risk sports which place this student at high risk for repeat brain injury. Contact sports considered unsafe are sports such as football, soccer, and competitive basketball.

Concerning noncontact sports, the student's ability to perform the sport safely from both a physical (e.g., coordination, strength) and judgment perspective must be evaluated by his parents and/or his coach or physical education teacher. If the student has the physical ability and the judgment to do the activity safely, then it is acceptable. Of course, protective gear should be worn, when appropriate (but is not required for everything). Acceptable activities include sports such as track and field (obviously eliminating activities such as the high jump or pole vault), swimming, bicycling in safe areas with helmet protection, racket sports, gymnastics (eliminating activities with potential for significant fall), noncontact martial arts, weightlifting (as appropriate for age), and softball (with appropriate headgear).

_____
Doctor's signature

- prepare materials for the lessons;
- stay with the class during special area classes such as music or art; or
- supervise the class while the teacher attends team meetings.

Instructional assistants are often asked to work with individual students, as needed and appropriate. In the case of your child, the instructional assistant may be the person who administers his tests on an individual basis, writes down his dictated answers to a test, checks to be certain that his homework assignments are copied correctly, helps him organize his notebook, or helps him prepare his materials for the day. Most children who receive special education services have some interaction with instructional assistants during their school day.

One-to-One Assistants. Depending on your child's needs, it may be necessary to have a one-to-one assistant assigned to him for part or all of the school day. This assistant would help only your child and be with him at all times. A one-to-one assistant might typically be recommended by the team if your child needs more assistance than can be provided by the classroom teacher and/or the instructional assistant. Examples of situations where a one-to-one assistant might be appropriate are if your child:

- requires constant prompts to initiate and/or complete tasks;
- requires ongoing assistance throughout the day to communicate with others within his school environment;
- requires immediate and consistent rewards and consequences as part of an intensive behavior management program;
- requires constant supervision for safety reasons;
- requires constant assistance with academic tasks and school materials; or
- requires frequent tracheostomy suctioning.

If the team agrees that your child requires a one-to-one assistant, it should be indicated on his IEP. Should your child become more independent in the future, the team may decide that a one-to-one assistant is no longer required and the requirement can then be removed from the IEP.

School Nurse. Another support person who may interact frequently with your child is the school nurse. She will administer medication, if needed, and monitor your child's general physical condition. Depending on the role that the nurse plays in your local school, she may provide tube feedings, tracheostomy care, or wound monitoring and/or care. If your child's school does not have a nurse on duty every day, some of these jobs will need to be assigned to other staff who are appropriately trained to carry them out.

Peer Buddies. Although other students cannot be considered support personnel, there are situations in which peer "buddies" can be helpful to your child. They are often used informally to provide copies of class notes, help manage school materials (books, notebooks, etc.), or accompany your child through the halls.

It is important that the team clearly identify who will be responsible for each portion of your child's care. For example, who will escort him to and from the bus, change his diaper, suction his tracheostomy, give him medication, do his tube feeding, provide his daily check-in and check-out, maintain his homework log and notebook, etc.? It should also be clear who will complete these tasks when the primary person is absent. This should be communicated to you, as well as to the support personnel who will be involved.

◼️ Your Child's Teacher

There are only a few graduate programs across the country that train educators with a specific emphasis in Traumatic Brain Injury. This makes it unlikely that your child's teacher will have had any extensive training in teaching students with TBI. Since TBI was added as an eligibility condition under IDEA in 1990, colleges and universities that prepare teachers have begun including some lectures and readings regarding teaching students with traumatic brain injury. Some even offer full courses or mini-courses on the subject, but many teachers have had little or no formal training in the education of students with TBI.

Special education conferences are increasingly offering sessions to train educators in aspects of TBI and this forum is the most likely place for teachers to get such exposure and training.

The level of teacher training in TBI is a legitimate question for you to pose while working with your school team. You can include provisions for teacher training in the IEP. For example, you can ask the team to agree that certain staff will be paid to attend a local conference. Sometimes you can ask the school to arrange training through a local brain injury rehabilitation facility. Some school systems have at least one staff member who has had training in TBI who can serve as a resource to your child's teachers. Such provisions can be included in the IEP or the minutes of the meeting, providing documentation that this is the school's plan.

Clearly, your child's primary teacher should have the most in-depth training in TBI. But it is also advisable for all staff who might encounter your child to have an orientation to TBI. This includes teachers of art, music, P.E., bus drivers, cafeteria workers, and aides. This type of overview can likely be provided by a rehabilitation facility or your state's Brain Injury Association. Typically these services would be provided free of charge or for a minimal fee that should be paid by the school. It is also a good idea to provide teachers with written handouts such as copies of this chapter or articles or brochures available from various organizations.

▪▪ Important Transitions

How your child's brain injury affects him may change over time. This is because the brains of children and adolescents are still actively developing. An injury to a developing brain can cause the brain to develop abnormally and new difficulties can arise unpredictably. With this in mind, there will likely be times in your child's life when re-evaluation might be desirable. Some indications that a re-evaluation is needed include:

- loss of skills,
- failure to acquire new skills,
- new behaviors, or
- significant changes in mood or personality.

Even if a full re-evaluation is not warranted, the brain injury rehabilitation team and the school team may need to redesign learning strategies, school accommodations and modifications, and other therapeutic services.

There are also other times when increased effort will be needed to plan for optimal school success. For example, it will be a good idea to prepare for each new school year. You might suggest that your child's current teachers share valuable advice with next year's teachers. A meeting toward the end of the school year is preferable to the beginning of the new year because any unresolved issues or concerns can hopefully be addressed over the summer.

Preparing to send your child to a new school would also be an especially important transition. Sometimes families send their child to a new school without informing the staff of their child's particular needs in hopes that a fresh start may be the answer to some of their child's difficulties. This is not recommended. It is better to alert the new staff to your child's history and prepare them with training and information than to set your child up for possible failure.

The regular transitions from elementary to middle school and from middle school to high school will require careful planning and coordination between the staffs of the two schools. Again, the teachers experienced in working with your child should offer insight into their successes so that the new teachers can use some of the same strategies for a smooth transition.

Transitions to higher levels of education are inherently difficult for all students. In middle school and high school, students are increasingly expected be more independent, self-motivated, and self-monitoring—all areas of potential difficulty for children who have sustained a TBI. If your child has difficulties in these areas, be aware that your child might need more supports than he did in elementary school.

■■ Procedural Safeguards

IDEA does not deal solely with your child's right to educational services. It also outlines procedural safeguards, which are your rights as the parent of a child with a disability, throughout the special education process. For example, you have the right to request an independent evaluation of your child, as discussed earlier in the chapter, and to have an evaluation conducted by a multidisciplinary team.

Your school system should give you a written copy of the procedural safeguards at the first team meeting and briefly review them with you. If you have questions or want to have them explained in more detail, feel free to ask. Depending on your school system, you may be given a copy at every meeting or you may have to sign a document at each meeting indicating that you have received a copy and explanation of the procedural safeguards. If you would like a copy to review before the first team meeting, just ask the team chairperson for one. Some of the most important safeguards are reviewed below.

Notice

Your child's school system, or local education agency (LEA), must give you written notice before every team meeting that is held to discuss your child. Whether the LEA wants to propose, change, or initiate the identification, evaluation, educational program, or provision of a free, appropriate public education for your child, you must be notified in writing at least ten days before the scheduled meeting. The meeting may be held with less than ten days' notice if you agree to that in writing. Agreeing to waive the ten-day notice often helps move the process along more quickly so that your child can receive services as soon as possible. If the scheduled meeting is not convenient for you, but you would like to attend, you may ask that it be rescheduled at a more convenient time.

Consent

The school system must get your consent before they evaluate your child for the first time or place him in a program that provides special education and related services for the first time. They also must attempt to get your consent before completing a reevaluation of your child. If you do not respond to the school system's written notice of their intent to reevaluate your child and they can show that they took reasonable steps to obtain your consent, they can complete the reevaluation without your consent. When you do not give your consent, the school system has the right to go to due process (see below) in order to get permission to go ahead with their proposed plan.

Parent Surrogate

A parent surrogate can be assigned by the local Superintendent of Schools to represent a student as a parent would in the educational decision-making process. This happens when:
   1. No parent can be identified,
   2. The whereabouts of the parent cannot be discovered after reasonable efforts, or
   3. The child is a Ward of the State.
The person chosen as a parent surrogate cannot be employed by any public agency that is involved in the care or education of the child and

cannot have any interests that conflict with the interests of the child whom they represent. The parent surrogate must have the appropriate knowledge and skills needed to represent the child adequately.

Educational Records

As the parent of a child with a disability, you have the right to review all educational records that relate to your child. This includes records used in the identification, evaluation, and educational placement of your child and the provision of a free, appropriate public education to him. Your local education agency is responsible for protecting the confidentiality of personally identifiable information, which includes: 1) your child's name, 2) parents' names, 3) family members' names, 4) address, 5) social security number, 6) student number, or 7) a list of personal characteristics or other information that makes it possible to identify your child with reasonable certainty.

As a parent, you have a number of rights related to your child's educational records. Some of them include:

- You may request and receive a list of the type and location of your child's educational records that are collected, maintained, or used by the school;
- You may review all of your child's educational records without unnecessary delay and before any due process hearing or IEP meeting. This must take place no more than 45 days after your request.
- You may have a person of your choice review your child's educational records.
- You may have copies of your child's educational records made without delay and the school may charge you a reasonable copying fee, as long as it does not effectively prevent you from exercising your right to review the records.
- You may have school personnel explain or interpret any item in your child's education record.
- You may see a list of individuals, other than yourself and authorized school employees, who have seen your child's educational records, and when and why they saw them.
- You should be asked to give your consent before your child's educational records are disclosed to anyone other than employees of the local education agency or

other agencies that participate jointly in providing your child's education

- You may refuse to give consent for access to your child's educational records.
- You may request a change in your child's educational records if you believe that the information contained in them is inaccurate, misleading, or violates your child's privacy or other rights. Once they receive your request to change the records, the local education agency must decide within a reasonable time period whether to change the information or refuse. If they refuse, they should notify you of your right to a hearing to review their decision.

Resolving Disagreements

When you and the local school system disagree about any step in the process of providing your child with a free, appropriate public education, the best option often is to discuss your disagreements at the team meeting. If you and the team members cannot settle the disagreement yourselves, IDEA offers several methods for resolving conflicts.

Mediation. One way to attempt to reach an agreement with the school system is to request a procedure known as mediation. During mediation, parents and school staff meet at a session that is moderated by someone (often another school employee) not directly involved in the dispute. All parties discuss the disagreement and attempt to reach a decision that is mutually acceptable. You can set this process in motion by sending a letter to your school district's special education office, explaining the nature of your complaint and requesting mediation. Mediation is voluntary for either party. That is, if you request mediation the school does not have to participate and vice versa.

Due Process. If you do not wish to go to mediation or if mediation doesn't work, you can request a due process hearing to try to resolve the disagreement. The specifics of your right to due process are too numerous to cover in detail in this chapter.

In general, however, a due process hearing is a more formal procedure than mediation. It is a procedure that allows both you and the school system to present your sides of the "case," to present evidence (such as the results of an independent evaluation, results of studies about children with TBI, your child's records), and to produce witnesses. You can be represented by a lawyer or a lay advocate (a parent or nonlegal professional with considerable knowledge about IDEA and students with disabilities). The school system will also use a lawyer or team of lawyers. Your goal will be to convince the Administrative Law Judge (ALJ) who is presiding over the case that what the school system is proposing will result in your child receiving an education that is not appropriate to his needs. The school system will attempt to convince the judge of the opposite—that what they are proposing *is* appropriate.

An example of how a due process hearing might work is as follows: You disagree with all or part of your school system's assessment of your child, so you request an independent evaluation at public expense. The school system doesn't want to pay for the independent evaluation, so they request a due process hearing to show that its evaluation is appropriate. If the Administrative Law Judge (ALJ) agrees that the school system's evaluation was appropriate, you still have the right to an independent evaluation at your own expense. If the ALJ decides that the school system's evaluation is not appropriate, the school system must then pay for the independent evaluation and your attorney's fees related to that hearing. (See below.)

Exactly how due process hearings work in your school system should be spelled out clearly in your local education agency's copy of procedural safeguards or parental rights, which you should receive at your first team meeting. Some of the books included in the Reading List for this chapter also provide an in-depth explanation of your rights in this area.

Attorneys' Fees. Under the Handicapped Children's Protection Act of 1986, parents or guardians may be able to recover attorneys' fees when they prevail in any dispute concerning educational services provided under IDEA for their child. That is, if you win a dispute with the school system, the school system may have to cover the costs of your lawyer (but not of a lay advocate). You should discuss this with your attorney because your right to recover fees is dependent upon meeting certain conditions set out in the Act.

:: A Brief History of Special Education Law

If you are planning to do any additional reading about special education issues, it may help to know the history of IDEA and the laws that preceded it. This is because the law has undergone several name changes and has been amended many times. If you are aware of some of the changes in special education law, it will be easier to recognize material that is not current.

The predecessor of IDEA was Public Law 94-142, the Education for All Handicapped Children Act (EHA) of 1975. This law established grants to states for the education of school-aged children with disabilities and entitled them to a free appropriate public education (FAPE).

The EHA has been amended several times. In 1986, the EHA was amended by Public Law 99-457. This law provided funding incentives for states to provide free appropriate education for preschool children with disabilities ages three through five. Further provisions, known as Part H, were added to help states develop early intervention programs for infants and toddlers with disabilities.

In 1990, the EHA was amended again by Public Law 101-476, which, among other things, changed the name to the Individuals with Disabilities Education Act, or IDEA. PL 101-476 also added the stipulation that if a child with a disability requires assistive technology devices or services to benefit from his or her education program, the local education agency (LEA) must make those services or devices available. In 1990, IDEA's reauthorization added the definition of traumatic brain injury as one of the designated disability codes warranting eligibility for special education services.

IDEA has been amended several times, most recently as Public Law 105-17 in 1997. Currently, Part B of the law guarantees a free appropriate education for children with disabilities aged three to eighteen (or older, in states that provide public education to all students beyond the age of eighteen) and Part C covers early intervention for infants and toddlers from birth through age two. Each amendment includes modifications, changes, and clarifications that guide school systems in how they design and implement their special education and related services programs.

∷ For Further Information about IDEA

You can obtain the latest copy of IDEA's regulations from the U.S. Government Printing Office at: Superintendent of Documents, U.S. Government Printing Office, Washington, DC 20402, or online at http://www.ed.gov/offices/osers/idea or http://www.ideapractices.org.

You should also know that IDEA outlines only the *minimum* requirements that states must meet in order to receive federal funds to assist in implementing special education and related services. Each state then writes its own regulations that must meet, but may go beyond, the federal requirements. You can contact your State Department of Education, Office of Special Education, for a copy of the state regulations or a parent guide to special education in your state.

■■ Educational Assistance for Students Who Are Not Eligible under IDEA

Not all students with TBI qualify for assistance under IDEA. To qualify for special education services under IDEA, the effects of a traumatic brain injury must have an impact on educational performance. A student therefore would not qualify if he has a mild or moderate TBI that does not have significant cognitive effects lasting more than a few weeks. A student also might not qualify if he has motor or sensory impairments, but no cognitive impairment, as a result of TBI. For example, your child might have a hand tremor that prevents him from taking notes in class, but otherwise function quite well at school.

If the school team finds that your child does not qualify for special education services under IDEA, for whatever reason, he may still be eligible for assistance under Section 504 of the Rehabilitation Act of 1973. Section 504 can be confusing because it contains gray areas and can overlap with IDEA. Essentially, it is a civil rights law that protects children and adults from discrimination due to a disability. It says that no individual can be excluded, solely because of his or her disability, from participating in any program or activity receiving federal financial assistance. That, of course, includes public schools and many colleges and universities.

To meet Section 504 requirements, schools must make "reasonable accommodations" for students with disabilities (as discussed previously in this chapter) so that they can participate in educational programs provided to other students. For instance, accommodations for the child with hand tremors above might be to provide a note taker or to allow him to tape lectures. Other examples of reasonable accommodations could include:

- modifying the general classroom program,
- special assistance from an aide,

- a behavioral management plan,
- counseling,
- monitoring medication,
- providing special study areas,
- use of assistive technology devices.

Do not hesitate to discuss any accommodation that you feel would assist your child with the school team.

Under Section 504, students may also receive related services such as speech-language pathology, occupational or physical therapy, or counseling, even if they are not receiving special education through IDEA.

To qualify for assistance under Section 504, your child must be found to have a physical or mental impairment that "substantially limits" one or more "life activities." Life activities include: walking, breathing, speaking and/or hearing, seeing, learning, performing manual tasks, and caring for oneself.

How individual schools document the services and accommodations to be provided under 504 varies widely. The school special education personnel can direct you or answer your questions.

❖❖ Americans with Disabilities Act

You might also have heard of the Americans with Disabilities Act (ADA). This is an antidiscrimination law that ensures individuals with disabilities have equal access to businesses and other public and private entities. It also mandates that businesses and public and private entities make "reasonable accommodations" for persons with special needs. In general, this means that an effort must be made to remove obstacles that prevent individuals with disabilities from participating in a program or using facilities, so long as making accommodations does not impose an undue financial burden on the entity. The question of whether an accommodation is reasonable is determined by the courts when there is a dispute. In addition, the law prohibits discrimination against persons with disabilities with respect to employment.

The ADA was not enacted specifically for students with disabilities, but there are two ADA provisions that affect the education of students. First, the ADA makes it illegal for nonsectarian private schools, including preschools, to discriminate against children with disabilities. So, private schools can't refuse to admit students with TBI just because they have a disability, but can deny admittance if they don't otherwise meet qualifications. Second, public schools are required to make reasonable accommodations for students with disabilities. Reasonable accommodations at school might include:

- making existing facilities accessible to, and usable by, students with disabilities,
- acquiring or modifying equipment or devices (e.g., a table of an appropriate height for a wheelchair),
- modifying examinations, training materials, and policies,
- providing qualified readers/interpreters, and other similar changes.

The ADA most often applies to making the school facilities accessible to students with disabilities by adding ramps, elevators, and other modifications to the building. Thus, a student with TBI who has physical impairments but attends all general education classes would fall under ADA protection.

ADA is also used to ensure that students with disabilities are able to participate in extracurricular activities. For example, they can't be excluded from the school play just because there isn't a ramp to the stage or can't be excluded from a field trip because the bus isn't wheelchair accessible. See Chapter 10 for more information on ADA.

:: Teaching Strategies for Children with TBI

Just as you have heard throughout the book, each child or adolescent who experiences traumatic brain injury has a unique outcome, so a cookbook of teaching strategies for every learning problem cannot be offered. As you have also read though, many students with TBI experience a similar constellation of problems. The general strategies offered here will apply to many students who have had a TBI, whether or not they qualify for educational assistance under IDEA.

Reduce Distractions. This can be accomplished in several ways. A smaller student-teacher ratio will reduce the distractions of other students. Preferential seating (e.g., away from door, near teacher, or away from windows), a quiet environment, or a classroom in which a limited amount of noise and activity are tolerated will reduce distractibility. Some students will need a schedule that involves fewer changes in classes; others will need to change classes when fewer people are in the hallways.

Provide Structure. The school team or administration should assist in selecting a teacher whose teaching style provides structure and routine. It will probably be important for your child to routinely know the expectations of the teacher. For example, the teacher should go over expectations for each assignment or class period, assignments should be posted in the same place, and transitions between activities should follow a predictable routine. Providing your child with written reminders or timelines for long-term assignments, going over assignment sheets daily, or breaking assignments down into steps are all ways to impose structure for success.

Use External Aids. A notebook that can aid your child's memory is often essential. Included in such a notebook might be the daily, weekly, or monthly schedule as appropriate; an assignment checklist; assignments or notes organized appropriately; or visual cues for study strategies. Your child will likely need instruction and consistent daily follow-up on the use of such a notebook. After sufficient practice, your child may be able to use it automatically.

If a memory or study strategy has worked well for your child, it would be appropriate to provide your child with an external aid such as a cue card with the steps in using the strategy. For example, your child might be allowed to use a card that has pertinent math formulas written on it. Not only does such an external aid provide the steps of the strategy, but its presence reminds your child to use the strategy.

Increase Self-Awareness. One of the hallmarks of TBI is the lack of insight that survivors typically have into their difficulties. Educators need to acknowledge this fact. That is, they need to understand that your child is not purposefully behaving in a certain way. Then, when opportunities arise, teachers can have private discussions with your child to increase his self-awareness, and, more importantly, to suggest strategies to change the problem behavior. For example, your child may tell the same story over and over to teachers or friends. A teacher who witnesses this behavior might speak to your child about it later and set up a signal to let him know when it is happening so that he can become more aware and try to change this behavior.

Focus on Process Rather Than Just Content. Your child's IEP goals and benchmarks should not just address the content material he is expected to learn. They should also address processes such as attention, acquisition, memory, and generalization and how they will be taught. For example, one of your child's IEP goals may be to increase reading comprehension for facts from a social studies text. However, if sustained attention is a problem area that ultimately affects academic tasks such as reading, then specific goals to increase sustained attention also need to be set.

Teach Strategies That Can Generalize. Students with TBI sometimes have trouble with *generalization*—that is, with using skills taught in one situation in a variety of different situations.

Generalizing is especially important if your child relies on external aids and strategies to become more independent. As teachers and therapists work with your child, they should offer several possible strategies and discover which ones work best for him. Then the basic components of the strategy should be generalized across learning environments so that your child is not required to use a fundamentally different strategy in each situation. For example, if step-by-step picture cues help your child remember his daily routine, then picture cues might also be used to prompt him for the correct steps of a mathematics process.

Provide Opportunities for Repetition. Variability is also common in students who have had a TBI. That is, a skill seems to have been acquired one day, only to be absent the next day. Opportunities for frequent review and repetition will be necessary.

Incorporate Active Learning. Students who have experienced TBI often think and act concretely, finding it hard to infer and/or abstract. For example, they may have trouble learning about fractions without using hands-on manipulatives such as a pizza or a pie. Multiple opportunities for hands-on active learning should be provided. New learning should be linked very concretely to old for the best possible chance of acquisition and retention. Continuing with the example of fractions, a child who learned the concept of ½ using a sandwich could use a sandwich to demonstrate ¼.

Provide Extra Time. Reduced processing speed is another hallmark of TBI. Even if school performance is accurate, it is often much slower. This is usually because it takes longer for the student to take in, organize, and act upon information. There may also be difficulties in motor speed when responding, either verbally or in writing. Allowing extra time for tests and class work will probably be necessary.

A related problem can be fatigue. Besides taking longer, some of these cognitive processes may also require more mental energy. Your child may therefore need an occasional rest period, or simply a periodic mental break.

Use Direct Language When Instructing. Students with TBI might also have difficulty processing complex language, particularly when it is lengthy or spoken rapidly. To help your child understand, teachers should:

- try to gain your child's attention before giving instructions,
- use shorter and more concrete language,
- avoid figurative speech,
- pair verbal information with signs or gestures and demonstrations, and
- teach your child to ask for clarification.

‖ Conclusion

Returning to school following traumatic brain injury can be challenging. This can be an emotionally trying time for you and your child, as you come face to face with learning or behavioral difficulties that can impede school progress and grapple with the need to make changes in your child's educational program.

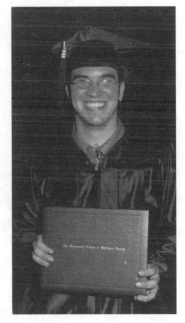

Fortunately, there are laws in place and information available to help you obtain appropriate educational services for your child. Arming yourself with knowledge of the special education process and information about strategies that can help students with TBI can make it easier for both of you. Working cooperatively as an active member of your school's team can also help a good deal.

Do not hesitate to seek help and information from the many resources that are available to you. Contact your local Brain Injury Association, individual members of your school's team or child's rehab team, and online resources such as those included in this book for suggestions of strategies that will help your child get the maximum benefit from his school experiences. Remember, as your child's parent, you will be the only constant on his school team throughout his school years. It is up to you to make sure that his best interests are kept in mind when making educational decisions.

▪▪ Parent Statements

I just can't even imagine her going back to school this way.

❧❀❧

I thought it was bad enough dealing with all of the medical doctors and insurance issues, but now that my son has gone back to school we are finding that it is just as frustrating.

❧❀❧

Just when I thought that I had her educational program all set, something had to change. Her physical therapist understood her and the problems from her brain injury. Now she has gone out on maternity leave and the new therapist doesn't seem to have had any experience with children with brain injury. I feel like I am telling her how to do her job.

❧❀❧

There are so many kids who are in special education, but none of them seem to be like my daughter. I wish there were other parents who knew what I was going through and could give me some advice.

❧❀❧

I am so glad that my son is back in school. When he left the hospital in June, we were left without any services. The school system seems to think that children only have needs between September and June.

❧❀❧

Since her brain injury, I have been teaching Kathleen and her brother, Mark, at home. There I can provide the best environment for her learning, adjusting our schedule around the times when she is most alert and attentive. I arrange for them to have lots of social interaction with other children. This has been the best decision for our family, and Kathleen loves the extra attention I can provide.

❧❀❧

I worry that he won't make it living away from home at college, but we have to let him try. If he fails, then we will just have to deal with it. In the meanwhile, all of us will get a little bit of a break from dealing with him every day.

❧

We were really struggling with our daughter's school program until we were hooked up with Mrs. Smith, the TBI specialist for our school system. Having another advocate for our child has really made a difference.

LEGAL ISSUES FOR FAMILIES OF CHILDREN WITH TBI

Nathaniel Fick

Look around you. Everyone you see is someone's child. Your child may now be six or sixteen, but one day he or she will cross the cusp of childhood/adulthood. As an attorney, I have been called upon to address legal issues surrounding children of all ages—even the forty-ish children of seventy-ish parents. That's why, for the purposes of this chapter, I am offering a global view of issues that should be considered by the families of people who have suffered brain injuries in childhood.

▪ A Lightning Strike That Changes Your Lives Forever— and Requires Timely Action

For children who sustain a brain injury—and their families—life changes in an instant. The earth seems to shift, and things are not as they were before. This sudden transition has broad legal implications.

First, it's essential that your family initiate as quickly as possible an immediate legal review of the actual event of your child's injury (the motor vehicle collision, assault, fall, etc.) or onset of harm (onset of symptoms, initial communication from health care professionals of harm). In addition, you should:

- Review existing family estate planning documents and discuss future estate plans;
- Review all insurance coverages (health, life, disability, automobile, catastrophic liability, homeowner's, and umbrella policies);
- Determine whether your child or family is entitled to government benefits at the federal, state, or local levels;
- Consider your child's competency to manage her own affairs; and
- Become knowledgeable about the important rights to education and freedom from discrimination guaranteed by federal laws.

In the first hours, days, weeks, and months following your child's injury, your family and rehabilitation team will have many opportunities to make sure that the legal system will work for your child, rather than against her. For example, keeping careful and current documentation and records is critical. This chapter will cover many of the actions that you can take to avert chaos, ensure that your child receives the best possible care, and clarify eligibility and access to other resources and benefits.

▪▪ Is a Lawyer Really Necessary?

While you are in the midst of coping with all the changes and emotions connected with your child's brain injury, seeing a lawyer may be the last thing on your mind. Already there are a dizzying array of medical professionals, therapists, and educators involved in your child's care—do you really need to consult a lawyer, too?

The short answer is "yes." In fact, you may need to consult with the lawyer throughout the course of your child's recovery. You may also need to consult with several types of lawyers on a range of issues, including analyzing fault, insurance benefits, special education issues, guardianship, power of attorney, and estate planning.

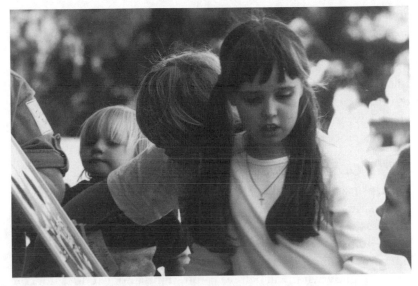

Should You Consider Litigation?

In general, there are two reasons that families of children with brain injury consider litigation. First, they may believe that someone or something is to blame for their child's injury and should pay some kind of financial compensation to their child or family. Second, they may have been unsuccessful in getting insurance companies to pay for services that they believe should be covered. In these circumstances, families hope that any additional money they receive through lawsuits will contribute to improving the quality of life for their child and their family. And indeed, one study of 238 adult patients with TBI found that *in cases where more financial resources were expended, independent living skills significantly improved.*

If you believe that your child may have been injured as a result of fault of some other person, you should consult an attorney with litigation experience. That is not to say that all families of children with TBI should or do get involved in lawsuits. Nevertheless, information gathering and investigation must be begun promptly to determine whether a lawsuit must be filed. Prompt investigation is essential if the lawyer is to obtain all significant evidence that would prove liability.

Battles Over the Cause of Your Child's Injury

When analyzed, almost all "accidents" are not accidents at all—*they are preventable events.* If the law is complied with or standards are met, "wrongs" usually do not occur. When a wrong occurs due to lack of compliance, tort law provides ways to call the wrongdoer to account and to compensate the victim. This requires the careful investigation and presentation of a claim, usually with the filing of a lawsuit. There are time limitations related to filing such a lawsuit, and the process is quite complex, making it essential to consult an experienced lawyer. The later section on "Working with a Neurolawyer" goes into this process in more detail.

Battles Over Insurance

Insurance companies (including health maintenance organizations, managed care organizations, and the like) are not in the business of giving away money or expending money if they can avoid doing so. All payments are governed by the language (contract provisions) of the policy, by governing law, and by public policy. Unfortunately, what you believe is fair, right, and just does not constitute "public policy." All services requested for your child are scrutinized for compliance with the policy terms, and limitations or exclusions. Families frequently have disputes with insurance carriers over which services are medically necessary. Even though you feel that a service is medically necessary and your physicians or health care providers agree completely, the insurance company may disagree or refuse to pay.

It is important to keep a copy of all correspondence to and from your insurance company. If letters to the insurance company do not result in the coverage you believe your child is entitled to, contact your state insurance department. State insurance departments are designated state agencies that act as go-betweens for consumers and insurance providers. These agencies are responsible for making sure that all policies and contracts issued by private insurers are within state insurance law guidelines for providing consumer education about insurance, and for investigating complaints against insurance brokers, agents, and companies. Additionally, these agencies may impose sanctions (including fines and revocation of licenses) against insurance providers found guilty of violating insurance laws and regulations.

If you feel that you have received unfair treatment from an insurance provider, you may file a written complaint with your state's insurance department, which can then investigate your claim. State insurance Departments are listed by state in the State Resources section of the Brain Injury Association's *National Directory of Brain Injury Rehabilitation Services*. (See the Resource Guide at the back of this book.)

Sometimes, your only recourse in a dispute may be to take the insurance company to court. For example, the terms of your insurance policy may not be in compliance with the law, but the company may deny it. For example, one family's policy stipulated that they were entitled to only $300,000 in coverage when by law they were entitled to $3,300,000 worth of coverage. The insurance carrier refused to provide this level of coverage, however, until the highest court in Maryland ordered them to pay.*

Usually the resolution of insurance disagreements hinges upon the contents of records created along the way—including medical records, insurance applications, insurance submissions, and correspondence. These are then analyzed against the contracts and the law. When your child's records are fragmented, and when relevant items are undocumented or incomplete, your family is much less likely to get the coverage you need. The next section therefore describes some strategies that will help you keep your child's records in order.

▪▪ Keeping Useful Records

Insurance disputes are only one reason why effective information gathering, record keeping, and timely and appropriate communication are essential. *Timely, complete, and directed documentation* are the bedrock for maximizing results for your child and your family. It can also bring order and sanity to all rehabilitation providers' record-based lives.

Don't assume that the professionals will provide you with all information needed or that their records will always be accurate. You should begin the task of maintaining objective, detailed records of your own.

Starting a Notebook

A marble composition book—you know, the bound kind you used in elementary school—is a great place to document what happens after your child's injury. This notebook is a tool for you, and should include the following types of information:

---

* *Staab v. American Motorist Insurance Co.*, 345 Md. 428, 693 A.2d 340 (1997).

Basic Information on the People Involved. Start with the full and complete personal and family history: names, addresses, ages, dates of birth and social security numbers of relevant individuals (e.g., injured child, parents, siblings). List all known hospitals, clinics, physicians, therapists, and others involved in caring for your child with TBI from the time of her injury. Include full names, titles, "alphabet soup" (R.N., M.D., Ph.D., C.R.R.N., C.P.C., C.R.C., C.C.M.), addresses, telephone numbers, and relevant dates. Remember to list all patient numbers or account numbers for each provider.

Personal Information. Add to the marble notebook your child's medical history. This includes hospital of birth, pediatricians(s), any hospitalizations, and vaccination history. Also include educational history (schools and dates of attendance, names of teachers who know your child well), and information on any jobs she might have held. Additional information that you should have readily available—but may want to segregate from the bound notebook—includes a complete psychological/psychiatric history for your child (listings of any counselors, social workers, psychologists, psychiatrists, past alcohol or drug counseling), prior injuries of any type, criminal record, and prior litigation of any nature and at any place.

Insurance Coverage. List *all* insurance policies—health, life, accident, disability, automobile, homeowners, catastrophic liability, and umbrella policies. Include the companies' full names, addresses, and telephone numbers, as well as policy numbers, claims numbers, agent's and agency's name, address, and telephone numbers. Locate the policies, declaration sheets, correspondence, booklets, advertising circulars, and other information relating to your child's insurance coverage.

Contacts with Professionals. Keep a record of all meetings, telephone calls, correspondence, and conferences. Each entry should include the date and notes about the participants and substance of each meeting/call/conference. Remember that you may have to make sense of these notes two or three years down the road. Each entry should cover the essential details. The reality is that "the shortest pencil is longer than the longest memory."

:: Working with a Neurolawyer

A *neurolawyer* is a lawyer who—through interest, education, and training— has developed a special expertise in representing clients with

TBI or spinal cord injury. This specialization requires education in the areas of neuroanatomy, neurophysiology, neurochemistry, neuropsychology, neurorehabilitation, and the biomechanics of neurotrauma. *Neurolaw* is recognized as a special field of jurisprudence and is listed as such in the authoritative *Martindale-Hubbell Law Directory*.

The neurolawyer plays no role in the medical care and treatment of the patient—except to try to make sure that the patient doesn't "fall through the cracks." He or she does, however, become an interested observer. There are many points at which the paths of medical and legal practitioners cross as they work toward their common aim of maximum improvement for the patient and family. For example, an experienced neurolawyer can spot holes in the documentation provided by your child's medical record that can create problems when you are seeking compensation from an insurance company or through a lawsuit.

The neurolawyer's first task is to evaluate the facts of your child's case and the applicable law. That is, he or she clarifies the five W's of the event leading to your child's brain injury—the who, what, when, where, and why. This is necessary to define the goals of representing your family and to determine the best course for achieving those goals. Obviously, many of the facts will be medical.

The second (and crucial) task is to gather evidence and preserve materials that substantiate the nature and extent of the injury and ongoing medical needs. During this stage, the neurolawyer also seeks to define the injury's impact on the lives of your child and her family. This requires close coordination with appropriate, qualified medical and rehabilitative experts.

The third task is to coordinate the presentation of the claim so that fact finders—such as an insurance case manager, a claims representative or manager, a claims committee or review board, or a judge or jury—can fairly and favorably consider the claim. Everything must be substantiated so that fact finders can understand and agree that the claim is legitimate.

A final, and ongoing task, is to communicate with health care providers and other professionals involved in the case so that all may work as a team toward the best possible outcome.

How to Select and Retain a Lawyer

DO NOT DELAY! Brain injuries change lives—forever. They draw a line that makes us measure everything in "before" and "after" terms. They create a complex and broad outflow of consequences for the individual, the family, and the community. *TIME is critical*, for legal as well as medical reasons. There are certain times and "windows of opportunity" that are essential for safeguarding the legal rights and entitlement of the individuals and families. Miss these times, and evidence disappears. Witnesses scatter. Facts grow hazy. Delay is always a serious enemy.

Despite the need for haste, however, you don't want to rush out and choose just any lawyer. As discussed below, the requirements are very complex, and you should take the time to find someone who is well qualified.

The Attorney's Qualifications

This is not the time to go to the lawyer who handled your cousin's divorce or the settlement of your home. You need a specialist with the knowledge, experience, and skills to bring the matter to a successful conclusion. You should look for:

- **Medical Knowledge.** "Neurolaw" is a recognized legal specialty area, and the attorneys who practice in it make a point of keeping up with medical developments. They read extensively; they attend professional conferences; they may even take or audit medical school courses or grand rounds. They have years of experience representing victims of brain and spinal cord injuries. To give just one example, they know which professionals are necessary and which are best to provide the expert testimony in court that is often the deciding factor in a case.

- **Financial "Avenues of Recovery" Knowledge.** Neurolawyers know which sources of reimbursement (Workmen's Compensation; all levels and aspects of first party or third party insurance coverages, including commercial general policies, umbrella coverage, uninsured and underinsured, and personal catastrophic coverages; as well as federal, state, and local benefits) are available in your child's case and how to deal with the companies, the bureaucracies, and the forums for determination involved. They also know how to structure trust funds and other financial arrangements to

maximize the value of settlements and awards your child
with TBI may receive.

- **Litigation Experience.** Neurolawyers routinely do
broader personal injury litigation, and you want someone with a good track record in this area. This does not
mean that you are going to take the matter to court, but
it does mean you have a lawyer who is fully capable of
winning the case in court if it does require a trial.

Personal Factors

Brain injury cases often take years. You and your attorney are
going to be working together for a long time, and it is essential that
your personalities mesh well. Look for a lawyer who believes in your
child's case and is sympathetic to the stresses involved. Look for someone you feel comfortable with and able to talk to.

Also look for someone who is a team player. Many different specialists in medicine, psychiatry, rehabilitation, and case management
will be involved in your child's case, and your attorney must be able to
work well with them.

Financial Factors

Legal costs for brain injury cases can run into the hundreds of
thousands of dollars—well beyond most families' resources. For this
reason, neurolawyers usually work on a contingent basis, receiving a
percentage of the financial award(s) as their fee. When handled on a
contingency fee basis, the family incurs no attorney fees if they do not
receive a financial award.

The contingency fee system makes first-class legal representation available to people who unquestionably need it but could not
otherwise afford it. Unfortunately, it also imposes a burden on the law
practice, which must cover up-front costs. These can amount to tens
of thousands of dollars or more, all of which the neurolawyer must
pay out of his firm's funds without any guarantee that he will win the
case and recover the money.

This makes neurolawyers understandably cautious about agreeing to take on a case. In your initial conversation with an attorney you
are thinking of retaining, you can expect that he or she will want to
know a great deal about your matter in order to determine the scope
of the problem and the available solutions.

Where to Find a Qualified Attorney

The Brain Injury Association's *National Directory of Brain Injury Rehabilitation Services* lists attorneys. BIA state associations, the Association of Trial Lawyers of America, and state and national Bar Associations can also provide names. So does the *Martindale-Hubbell Law Directory,* available at local libraries.

Finally, you might ask for recommendations from attorneys you have worked with before, medical and rehabilitation professionals, and people with brain injury and their families.

The Initial Interview

Every contact with your attorney will usually be fact- and issue-specific. Make sure you know ahead of time what information your attorney is interested in. Organize the information for discussion so that the conversation can be as productive as possible for all parties.

Much of the information you'll be asked for falls into the traditional categories: WHO, WHAT, WHEN, WHERE, and WHY.

1. **WHO** means the family's full names, correct addresses and telephone numbers, dates of birth, social security numbers, marital status and family relationships. Also employment information, if your child was employed (since this figures into lost wages/income)—including the full name of the employer, address, employee's title and duties, rates of pay, and dates of employment—and similar facts.

2. **WHAT** covers event information. For example, discussion of a motor vehicle accident would focus on how it happened, witnesses, police investigation, and news coverage.

3. **WHEN** includes all relevant dates: dates of injury or onset of complaints and dates of all hospitalizations and other diagnostic or health care activities, such as neuropsychological evaluation.

4. **WHERE** includes the location of the event and subsequent care and treatment, in as much detail as possible.

5. **WHY** covers interpretive information. What do you *think* happened? What do you *think* caused or contributed to this situation? Since your child and family have lived with this problem, you may have impressions that are important for the investigation and case presentation.

What the Lawyer Does with the Information

As mentioned above, not all injuries become legal cases. The lawyer's primary function is to assess whether or not there is a basis of responsibility on the part of another party. That is, he or she needs to determine whether any individual, group, or object is at fault for your child's injury. If such responsibility seems to exist, the lawyer's role is to "pin it down" by securing and safeguarding the necessary evidence for later review and analysis.

The lawyer will also be concerned with pinning down and documenting all the ways that your child's brain injury has changed her own and your family's life. Some of these changes might include:

- There is a new "vesting" of legal responsibility where there was no legal responsibility before the brain injury. (For example, your child is approaching the age when she would be expected to be fully independent and earn her own living, but is now a "destitute, disabled" member of the family who requires parental care and support.)
- There is a need to have a guardian appointed, when there was previously no need. (See the section on Guardianship below.)
- Changes in your family's estate planning are now necessary due to increased needs to safeguard your injured child's future.
- There is a need to set up a Special Needs Trust or some other appropriate trust to protect assets and safeguard your child's entitlement to federal, state, or local benefits.
- There is a need for "family law advice" due to pre-existing custody, visitation, or support issues.
- There is a need for representation in criminal proceedings or other parts of the juvenile justice system, within the education system, or other administrative bodies due to psychosocial or other issues and other events that are affected by some of the consequences of the injury.

Again, even if such problems have arisen, that does not automatically translate into the filing of a lawsuit. And if a decision is made to file a lawsuit, the mere filing of the lawsuit does not catapult you into court. Greater than 90 percent of all cases filed in court are resolved without the necessity of trial! Filing a lawsuit ensures that your claim will not be found invalid merely because a statute of limitations has run out. It also creates a *forum for discovery*—being able to formally pursue evidence with subpoena power of the court.

It is best to always think in terms of one day having to present the entire life and event history in a formal setting—whether in a court, at some administrative hearing, or in another dispute resolution forum. Even when things are progressing smoothly, do not be lulled into complacency.

Whether presenting your child's "case" for evaluation of responsibility for the injury, for a determination of entitlement to benefits, or for any other issue resolution, the only way to properly prepare is with the core information discussed throughout this section.

Educational Rights and Benefits

As Chapter 9 explains, there is a federal law that provides children with TBI with some very important educational rights. This law, the Individuals with Disabilities Education Act (IDEA), guarantees a free, appropriate public education to students with disabilities from birth through high school. Among the rights granted to qualifying children under this law are:

- The right to an *evaluation* by a team of professionals with different areas of expertise to determine whether they are eligible or ineligible for services.
- The right to a *"free appropriate public education"*—that is, to an education program provided entirely at public expense that meets your child's special learning needs.
- The right to *special education and related services.* Under the law, "special education" refers to instruction specially designed to meet the unique learning needs of a child with disabilities, which may be provided by regular education teachers, special education teachers, or other professionals. "Related services" refers to physical, occupational, or speech-language therapy, transportation, the assistance of an aide, or any other service necessary for your child to benefit from her educational program.
- The right to be educated to the maximum extent appropriate in the *"least restrictive environment"* (LRE). The

LRE is the educational setting that enables your child to have the maximum contact with typical children and the general education curriculum while still making progress toward her individual education goals.

- The right to have an *Individualized Education Program (IEP)* or *Individualized Family Service Plan (IFSP)*. For children three and older, the IEP is a written plan that describes long-term goals and short-term objectives for learning, as well as the services that will be provided to help the child reach those goals, and the setting where the services will be provided. The IFSP is a similar plan for children under age three, with the distinction that goals for family members may also be included. IEPs and IFSPs are both developed by teams consisting of school personnel, parents, and the child herself, if she chooses to participate.

- The right to be considered for an *extended school year (ESY)*. Children who lose a significant amount of progress during the summer may be eligible to receive educational services during the summer at public expense.

- The right to *written notice* whenever changes to your child's eligibility, placement, or education program are proposed.

- The right to *disagree* with the school about any matter "relating to the identification, evaluation, or educational placement of the child, or the provision of free appropriate public education" to the child. Parents are allowed to disagree both informally—such as by writing a letter of complaint to the special office of your school district—or formally, by requesting an impartial due process hearing before a hearing officer, with the right to have counsel, to present evidence, to cross-examine witnesses, and to receive from the hearing officer a written statement of findings of facts and determinations.

Each of these rights is discussed in more detail in Chapter 9.

The law is ever-evolving. Periodically there are changes in benefits, programs, due process rights, eligibility, funding, or access to supplementary aids and services. There are amendments and court determinations that call us to review and reconsider what is "old law" and what is "new law." This makes it crucial for you to stay abreast of changes that may affect your child's education. Get to know and use available resources—the public library, the special education director of your local school district, your local P & A (protection and advocacy) office, resources of the Brain Injury Association, legislators, department of legislative reference, and your attorney.

In addition, there are a number of print and online sources of information about proposed and actual changes to IDEA. See, for example, the FedLaw website, the National Council on Disability, and other organizations listed in the Resource Guide at the back of the book.

■■ Protection from Discrimination

In the United States, there are several laws that protect children with TBI and other individuals with disabilities from discrimination. The most far-reaching of these is the Americans with Disabilities Act (ADA), but the Rehabilitation Act of 1973 also provides important protections.

Americans with Disabilities Act (ADA)

The Americans with Disabilities Act (ADA) was signed into law on July 26, 1990. It prohibits discrimination on the basis of disability, much as earlier civil rights laws made it illegal to discriminate against people on the basis of sex, race, or religion. The ADA is divided into five titles or sections:

Title I: Employment. This section pertains to all employers with fifteen employees or more. It prohibits employers from discriminating against qualified individuals with disabilities during the application or hiring process, or when determining salary, benefits, or other aspects of employment. It prohibits employers from asking about the presence of a disability and refusing to hire someone solely because they have a disability. If an employee chooses to disclose her disability to her employer, however, then the employer is required to provide "reasonable accommodations" to help the employee succeed—provided the accommodation does not impose an "undue hardship" on the employer.

Under ADA, a reasonable accommodation is defined as any modification or adjustment to a job, an employment practice, or the work environment that makes it possible for a qualified employee with a disability to have an equal employment opportunity. For your child, reasonable accommodations on the job might include job sharing or a shortened work schedule, if she has difficulty concentrating for eight hours, or job checklists or memory log books to help her remember the requirements of her job.

Title II: Public Services. This section of the ADA prohibits discrimination against individuals with disabilities by state and local public agencies that provide services such as transportation. For example, all buses, trains, or other forms of public transportation must be accessible to people with disabilities.

Title III: Public Accommodations. A public accommodation is a business, program, or agency that provides services or goods to the public. The ADA lists twelve categories of public accommodations, including: places of lodging (inns, hotels, motels); establishments serving food or drink; places of exhibition or entertainment (movie theaters, stadiums, concert halls); sales or retail establishments (stores of all kinds, shopping centers); places of public display or collection (museums, libraries); schools serving students of all ages; places of exercise or recreation (gyms, health spas, bowling alleys); places that provide testing services. (Facilities run by religious entities and private clubs are excepted.)

Under ADA, individuals with disabilities are entitled to "full and equal enjoyment of the goods, services, facilities, privileges, advantages, or accommodations" of any place of public accommodation. Furthermore, public accommodations are specifically prohibited from forcing people with disabilities into separate or unequal facilities or programs. All new construction and modifications to existing buildings must be accessible to people with disabilities. And existing facilities must remove all barriers to service, if readily achievable. (This means that the cost of making the change should not be too great given the overall financial resources of the facility and the impact of the alteration upon the business's operation.)

For your child with TBI, this section of the ADA means that she should not be denied the opportunity to go anywhere or do anything because she is considered disabled. For example, a summer camp or a swimming class could not exclude her just because she has a TBI, or because there is a separate recreation program for children with disabilities that they think might be more appropriate. (If there are legitimate safety concerns, however, they are allowed to have specific criteria for participation or require modifications.) Your child is also entitled to aids and supplementary services when she needs them in order to be a full and equal participant in using a public accommodation. For example, if she is taking a college entrance exam, she might be entitled to take extra time to take the test, use a large-print format, or take the exam in a room with few distractions.

Title IV: Telecommunications. This title guarantees the rights of individuals with hearing impairments to be able to communicate by telephone. Telephone companies must provide telephone relay services to people who use telecommunication devices for the deaf (TTYs) or similar devices.

Title V: Miscellaneous. This section covers a variety of protections for individuals with disabilities. Perhaps the most important are provisions making it illegal to coerce, threaten, or retaliate against individuals with a disability, or people who are attempting to help individuals with disabilities, for asserting their rights under the ADA.

If you believe your child has been discriminated against under Titles II or III of the ADA, you can send a letter of complaint to The U.S. Department of Justice, Civil Rights Division, Coordination and Review Section. For complaints about discrimination under Title I, send a letter to the Equal Employment Opportunity Commission. (See the Resource Guide for addresses.) You may also bring a lawsuit against any business or program that you feel has discriminated against you or your child under ADA. Your state P&A office can provide information and help you in a discrimination complaint.

The Rehabilitation Act of 1973

Before the ADA was enacted, the Rehabilitation Act of 1973 was the only federal law prohibiting discrimination against individuals with disabilities. And it only prohibited discrimination by programs that received federal funding from the U.S. government. Still, because so many entities, including public schools, receive federal funds, the law provides many useful protections.

The heart of the Rehabilitation Act is Section 504, which states: "No otherwise qualified individual with handicaps . . . shall solely by reason of her or his handicap, be excluded from participation in, denied the benefits of, or be subject to discrimination under any program or activity receiving Federal financial assistance."

As Chapter 9 discusses, Section 504 can protect the rights of children with TBI in schools that receive federal funding. For example, your child may be eligible for a 504 plan if she is not eligible for an individualized education program (IEP) under IDEA. Like an IEP, a 504 Plan specifies goals and objectives for your child, and explains what the school will do to help your child reach those goals. Your child is less likely to receive therapies and other direct services with a 504 plan, and more likely to receive "accommodations" or changes to the learning environment, than she is with an IEP. For example, she might be given preferential seating, or extra time to complete assignments and tests.

Another program created under the authority of the Rehabilitation Act of 1973, as amended, Title 1, Part B, Section 112, is the Client Assistance Program, discussed below.

■ Governmental Programs and Benefits

There are a variety of federally funded programs and benefits in the United States that families of children with TBI are often eligible for. Sometimes if you qualify for one program you automatically qualify for another. For example, children who qualify for Supplemental Security Income (SSI) benefits also qualify for Medicaid. Often, however, programs have their own eligibility criteria (and red tape!), so it will likely require quite a bit of work to first determine which programs can benefit your child and then to apply for them.

Client Assistance Programs and Protection and Advocacy Systems

Each state offers Client Assistance Programs (CAP) and Protection and Advocacy (P & A) Systems. These offer valuable resources to people with traumatic brain injury and their families who meet eligibility criteria. In the event your child is not found eligible for services, the CAP or P & A System will provide assistance to locate other resources.

Client Assistance Programs and Protection and Advocacy Systems investigate, negotiate, and mediate solutions to problems experienced by qualifying people with disabilities, their families, or agency representatives. They offer technical assistance to attorneys, government representatives, and service providers. They also provide legal counsel and litigation services to eligible individuals who are unable to obtain adequate legal services in their communities. Training for advocate, consumers, volunteers, professionals, and others is also provided.

Client Assistance Programs and Protection and Advocacy Systems are listed in the state resources section of the Brain Injury Association's *National Directory of Brain Injury Rehabilitation Services*. You can also locate your local CAP or P&A office by contacting the National Association of Protection and Advocacy Systems, as listed in the Resource Guide at the back of this book.

Client Assistance Programs

Client Assistance Programs (CAP) provide services to individuals seeking or receiving services under the Rehabilitation Act (including federally funded vocational rehabilitation and independent living services).

The goal of CAP services is to help people with disabilities obtain information and access to the array of services available through programs, projects, and facilities funded under the Rehabilitation Act. CAP is administered by the U.S. Department of Education, Office of Special Education and Rehabilitative Services, Rehabilitation Services Administration.

Protection and Advocacy for Persons with Developmental Disabilities

Protection and Advocacy Systems for persons with developmental disabilities (PADD) were established to provide advocacy services to people with developmental disabilities. Developmental disabilities are defined by the federal government as chronic and attributable to mental and/or physical impairments that are evident before the age of twenty-two. Such disabilities tend to be life-long and result in substantial limitations in three or more of the following major life activities: self-care, receptive and expressive language, learning, mobility, self-direction, the capacity for independent living, and/or economic self-sufficiency.

Services available from state PADDs usually include: information and referral to other sources of assistance; peer and self-advocacy training; representation in administrative and judicial proceedings; investigation of abuse and neglect; and legislative advocacy.

PADD is administered by the U.S. Department of Health and Human Services Administration on Developmental Disabilities. State PADD offices are called by different names—Disability Law center; Protection and Advocacy, Inc.; [State Name] Disability Law Project;

[State Name] Protection & Advocacy. To locate the protection and advocacy office in your state, check with the Department of Public Health or the Office of the Governor, or contact the National Association of Protection and Advocacy Systems in the Resource Guide.

Protection and Advocacy for Individuals with Mental Illness

The Protection and Advocacy system for persons with mental illness (PAIMI) was established to protect the rights of persons with mental illness under federal and state statutes, and to investigate allegations of abuse and neglect of individuals residing in facilities. Individuals eligible for services must reside in facilities that provide twenty-four-hour care and treatment, or have been discharged from such a facility within the previous ninety days. Programs also represent individuals in certain situations involving prisons and jails, and transportation to and from facilities.

The PAIMI system is administered by the U.S. Department of Health and Human Services, National Institute of Mental Health.

Protection and Advocacy for Individual Rights (PAIR)

Protection and Advocacy program for individual rights (PAIR) was established to help enforce the Americans with Disabilities Act (ADA) and the 1988 Fair Housing Act Amendments. Through the PAIR programs, P & A systems nationwide protect and advocate for services to people with disabilities who are not eligible for PADD or PAIMI programs, or whose issues do not fall within the jurisdiction of the Client Assistance Program.

PAIR is administered by the U.S. Department of Education, Office of Special Education and Rehabilitative Services and Rehabilitation Services Administration (RSA). In your state, check with the Department of Public Health or the Office of the Governor, or contact the National Association of Protection and Advocacy Systems in the Resource Guide.

Social Security Disability Insurance (SSDI) and Supplemental Security Income (SSI)

Social Security Disability Insurance (SSDI) and Supplemental Security Income (SSI) are federal programs that provide additional income to eligible individuals with disabilities in the form of a monthly check. Both programs are administered by the Social Security Administration.

Children can qualify for assistance if they meet Social Security's definition of disability and if their income and assets fall within the eligibility limits.

Most children do not have their own income and do not have many assets. However, when children under age eighteen live at home (or go away to school but return home occasionally and remain their parents' dependents), the parents' income and assets are considered in determining eligibility. This process is referred to as "deeming" of income and assets. You will need to check with your Social Security office for information about your state's deeming process.

When a child turns eighteen, the parents' income and assets are no longer taken into consideration in determining eligibility. A child who was not eligible before her eighteenth birthday because parental income or assets were too high may become eligible at eighteen.

On the other hand, if a child with a disability who is receiving financial assistance turns eighteen and continues to live with her parents, but does not pay for food or shelter, a lower payment rate may apply.

Social Security Disability Insurance (SSDI)

Social Security Disability Insurance (SSDI) provides basic protection against the loss of income due to disability. Its benefits may extend to both the worker with a disability and to family members (including children). SSDI provides a monthly payment to eligible persons. SSDI defines disability as:

> *A physical or mental impairment that prevents an individual from doing any substantial gainful activity and that is expected to last (or has lasted) at least one year or to result in death.*

The law states that a child will be considered disabled if she has a physical or mental condition (or a combination of conditions) that results in "marked and severe functional limitations." This condition must last or be expected to last at least twelve months or be expected to result in a child's death. And, the child must not be working at a job that is considered substantial work.

To determine whether a child meets the criteria, a disability evaluation specialist first checks to see if the child's disability can be found in a special listing of impairments that is contained in the

Social Security's regulations, or if the condition is medically or functionally equal to an impairment that is on the list. These listings are descriptions of symptoms, signs, or laboratory findings of more than 100 physical and mental problems, such as cerebral palsy, mental retarda-

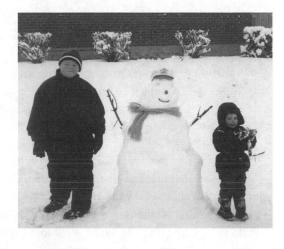

tion, seizure disorders, or communication impairments that are severe enough to disable a child. Traumatic brain injury is not one of the conditions currently on the list. However, if the symptoms, signs, or laboratory findings of your child's condition are the same as, or medically equal in severity to a condition on the list, your child is considered disabled for SSI purposes. Your child will also be considered disabled if the functional limitations from her condition or combination of conditions are the same as the disabling functional limitations of any listed impairment.

To determine whether your child's impairment causes "marked and severe functional limitations," the disability evaluation team will obtain evidence from a wide variety of sources who have knowledge of your child's condition and how it affects her ability to function on a day-to-day basis and over time. These sources include, but are not limited to, the doctors and other health professionals who treat your child, teachers, counselors, therapists, and social workers. A finding of disability will not be based solely on your statements or on the fact that your child is or is not enrolled in special education classes.

Supplemental Security Income (SSI)

Supplemental Security Income (SSI) provides monthly payments to people who are elderly, disabled, or blind and who do not have enough income to support themselves. The federal government establishes a basic amount annually for SSI payments. Some states add money to the basic federal amount.

Determining whether your child qualifies for SSI is a two-step process. First, your local Social Security Office will decide if your child's income and assets are within SSI limits. Next, all documents and evidence pertaining to your child's disability are sent to a state office, usually called the Disability Determination Service (DDS). There a team made up of a disability evaluation specialist and a doctor reviews your child's case to decide if she meets SSI's definition of disability, which is:

> *A physical or mental problem that is expected to last at least one year or to result in death.*

If the available records are not thorough enough for the DDS team to make a decision, you may be asked to take your child to a special examination that Social Security will pay for. It is very important that you do this, and that your child puts forth her best effort during the examination. Otherwise, the results of the examination will not be considered valid. Failure to attend the examination or invalid results due to poor effort could result in your child being found to be ineligible.

People who receive SSI are usually eligible for Medicaid (see below) and food stamps. Application for these is made separately at the agencies administering Medicaid or food stamps in each state. SSI personnel will help people apply.

SSI offers incentive programs to individuals with disabilities who want to work, including Plans for Achieving Self Support (PASS) and Impairment-Related Work Expenses (IRWE). Under the PASS system, an individual can have more income or assets than SSI recipients are usually allowed, provided the extra money will be used to enable the recipient to work in the future or to establish a business to help her become gainfully employed. Under the IRWE program, the cost of special items and services an individual with disabilities needs in order to work can be deducted from her earnings when determining financial eligibility for SSI.

When applying for SSI, you will need: your child's Social Security number and proof of age, income and asset information (i.e., bank book, payroll slips, etc.), mortgage or lease information, and medical records.

Applying for SSI and SSDI

To apply for Social Security Disability Insurance (SSDI) or Supplemental Security Income (SSI), contact the Social Security Administration (SSA) at: 1-800-772-1213 or visit their website at http://www.ssa.gov.

You can also check the Blue Pages of the telephone book under "U.S. Government" for information about the local Social Security office. The Social Security Administration suggests avoiding these busy times: the first Monday of the month, days after holidays, and between 10:00 a.m. and 3:00 p.m.

Medicare and Medicaid

Medicare and Medicaid are federal programs that can help pay for the medical expenses of children and families who meet the eligibility criteria.

Medicare

Medicare is a federal health insurance program that provides acute-care coverage for people over age 65, as well as some individuals who are covered by Social Security Disability (SSDI) benefits (see above). Medicare has two parts: Hospital Insurance (Part A) and Medical Insurance (Part B).

Hospital Insurance (Part A) Medicare coverage is limited to services considered "reasonable and necessary" for the diagnosis and treatment of illness or injury. Services include inpatient hospital stays, nursing facility care, home health care services, and hospice care. If your child qualifies for SSDI, she will automatically be eligible to receive this coverage.

Medical Insurance (Part B) Medicare pays for physician services, hospital outpatient services, ambulatory surgery, and diagnostic and laboratory tests. Coverage is also provided for limited outpatient physical, occupational, and speech therapy services and medical equipment and supplies. Most Medicare recipients have to pay a premium to receive Part B coverage. However, if your child qualifies for Medicaid (see below), Medicaid may pay the Part B premium for her.

For more information, contact the local Social Security office (listed in the telephone book Blue Pages under "U.S. Government") or the Social Security Administration at 800-772-1213.

Medicaid

Medicaid is a joint federal/state program that provides basic health care insurance for people who are disabled, poor, or receive certain governmental income support benefits (such as SSI), and who meet income and resource limitation tests.

Services that may be covered by Medicaid include hospital inpatient and outpatient services, physician services, custodial care services (both in institutional or community settings), rehabilitation services, prescription drugs, and dental care.

For more information, or to apply for Medicaid, contact the state Medicaid office listed in the State Resources section of the Brain Injury Association's *National Directory of Brain Injury Rehabilitation Services*. (See Resource Guide.) You can also visit the Medicaid information page on the Health Care Financing Administration's website at http://www.hcfa.gov/medicaid or call them at 410-786-3000.

Defense and Veterans Head Injury Program

If your child's brain injury occurred while she was in the military or working for the Department of Veterans' Affairs (DVA), she qualifies for services through the Defense and Veterans Head Injury Program (DVHIP).

The principal goals of the DVHIP are to ensure that all military and DVA personnel with traumatic brain injury receive appropriate evaluation and follow-up of their injuries. The program also helps locate and coordinate needed services for eligible individuals. In addition, the program is designed to collect data about the relative efficacy and cost of various TBI treatment and rehabilitation strategies, and to help define optimal treatment for persons with TBI.

Seven regional military and Veterans TBI Centers have been established:

1. Walter Reed Army Medical Center - Washington, DC
2. Wilford Hall Air Force Medical Center - San Antonio, TX
3. Tampa VA Medical Center - Tampa, FL
4. Minneapolis VA Medical Center - Minneapolis, MN
5. Palo Alto CA Medical Center - Palo Alto, CA
6. Richmond VA Medical Center - Richmond, VA
7. Balboa Naval Medical Center - San Diego, CA

For more information on the DVHIP, contact:
Defense Veteran's Head Injury Program
Walter Reed Army Medical Center
Building 1, Second Floor
Washington, DC 20307-5001
Fax: 202-782-4400

Guardianship

Time passes quickly and children become adults. Once your child with TBI reaches age eighteen, the law presumes that she is competent and independent—capable of caring for herself and making her own decisions. If your child is not capable of managing her own life, you should consider formally appointing a legal guardian for her.

Guardianship may be of the person, of the estate, or both. A guardian of the person assumes responsibility for the personal welfare of that individual. This usually includes decisions about medical care, vocational development, education, assistive and supplemental services, residence, diet, and leisure activities. A guardian of the estate cares for and manages the property of the person with a disability, controlling and making decisions with regard to investments, assets, and disposition of property.

To appoint a guardian for your child, you will need to initiate a court proceeding in which you present evidence setting forth the need for a guardian. Guardianship proceedings deal with the issue of competency. Although there is some variability from state to state, the central issue is always whether the individual is capable of managing his or her own affairs, or instead is *"suffering from a disability by reason of which (he/she) is not mentally capable of managing (his/her) personal affairs, as shown by the certificates of two (2) physicians attached to the Petition for Appointment of a Guardian."*

Each state has strict rules governing the role and the responsibilities of guardians. These are usually readily available at the public library.

Estate Planning

Everyone, no matter how modest their means, has an estate. An estate is simply whatever property and entitlement a person may have. Planning out what will happen to your estate after your death is especially important for parents of a child with TBI if there are doubts that she will be able to support herself independently as an adult. It is your best guarantee that your hope and plans for your child's future will be realized.

An estate may be "planned" and administered through the use of various devices. Estate planning devices include, but are not limited to:

- Last will and testament
- Trusts (living, supplementary, or special needs, testamentary, and others)
- Durable power of attorney
- Appointment of health care agent (also known as a *medical power of attorney* or a *durable power of attorney with medical provisions*)
- Advanced medical directive (also known as a *living will*)

The sections below offer some general guidance on using these estate planning devices. However, the best way to make sure that your estate plan provides adequately for your child with TBI is to consult an attorney who is experienced in estate planning for families of children with disabilities. Individualized estate planning is vital because of the uniqueness of each child, that child's needs, the finances and assets of each family, and the fact that each state's laws are different.

Last Will and Testament

A Last Will and Testament is a written directive of how you want your estate to be handled. It may include instructions on:

- how to dispose of your remains;
- who is to handle your affairs after your death (the Executor or Personal Representative);
- who is to be the guardian of any minor children (if no other parent is living or responsible for the children);
- who to give your assets to (naming the Beneficiaries); and
- other potentially important instructions.

Having a well-written will is particularly important to parents of children with disabilities. An improperly made-out will can jeopardize your child's entitlements to federal, state, and local benefits. A poorly written will can also subject your child's assets to "cost of care liability," depending on what services she needs as an adult. In many states, people with disabilities who are receiving residential services or even daytime or vocational services are "liable" to pay for the cost of their services, if they are able to do so. This means the state may tap into funds your child inherits if your will is not constructed so as to specifically prevent funds from being used for cost of care.

Trusts

A trust is a powerful estate planning tool that can provide a secure financial future for your child with TBI while safeguarding other family assets and distributions. Through a trust, property is held by an individual or institution (known as the trustee) for the benefit of the disabled person (the beneficiary).

A full chapter could be written on this topic alone because a poorly structured trust can pose a great risk to your child or her caregiver. The most important thought you must come away with about trusts is this: **Never use a "boilerplate" or attempt to self-draft a trust.**

Every individual's situation is different. *Every* family's situation is unique. There are so very many types of trusts, and the consequences of a failed trust can be so expensive and disruptive that the consideration of and creation of a trust always requires special and careful professional advice. You *must* meet with a knowledgeable lawyer to determine which types of trusts will best address the particular needs of your family.

Special Needs Trust

The Supplemental or Special Needs Trust (SNT) is an excellent way for families to leave funds for children with TBI without disqualifying them from federal, state, and local benefit and assistance programs. You should always consider an SNT as a financial and investment management tool if your family receives any funds through a settlement or judgment.

The key characteristic of an SNT that distinguishes it from other tools that can be used to manage funds for your child is that funds in the trust are not considered your child's assets, nor considered available to your child. The individual named as the beneficiary of the SNT has no right to demand distribution or payments of any kind, has no ownership interest, and has no authority or control over administration of the trust. This means that agencies such as the Social Security Administration (SSA) do not consider the trust funds "available resources" in determining your child's eligibility for benefits.

Private funds are safeguarded in an SNT and used to enhance the quality of life for your child while she remains entitled to other benefits, such as Medicaid, Aid to Families with Dependent Children (AFDC), and Supplemental Security Income (SSI). Considering the vast array of services and care that are often important to the quality of life of TBI survivors, preserving access to these programs is critical. For example, Medicaid coverage is not limited to traditional medical services. Medicaid eligibility is often the factor that determines what is available to the individual in the way of residential care alternatives, rehabilitation, and case management services. Although the services available within any given program are ever changing, services available via Medicaid in the past have included long-term care and rehabilitation, group home and other care facilities, sheltered workshops, work activity rehabilitation and training, various therapies, and other client-centered services.

Durable General Powers of Attorney

A Durable General Power of Attorney is a written document that allows another person (the "attorney-in-fact") to act on behalf of the principal (the person granting the power of attorney). The instrument creating the relationship defines the scope and duration of the powers conferred upon the attorney-in-fact. Unlike a Limited Power of Attorney, the Durable General Power of Attorney, as the name implies, permits the attorney-in-fact to perform virtually every act that the principal could perform if present and competent. It is "durable" because the power of attorney persists even if you become incapacitated.

As children reach adulthood, parents lose "voice"—the standing and authority to actually act and speak for their adult child. Some children with brain injuries are not profoundly incapacitated or under guardianship, but still may wish to empower others (such as parents) to act on their behalf under certain circumstances. Likewise, parents of a child who requires more care might want to appoint someone to make decisions for their child if they become incapacitated. Power of Attorney should only be granted after a careful discussion with a lawyer.

NOTE: A Durable General Power is *not* recommended for everyone. If you have been married less than five years, are experiencing marital difficulties, or have less than *absolute* trust in the person to whom you would grant such a power, *don't do it.*

Individual situations and state guidelines should be taken into consideration, along with the current age of your child, in determining whether a Durable General Power of Attorney might be advisable. Again, talk to an attorney knowledgeable in issues related to children with disabilities about whether a Durable General Power might be right for your family.

Appointment of Health Care Agents

An Appointment of Health Care Agent (formerly called a Durable Health Care Power of Attorney) is a written document that gives another person, as a substitute for the patient, the power and authority to make decisions about health care and treatment.

The holder of the appointment can make medical decisions in place of the patient when the patient is disabled and cannot make such decisions. The holder can both authorize medical care and treatment and also direct the withdrawal of care and treatment.

An Appointment of Health Care Agent is considered a broader and more desirable grant of authority than an Advance Medical Directive, or "living will," since the Advance Medical Directive authorization is limited to situations where the patient has a terminal condition and death is imminent. With an Appointment of Health Care Agent the holder of the appointment is empowered to make specific health care decisions based on the then-known facts and some knowledge of what the patient wants.

A minor cannot hold an Appointment of Health Care Agent. However, as a minor comes of age, consideration of an Appointment of Health Care Agent is appropriate.

Advance Directives

An Advance Medical Directive (formerly called a living will) is a document in which someone, while competent to do so, expresses a wish that her life not be prolonged by artificial, extraordinary, or heroic measures. This type of directive does not involve disposing of one's property.

Through an Advance Directive, an individual can elect that under certain circumstances life not be extended by life-sustaining procedures, including the artificial administration of foods and liquids. The individual can also specify whether she would like medication administered to alleviate pain and suffering. Women can further stipulate any modifications that would be acceptable if they are pregnant at the time medical decisions need to be made.

Normally, an Advance Directive (or Living Will) becomes effective when the individual's condition is determined to be "terminal"—meaning that death is imminent and that there is no reasonable expectation of recovery, even if life-sustaining procedures are used. An Advance Directive would also clarify the patient's wishes if:

- she is in a persistent vegetative state;
- she is not conscious or aware of the environment or able to interact and there is no reasonable expectation of recovery; or
- she has an irreversible, end-stage condition caused by injury, disease, or illness for which treatment would be medically ineffective.

The laws applying to Advance Directives vary from state to state, so it's important to check the law of the state in which the individual resides.

An Advance Directive cannot be executed by a minor. However, as a minor comes of age, discussion about an Advance Directive may be appropriate.

▪▪ Life Care Plans

All of the tools described in the section above are broadly a part of estate planning for any family. A completely separate device, specifically to help plan for the lifetime needs of someone with a catastrophic injury, is a Life Care Plan.

A Life Care Plan can create a global view of your child's future. This view is presented in a document that summarizes the medical, psychosocial, educational, vocational, and daily living needs of your child with TBI.

The Life Care Plan addresses goals for rehabilitation, assesses your child's current needs, and projects future needs. It lends structure to the future and provides a coordinated approach for providers, consultants, and your family to create a foundation for the best possible care—care that will minimize medical complications and maximize your child's ability to function and care for herself. A properly prepared, complete Life Care Plan can be used to present your child's specific needs to decision makers such as insurance adjusters, case managers, lawyers, judges, and jurors. It helps them evaluate appropriate damages in the case, and it provides a rational, objective basis for negotiating for benefits or negotiating a structured settlement. Having a Life Care Plan can also make family-level estate planning easier.

If you are seeking damages for your child's injury, the plan can clarify your child's pain and suffering, loss of the enjoyment of life, and other noneconomic aspects of the claim. It adds depth and coloration to descriptions of your child's condition and of the impact of injuries, limitations, and disabilities.

Creating the Life Care Plan

To develop a Life Care Plan for your child, you may want to meet with a Life Care Planner. Usually this is someone who holds the degree of M.S., Ph.D., or R.N./B.S.N. and has extensive rehabilitation credentials, or a physician with the specialty of life care planning who has added training and experience.

The Life Care Planner can assess your child's current needs and goals for rehabilitation. He may also project your child's future needs.

A comprehensive and well-prepared Life Care Plan requires that the Life Care Planner:

- Become familiar with the nature and extent of your child's injury and the progress made toward recovery.
- Review all records regarding medical care to date.
- Consider the medical aspects of the disability. (See Chapter 2.)
- Consider the psychological aspects of the disability. (See Chapters 5 and 7.)
- Review all records relevant to your child's work history and assess the ability to function in the area of previous employment (if any).
- Consider all of your child's other skills.
- Assess your child's ability to work and hold a job.
- Administer whatever tests are necessary to assess your child's ability to work.
- Become familiar with the workplace in order to consider other types of employment for your child.
- Become familiar with pay scales for positions your child is capable of holding.
- Determine (reach an opinion on) your child's work-life expectancy, considering her current health.
- Project the amount of wages your child would have been likely to earn.
- Consider your child's current health status and determine future medical and rehabilitative needs.
- Address each area of need fully, so that the Life Care Plan can be offered into evidence at a trial, if need be.

∷ Assessing the Effects of TBI

Sometimes it might be necessary to show a cause-and-effect relationship between a certain event and your child's brain injury. Most often this occurs because you are considering litigation to establish fault (e.g., your child was injured in a motor vehicle collision, by a particular product, playing a particular sport, or during an assault). You might also need to make such an assessment to help your child access healthcare or other insurance benefits or government entitlements.

In conducting this assessment, you will need to carefully document the differences in your child's physical, cognitive, and psychosocial functioning before and after the incident. This chart lists areas that are frequently focused on in an attempt to document deficits your child might have subsequent to a particular event.

Decreased Physical Abilities

- Decreased functional capacity
- Decreased safety awareness
- Lack of endurance or strength
- Problems with walking, coordination, or use of limbs or body
- Problems seeing, hearing, or tasting
- Loss of feeling or sensation
- Loss of bowel or bladder control
- Difficulty speaking clearly
- Continuing medical problems such as seizures

Decreased Cognitive Abilities

- Problems with attention, concentration, memory
- Inability to self-regulate
- Impaired judgment
- Decreased processing skills
- Impaired organizational skills
- Problems with basic academics
- Difficulties handling money
- Difficulties beginning or following through on tasks

- Inability to reason clearly and solve problems
- Slower thought process
- Inability to say what is meant
- Difficulty understanding others
- Trouble following directions
- Inability to manage time
- Poor insight into problems

Changes in Behavior and Emotional Control

- Irritability
- Anxiety
- Depression/withdrawal
- Changes in control of temper
- Impulsivity
- Lack of initiation
- Lowered frustration tolerance
- Lack of energy
- Poor social interactions
- Strained family relations
- Anger, aggression, verbal outbursts
- Fear of the future
- Problems controlling behavior in social situations

Psychosocial Changes

- Inability to sustain relationships
- Inability to generalize (apply a skill learned in one situation to another similar situation)
- Denial of deficits

Potential Consequences of TBI

- Breakdown of family support systems
- Withdrawal of friends
- Physical deterioration
- Isolation
- Substance abuse
- Unemployment
- Increased health risk
- Increased risk of repeat hospitalization

∷ Balancing Your Child's Rights with What Is Right for Her

When a child has a brain injury, there is a tremendous desire to return to the life she had before the injury. Often this is accompanied by a belief that your child has a "right" to do certain things or participate (again, perhaps) in certain activities. Powerful desires on the part of your child and on your part, if you are too accommodating, can sometimes override wisdom or safety.

Getting a Driver's License. One area where parents and children frequently clash is over the right to drive. However, whether your child has previously been licensed, or is now approaching driving age and expressing a desire to get a license, safety is the first concern. Safety for your child (from reinjury), safety of others, and the legal consequences arising because of known deficits, limitations, or concerns must always be assessed.

In general, states do not specifically prohibit licensing or relicensing of drivers who have had a TBI. However, some states require that physicians inform the Motor Vehicle Administration about patients who have had injuries that may impair driving skills. Also, during the initial licensing or renewal process, some states ask questions as to whether

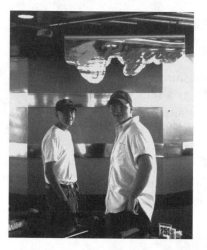

there are any conditions (such as seizures, blackouts, or physical or mental impairments) that may affect driving abilities.

If your child was previously licensed, it is best to have her driving skills retested. There are driver evaluation programs associated with some rehabilitation centers, and the Motor Vehicle Administration can also do retests. This retesting reduces the likelihood of an issue of "negligent entrustment" being raised if there were a later accident. (It also increases the likelihood that your child will not be back on the road before it is safe!) Children who have not previously been licensed should likewise be evaluated by an instructor who has worked with drivers with disabilities to ensure that perceptual and cognitive skills are adequate.

:: Subpoena, Summons, and Official Notices

Do not ignore any subpoena, summons, or official notices; do not ignore even what you view as "unofficial" notices! Whatever it is—*read it carefully*...and then *read it again*. Usually there are rather specific instructions, although they may be unsettling because they usually use some type of "command" language. Follow up right away. Delay can cause problems, even a shift in status from "entitled" to "unentitled" and create new complications or hurdles not previously anticipated.

Example: Parents of a now-adult with TBI had previously sought and obtained guardianship for him in their state of residence. But when they moved from state to state, they failed to take the steps necessary to maintain the guardianship. Eleven years after their child's injury, the county sought and obtained guardianship against the will of the parents due to behavioral issues. The county then had the adult child admitted to a psychiatric hospital and authorized treatment with drugs—all of which the parents were vociferously opposed to. This was only able to occur because the parents had failed to attend to official notices in a timely manner.

:: In Closing

Learning about all the legal issues that confront you when your child has a head injury can be overwhelming—especially if you feel that your hands are already full taking care of your child's medical, educational, and emotional needs. But if your child is going to have the best quality of life possible, you *must* understand her rights, benefits, and entitlements, as well as how to obtain them. Fortunately, there are many individuals—including attorneys and staff at advocacy and disability organizations—who can help you understand the right course of action for your child and your family. You can do it if you take it day by day, a step at a time.

:: Reference

Mark J. Ashley, Craig S. Persel, David K. Kruch. "Changes in the Reimbursement Climate: the Relationship among Outcome, Cost and Payor Type in the Postacute Rehabilitation Environment," Fourth Conference of the International Association for the Study of Traumatic Brain Injury (IASTBI), 1994.

▓▓ Parent Statements

I never imagined that I would have to be an expert in special education and the law.

⋖⊱⊰⋗

I worry the most about his future. How will he survive as an adult? Who will take care of him if and when he's on his own?

⋖⊱⊰⋗

Parents are supposed to be equal partners with teachers at IEP meetings, but it can be really intimidating to sit around a table of school professionals. I just had to convince myself and them that I knew my child the best.

⋖⊱⊰⋗

I feel very fortunate that I live in a state that has a law prohibiting health insurance companies from excluding people from coverage due to "pre-existing conditions." At least I don't have to worry about what would happen if I ever changed jobs and lost my insurance.

⋖⊱⊰⋗

It really stinks to find out that you make too much money for your child to qualify for government benefits like Medicaid, when you know how much you could use the financial assistance. To make matters worse, I know from e-mailing parents in other states that some states have waivers to let families qualify even if their income exceeds the limit. Of course, my state is not one of them.

⋖⊱⊰⋗

I feel like I want to wait and see how independent our son might be as an adult before we disinherit him or appoint a guardian or anything like that. I know this is not good estate planning, but that's the way I am.

⋖⊱⊰⋗

Before we had children, we had a will drawn up that said my sister and her husband would be the guardians of any children we might have in the event of our deaths. Now I feel as if I ought to go back to my sister and ask her if it's still OK for her to be listed as the guardian, but I'm afraid to ask. What if she says "no"?

✦

I'm glad to know that there are federal laws prohibiting various types of discrimination against people with disabilities. I sure do wish they didn't apply to any members of my family, though.

✦

I feel so much more confident at IEP meetings than I used to. Once you have a good grip on your child's needs and what the school is obligated to provide, it's much easier to ask them to add specific goals and services to the IEP. The worst they can do is say "no," and even if they do, you can still argue with them and try to make your case. The more information you bring along to back up your point, the better. It helps a lot if you can pass around photocopies from books that back up what you say.

APPENDIX

SCALES USED TO ASSESS PATIENTS WITH TRAUMATIC BRAIN INJURY

■ Glasgow Coma Scale

(Usually administered within the first 24 to 48 hours.)

1. Eye opening response to stimulation [opens eyes]
   Spontaneously 4
   To sound 3
   To pain 2
   Never 1

2. Movement response to stimulation [best motor/physical response]
   Follows commands 6
   Localizes pain 5
      (attempts to remove painful stimulus)
   Withdraws in response to pain 4
   Abnormal flexion (bending)in response to pain 3
   Abnormal extension (straightening) in response to pain 2
   No response 1

3. Spoken response to stimulation [best verbal response]
   Oriented (normal conversation) 5
   Confused conversation 4
   Inappropriate words 3
   Incomprehensible sounds 2
   None 1

■ Modified Glasgow Coma Scale

(For children age 3 and younger, the spoken response may be scored as follows.)

3. Best verbal response to stimulation
   Oriented (social smile, oriented to sound, follows objects) 5

Confused/disoriented (crying, consolable) 4
Inappropriate words/crying 3
Restless, agitated 2
No Response 1

Using the Glasgow Coma Scale, severity is rated according to the following scores:
- Mild - GCS 13-15;
- Moderate - GCS 9-12;
- Severe - GCS 3-8.

■■ Rancho Los Amigos Cognitive Scale

Goals
1. To document systematically the TBI patient's behavioral responses to people and things in the environment.
2. To allow some limited ability to predict what types of behaviors can be expected from the patient in the future.
3. To allow for suggestions as to how to help the patient interact and communicate with the family, friends and medical staff more effectively and consistently.

Scale
Level I: No response to pain, touch, sound, or sight.
Level II: Generalized reflex response to pain.
Level III: Localized response. Blinks to strong light, turns toward/away from sound, responds to physical discomfort, inconsistent response to commands.
Level IV: Confused—Agitated. Alert, very active, aggressive or bizarre behaviors, performs motor activities, but behavior is non-purposeful, extremely short attention span.
Level V: Confused—Non-agitated. Gross attention to environment, highly distractible, requires continual redirection, difficulty relearning new tasks, agitated by too much stimulation. May engage in social conversation but with inappropriate verbalizations.
Level VI: Confused—Appropriate. Inconsistent orientation to time and place, retention span/recent memory impaired, begins to recall past, consistently follows simple directions, goal-directed behavior with assistance.
Level VII: Automatic—Appropriate. Performs daily routine in highly familiar environment in a non-confused but automatic robot-like manner. Skills noticeably deteriorate in unfamiliar environment. Lacks realistic planning for own future.
Level VIII: Purposeful—Appropriate.

Note: As patients improve after a brain injury, they may move from one level to the next, but often demonstrate characteristics of more than one level at a time. Depending on the extent and type of injury, they may remain at any one level for an extended period of time.

GLOSSARY

ABC Method—technique for evaluating and tracking undesirable *target behaviors* that analyzes: A—*Antecedent*, or what happens prior to a behavior; B—*Behavior*, or what happens as a result of *A*; and C—*Consequence*, or what happens as a result of *B*. *See also* Duration Method; Frequency Count.

Abducens—One of the three *cranial nerves* involved in movements of the eyeball and pupil. *See also* Oculomotor; Trochlear.

Abnormal—Not typical or average.

Accommodation—An adaptation of the classroom environment, format, or situation made to suit the *special needs* of a student. The adaptation does not alter the content or level of the material, or expectations of the student. *See also* Modification.

Active Ignoring—Briefly removing all *reinforcement* (attention, scolding, eye contact) when your child is engaged in a mildly annoying *behavior* in an effort to avoid accidentally reinforcing a behavior you wish to eliminate. Also known as *planned ignoring*. *See also* Extinction Burst.

Activities of Daily Living (ADL)—The accumulation of knowledge and the ability to perform the self-care tasks required to live independently in the natural environment. Such life skills include eating, dressing, grooming, and bathing. Also called *functional abilities*, functional life skills, or self-help skills.

Acuity—Keenness of vision; refers to the ability to see clearly.

Acute—Refers to the most severe and critical period of a disease or injury.

Acute Care Hospital—A medical facility whose primary goals are to provide diagnosis of disease and to stabilize patients. *See also* Initial Course; Intensive Care Unit.

Acute Management Stage—Care provided to a patient during the initial period of hospitalization.

ADA—*See* Americans with Disabilities Act.

Adaptive Equipment—Devices that assist in and promote the recovery process by optimizing your child's physical and psychological independence, energy, efficiency, and safety, and preventing secondary problems. Also known as *assistive devices* or *assistive technology*.

Adaptive Physical Education Teacher—A physical education teacher with special training or knowledge in adapting activities for children with *disabilities*. Also known as *motor teacher*.

ADH—*See* Antidiuretic Hormone.

ADL—*See* Activities of Daily Living.

Administrative Law Judge (ALJ)—An impartial hearing officer who presides over a *due process hearing*.

Admission, Review, and Dismissal (ARD)—A group or committee made up of teachers and other professionals responsible for the admission of children to *special education*, review of the progress of children in special education programs, and dismissal of children from special education.

Advance Medical Directive—A document in which someone, while competent to do so, expresses a wish that his life not be prolonged by artificial, extraordinary, or heroic measures. This type of directive does not involve the disposing of one's property. Formerly called a *living will*.

Advocacy—Supporting or promoting a cause. Speaking out.

AED—*See* Antiepileptic Drug.

AFO—*See* Ankle Foot Orthosis.

Age Equivalent Score—In formal testing, a converted score that expresses the child's score in terms of chronological age equivalency. *See also* Formal Assessment; Percentile Rank; Standard Score.

Alternating Attention—The ability to shift focus from one task to another. *See also* Attention; Divided Attention; Selective Attention; Sustained Attention.

Americans with Disabilities Act (ADA)—A federal law that prohibits *discrimination* against people with *disabilities* in employment, public accommodations, and access to public facilities. It also mandates that businesses and public and private entities make *reasonable accommodations* for persons with *special needs*.

Amnesia—*See* Amnestic Syndrome.

Amnestic Syndrome—A relatively rare condition that results in persistent, severe impairment in the ability to acquire (store) and retrieve new factual information with otherwise preserved *cognitive* function. Also known as *amnesia*. *See also* Post-traumatic Amnesia.

Anesthesia—Administering drugs to induce loss of *consciousness* and sensation.

Ankle Foot Orthosis (AFO)—An *adaptive device* made of lightweight plastic that is worn inside the shoe to provide support to the ankle and foot.

Annual Goal—An educational or developmental goal set for a child with *disabilities* and outlined in their *IEP*. Progress toward these goals is discussed during the *annual review* meeting.

Annual Review—Yearly meeting to review a student's *IEP*.

Anomia—Word-finding difficulties.

Antecedent—The conditions (actions, locations, people, time of day, interactions, emotions, and thoughts) that occur immediately prior to occurrence of a *target behavior*. *See also* ABC Method.

Antecedent Strategy—A tactic designed to prevent the occurrence of an undesirable *target behavior*. *See also* ABC Method; Antecedent.

Antibody—A protein produced by the *immune system*, which fights infection, keeping the body healthy.

Antidiuretic Hormone (ADH)—The *hormone* secreted by the *pituitary gland* that tells the kidneys to conserve free water in the body. *See also* Syndrome of Inappropriate ADH.

Antiepileptic Drug (AED)—Medication administered to prevent *seizures*. *See also* Carbamazepine; Epilepsy; Phenobarbital; Post traumatic Epilepsy; Valproic Acid.

Appointment of Health Care Agent—A written document that gives another person, as a substitute for the patient, the power and authority to make decisions about their health care and treatment. Formerly called *Durable Health Care Power of Attorney*.

Apraxia—The inability to make or plan the movements needed to produce sounds or words. *See also* Dyspraxia.

Arachnoid—The protective *membrane* that is attached to the surface of the brain. *See also* Dura Mater; Meninges; Pia Mater.

Arousal—One's general state of alertness, ranging from *coma* to extremely focused vigilance.

Articulation Therapy—Therapy administered by a *Speech-Language Pathologist* to help a child produce more precise *speech* sounds. *See also* Motor Speech Disorders.

Assessment—The process used to determine a child's strengths and weaknesses, either to develop a treatment plan or a plan to address the child's needs for special education. Includes informal and formal testing and observations performed by one or more professionals. Term may be used interchangeably with Evaluation.

Asset—Anything owned that has marketable value. *See also* Estate Planning.

Assistive Devices—*See* Adaptive Equipment.

Assistive Technology—A device that is used to maintain or improve the function of a child with special needs.

Assistive Technology Specialist—Someone with expertise in selecting, obtaining, and using *assistive technology* for children with special needs.

Atrophy—Shrinkage, wasting away.

Attention—Mental alertness and concentration; a prerequisite to all *conscious* and voluntary *cognitive* activity. *See also* Alternating Attention; Divided Attention; Selective Attention; Sustained Attention.

Attention Deficit Disorder (ADD)—This term is sometimes used to refer to AD/HD without hyperactivity. *See also* Attention-Deficit/Hyperactivity Disorder (AD/HD).

Attention-Deficit/Hyperactivity Disorder (AD/HD)—A condition characterized by distractibility, restlessness, short *attention* span, *impulsivity*, and sometimes *hyperactivity*.

Audiologist—A professional who assesses and treats hearing loss.

Auditory—Relating to the ability to hear.

Augmentative Communication Device—A piece of equipment that allows a person to communicate without using *speech*.

Aura—An unusual sensation (through any of the senses) that may alert a person to an impending *seizure*.

Autonomic—Describes processes within the body that occur without deliberate thought or action.

Aversive—An unpleasant *stimulus* that follows an undesirable *target behavior*. *See also* Behavioral Contingency.

Axon—The part of a *neuron* (nerve cell) that conducts impulses, resulting in the stimulation of another *cell* (neuron, gland, or muscle fiber). *See also* Myelin.

Baclofen—Medication used to relax rigid, tight muscles throughout the body. *See also* High Tone. Also known as *Lioresal*™.

Basal Ganglia—Areas located below the *cerebral hemispheres* which helps control habitual movements and posture.

Behavior—The way a person acts or conducts himself. *See also* Target Behavior.

Behavioral Contingency—Refers to a principle of learning that states that *behavior* is determined by its *consequence*: if a child likes the *consequence* of his behavior, he will continue practicing that behavior, and visa versa. *See also* ABC Method; Aversive.

Behavioral Observation—Watching and assessing a child's *behavior* in a variety of settings and contexts. *See also* Informal Assessment.

Behavioral Psychologist—A psychologist who assists parents and teachers in decreasing problem *behaviors* and increasing appropriate behaviors in children.

Benchmark—*See* Short-term Benchmark.

Beneficiary—A person indicated in a *trust* or insurance policy to receive any payments that become due. *See also* Trustee.

Blind Spot—Loss of vision in the specific area of the *retina* that is connected to an area of damage in the brain. Condition results from localized injury to the *primary zone* of the *occipital lobe*. Also known as *scotoma*.

Blindsight—A *visual* system, second to the primary *occipital lobe,* that perceives an object's presence and location, without actual awareness of its existence, but provides no information about its specific features or identity.

Bolus—The clump or mass of chewed food formed in the mouth during the *oral phase* of swallowing and delivered to the stomach during the *pharyngeal phase*.

Botox™—A trade name for *botulinum toxin*.

Botulinum Toxin—A drug injected directly into muscle with *high tone,* in order to relax and lower the tone of that muscle. Also known as *Botox™*.

Brainstem—Made up of the *midbrain* and *hindbrain* (not including the *cerebellum*), the brainstem is the pathway between the *diencephalon* and *spinal cord* and is responsible for basic bodily functions such as breathing and heart rate.

Brainstem Arousal Unit—One of the three functional units of the brain responsible for regulating the level of alertness of the entire brain; a certain level is necessary for any organized mental activity to occur. *See also* Response Output Unit; Sensory, Reception, Processing, and Storage Unit.

Carbamazepine—One of the most commonly prescribed *antiepileptic drugs* used to control *post-traumatic seizures*. Also known as *Tegretol™*.

Care Manager—A qualified coordinator of services and equipment for a patient who has sustained a *TBI*; provides a link between health care providers, patient, and insurance carrier.

Case Manager—An individual designated to oversee the education and *related services* for a child with *disabilities* and the services provided to his family. Also known as *service coordinator*.

Catheter—A hollow tube inserted into an opening in the body that allows for the passage of fluids.

CBLA—*See* Curriculum Based Language Assessment.

Cell—The smallest unit of a living organism; the basic structure for tissue and organs.

Cellular—Consisting of or pertaining to *cells*.

Central Nervous System (CNS)—Made up of the brain and *spinal cord*, this system is responsible for controlling what we think and do.

Cerebellum—The part of the *hindbrain*, located under the *occipital lobes*, which connects to the rest of the brain by tracts that enter the *brainstem*. Responsible for *equilibrium* and the coordination of *voluntary muscle activity*, it also plays a role in the modulation of *muscle tone*.

Cerebral Hemispheres—The right and left sections of the *cerebrum*, separated by a deep crevice and subdivided into four *lobes* each. *See also* Dominant Hemisphere; Left Cerebral Hemisphere; Limbic System; Nondominant Hemisphere; Right Cerebral Hemisphere.

Cerebrospinal Fluid (CSF)—Fluid in the *subarachnoid* space that cushions the brain during movement. *See also* Ventricular System.

Cerebrum—Made up of the *right* and *left cerebral hemispheres*, it is the part of the brain that controls *conscious* and voluntary processes. The cerebrum and *diencephalon* make up the *forebrain*.

Chaining—A process in which a child masters a complex skill by learning its components step by step and then putting them together. *See also* Task Analysis.

CHI—*See* Closed Head Injury.

Chunking—Grouping related information together for the purpose of storing more information in *short-term memory*. This process increases the likelihood that the information will make it into *long-term memory*.

Circumlocute—To talk "around" a topic without ever getting to the point.

Client Assistance Programs (CAP)—Programs that help people with *disabilities*, their families, or agency representatives obtain information and access to the array of services available through programs, projects, and facilities funded under the *Rehabilitation Act of 1973, Title V*.

Closed Head Injury (CHI)—The most common type of *head injury*. It does not involve penetration of the *dura mater*.

CNS—*See* Central Nervous System.

Cognition—The ability to know and understand the environment and to solve problems.

Cognitive—Relating to *cognition*.

Coma—A state of decreased responsiveness to external or internal *stimuli* following injury to the brain; characterized by lack of voluntary eye opening, response to simple commands, and comprehensible *speech*. *See also* Comatose.

Comatose—The state of being in a *coma*.

Compensate—To adopt or design new techniques to solve problems and make up for inabilities.

Compliance—When a child meets the terms of your request with no more than a brief delay.

Computerized Tomography Scan (CT Scan)—A procedure that uses computerized X-rays to show pictures of cross sections of the brain or body.

Conceptual Organization—Refers to the process of categorizing information so that concepts can be stored in the brain and retrieved when needed.

Concussion—A mild *head injury*, with or without short loss of *consciousness*. *See also* Postconcussion Syndrome.

Confabulation—Sometimes mistaken for intentional lying, this is a *compensatory* process of filling in gaps in memory with fictitious information. *See also* Expressive Language; Irrelevant Conversational Speech; Tangential Conversational Speech.

Congenital—Inherent; born with.

Consciousness—The state of being aware of one's feelings and surroundings.

Consequence—The conditions, either positive or negative, that take place immediately following a *behavior*; believed to determine whether or not the child will repeat the same behavior in the future. *See also* ABC Method.

Contingency Contract—A type of *positive reinforcement*, in the form of a contract, designed for older children and adolescents, that spells out all of the events (contingencies) that will occur if the child performs certain *behaviors*.

Contingency Fee System—A system of compensation in which a lawyer receives a percentage of the financial award(s) as his or her fee for successful representation. The injured party's family do not pay attorney fees if they lose in court.

Contracture—Limitations in range of motion of body parts and joints due to muscle and soft tissue shortening. *See also* High Tone.

Contrecoup Contusion—A bruise on the brain 180 degrees from the place where an individual's head has been struck; where the opposite side of the brain has hit against the inside of the skull with speed. *See also* Contusion; Coup Contusion.

Contusion—A bruise. A brain contusion can result in the death or disruption of *cells*. *See* Coup Contusion; Contrecoup Contusion; Immediate Injury.

Coordinated Rehabilitation Continuum—A system of care that provides *rehabilitation* therapies in various settings and at various intensities, allowing the person served to move from one setting to another as dictated by their changing needs and abilities.

Corporal Punishment—Physical punishment that includes spanking, paddling, swatting, and other forms of striking a child, generally across the buttocks.

Cortex—The part of the brain made up of *gray matter.* It makes up the outer area of the *cerebral hemispheres* where the *cell* bodies of the nerve cells (*neurons*) are located. *See also* Cortical.

Cortical—Referring to the *cortex* of the brain.

Cost-of-Care Liability—The right of a state providing care to a person with *disabilities* to charge for that care and to collect from that person's *assets.*

Coup Contusion—A bruise on the *cortex* of the brain at the point of contact where the individual's head has been struck. *See also* Contrecoup Contusion; Contusion.

Cranial Nerve Dysfunction—Disruption of the *cranial nerves* due to swelling, bleeding, or other sources of pressure in the brain caused by *TBI.*

Cranial Nerves—Twelve pairs of nerves arising in the brain or *brainstem* that control muscles located in the head, such as those for eye movement, talking, swallowing, and smiling. Cranial nerves also receive *sensory* information from the head.

Critical Life Skill—Any skill on your child's *IEP* that the *multidisciplinary team* deems critical to his overall educational progress.

CSF—*See* Cerebrospinal Fluid.

CT Scan—*See* Computerized Tomography Scan.

Cue—Gestures or words that prompt a person to perform a *behavior* or activity. Also known as *prompt.*

Curriculum Based Language Assessment (CBLA)—An *informal assessment* used to identify the *language* demands of your child's school curriculum and how well your child handles those demands. Recognizing what strategies your child is employing and what *modifications* can be made to minimize language challenges through this method is useful in developing instructional goals that are meaningful to your child.

DAI—*See* Diffuse Axonal Injury.

Dantrium™—A trade name for *dantrolene.*

Dantrolene—*Oral* medication used to reduce *high tone* in muscles throughout the body. Also known as *Dantrium*™.

Declarative Memory—Memory for facts and episodes of personal experience. *See also* Hippocampus.

Defense and Veterans Head Injury Program (DVHIP)—A program whose goal is to ensure that all military and Department of Veterans' Affairs personnel with *TBI* receive appropriate evaluation and services for their injuries.

Deficit—A lack of something necessary or fundamental.

Delayed Injury—A secondary injury that occurs after a *TBI*, such as *edema, hemorrhage, herniation syndrome, hypoxic ischemic injury*, and damage from the *neurotoxic cascade. See also* Immediate Injury.

Delusion—A false belief.

Depakene™—A trade name for *valproic acid*.

Developmental Delay—A term used to describe an infant or child who is not exhibiting age-appropriate *behaviors* or acquiring skills at the same rate as other children. Developmental delays may or may not be outgrown.

Developmental Disability—A condition originating before the age of eighteen that may be expected to continue indefinitely and that impairs or delays development of skills and impairs the child's ability to function independently in society.

Dexedrineä—A trade name for *dextroamphetamine*.

Dextroamphetamine—A stimulant medication sometimes prescribed to treat *AD/HD*. Also known as *Dexedrineä*.

Diabetes Insipidus (DI)—A condition that *can* but rarely does occur after very severe *TBI*, in which too little *antidiuretic hormone* is secreted, resulting in rapid, large losses of water in the urine, leading to dehydration. Not related to "sugar" diabetes.

Diencephalon—A part of the *forebrain* made up of the *thalamus* and *hypothalamus*. *See* Cerebrum.

Differential Reinforcement—A process in which *positive reinforcement* is withheld in an effort to diminish or eliminate a child's undesirable *behaviors. See also* Reinforcement.

Diffuse—A spreading out. In relation to *TBI*, it refers to a *head injury* affecting multiple areas throughout the brain. *See also* Focal.

Diffuse Axonal Injury (DAI)—Injury to the *axons* throughout the brain. Also known as *shearing injury. See also* Immediate Injury.

Dilation—Becoming wider or larger.

Disability—A term used to describe a delay in physical or *cognitive* development. The older term *"handicap"* is also sometimes used.

Disability Determination Service (DDS)—A state office that reviews all documents and evidence pertaining to a child's *disability* and decides whether he is eligible for *SSI* based on its definition of disability.

Discrimination—Showing favor toward one person, race, or group and prejudice toward another.

Disinhibition—Speaking or acting without thinking it through first, resulting in socially unacceptable *behavior*.

Dislocation—When a bone comes out of its socket at a joint.

Divided Attention—The ability to attend to multiple tasks, or multiple components of a task, simultaneously. *See also* Alternating Attention; Attention; Selective Attention; Sustained Attention.

Dominant Hemisphere—Either the right or left section of the *cerebrum*, depending on the individual, which usually controls the dominant hand and *verbal* functions: *speech* and *language*, including reading and writing, and calculations. *See also* Cerebral Hemispheres; Nondominant Hemisphere.

Due Process Hearing—The first step in an appeal process, under *IDEA*, that allows both the parents and the school system to present their sides of the "case" concerning the child's *special education*. An *administrative law judge* is required to review the evidence, hear witness testimony, and then render a decision.

Dura—Abbreviation of *dura mater*.

Dura Mater—The tough *membrane* attached to the inner surface of the skull that helps protect the brain. *See also* Arachnoid; Meninges; Pia Mater.

Durable General Power of Attorney—A written document that allows an individual to perform virtually every act that the person granting the power of attorney could perform if present and competent.

Durable Health Care Power of Attorney—*See* Appointment of Health Care Agent.

Duration Method—A means of tracking an undesirable *target behavior* by noting the length of time a child engages in that behavior. *See also* ABC Method; Frequency Count.

Dysarthria—Slow and labored *speech*, sometimes with imprecise *articulation*, that can occur in the initial phases of recovery from *TBI*.

Dysfluency—*Speech* that is characterized by repetitions of sounds, syllables, words, or phrases, which impair its overall flow. Also known as *stuttering*, dysfluent speech often occurs in the initial phases of recovery from *TBI*.

Dyspraxia—Difficulty making the movements needed to produce sounds or words. *See also* Apraxia.

ED—*See* Emotionally Disturbed.

Edema—Swelling due to accumulation of fluids. In relation to *TBI*, it is a swelling of the brain. *See also* Delayed Injury; Syndrome of Inappropriate ADH; Transependymal Edema.

EEG—*See* Electroencephalogram.

Electroencephalogram (EEG)—A noninvasive, painless test that records the brain's electrical activity (brainwaves) and may show *abnormal* patterns associated with injuries or *seizures*.

Electrolytes—Compounds (or salts) in the body, such as sodium, potassium, and chloride, which play a basic role in the health and activity of *cells*, and are easily measured in the blood.

Emotional Lability—Describes dramatic mood swings, common in individuals with *TBI*, caused by damage to the *frontal lobes*. *See also* Flat Affect.

Emotionally Disturbed (ED)—Having a *learning disability* or *behavioral* disturbance characterized by an inability to learn, or maintain normal relationships with peers and teachers. Children with *TBI* were frequently categorized as being emotionally disturbed before *IDEA* included TBI as a *disability*. Formerly known as *seriously emotionally disturbed*.

Endocrine System—The system of internal glands of the body (such as *pituitary*, thyroid, and adrenal), which make and secrete *hormones* that then produce specific effects in the body.

Endoscope—A tool consisting of a lighted tube with a camera at the end that is inserted into the body to enable a doctor to examine the inside of a body cavity.

Environmental Modifications—Adaptations to a child's surroundings that allow him to function more easily and appropriately according to his physical and *behavioral* needs.

Environmental Prompt—A reminder (such as a note) placed in a child's environment to *cue* him to perform a particular action.

Epidural Hematoma—Bleeding between the skull and *dura mater*.

Epilepsy—A chronic condition in which abnormal electrical activity in the brain causes *seizures*.

Equilibrium—A state of balance and stability.

Esophagitis—Inflammation of the *esophagus*.

Esophagus—The tube leading from the throat to the stomach, through which food and fluids pass. *See also* Pharyngeal Phase.

Estate Planning—Formal written arrangements for handling the possessions and *assets* of people after they have died. *See also* Estate.

ESY—*See* Extended School Year.

Evaluation—*See* Assessment.

Executive Function—*Cognitive* or thinking abilities that allow us to have self-regulated, goal-directed *behavior*.

Expressive Language—Using *language* in the form of gestures, words, and written symbols to express oneself. *See also* Language; Receptive Language.

Extended School Year (ESY)—Extension of *special education* or *related services*, provided for your child by the school district, beyond the regular school year.

Extinction Burst—A brief, but significant, increase in the frequency or intensity of a *target behavior* that can occur after the technique of *active ignoring* is employed.

Fading—A process of steering a child through the steps of a task, then gradually withdrawing, or fading physical guidance and *verbal prompts* as he learns the new *behavior*.

FAPE—*See* Free Appropriate Public Education.

Fine Motor—Related to the use of the small muscles of the body, such as those in the hands, feet, fingers, and toes. *See also* Gross Motor, Motor.

Fissure—Deep crevice or gap.

Flat Affect—Describes apparent emotional indifference, common in individuals with *TBI*. *See also* Emotional Lability.

Focal—Refers to a *head injury* that affects only a localized or contained area of the brain. *See also* Diffuse.

Focal Seizure—*See* Partial Seizure.

Foot Drop—A term used to describe the inability to lift up the toes and foot while walking.

Forebrain—The most highly developed of the three major sections of the brain, it is made up of the *cerebrum* and *diencephalon*.

Formal Assessment—A battery of *standardized* tests, based on norms, administered in a low-distraction, one-to-one setting. The overall purpose of this type of testing is to compare performance after *TBI* to performance before TBI and to determine areas of strength and weakness. The results of these tests will be expressed as *age equivalent scores, percentile rank*, or *standard scores*. *See also* Informal Assessment.

Fracture—A crack, split, or break in a body part, especially bone.

"Free Appropriate Public Education" (FAPE)—The right, under *IDEA,* of every child with *disabilities* to an education provided at public expense that is appropriate to the child's developmental strengths and needs. *See also* Public Law 94-142, Education for All Handicapped Children Act of 1975.

Freedom From Distractibility—*See* Selective Attention.

Frequency Count—A means of tracking an undesirable *target behavior* by counting the number of times it occurs during a defined period of time. *See also* ABC Method; Duration Method.

Frontal Lobe—One of the four *lobes* in each *cerebral hemisphere*, which assist in coordinating fine movement, the *motor* aspect of *speech*, *executive function*, motivation, social skills, and certain parts of what we call personality.

Frustration Tolerance—The ability to accept merely the *anticipation* of a desired goal (represented in *working memory*) as an effective stand-in for the actual thing.

FSIQ—*See* Full Scale IQ.

Full Scale IQ (FSIQ)—The combined results of the *Verbal IQ* and *Performance IQ* subtests of the *Wechsler Intelligence Scale for Children-Third Edition*, which yield an estimate of overall intellectual ability.

Functional Abilities—*See* Activities of Daily Living.

G Tube—*See* Gastrostomy Tube.

Gastroesophageal Reflux (GER)—Regurgitation of food from the stomach up through the *esophagus*, which can cause heartburn, *esophagitis*, and increased chance of stomach contents going up and then down the wrong way into the lungs.

Gastrostomy Tube (G Tube)—A tube used to feed and provide fluid and nutriment to an individual who is unable to adequately maintain their own hydration and nutrition. The tube is inserted through an artificial opening on the surface of the abdomen into the stomach. *See also* Nasogastric Tube; Percutaneous Endoscopic Gastrostomy Tube.

GCS—*See* Glasgow Coma Scale.

Generalization—The application of learned information to a novel situation.

Generalized Seizure—A *seizure* that affects the function of the entire brain.

GER—*See* Gastroesophageal Reflux.

Glasgow Coma Scale (GCS)—A scale developed by *neurosurgeons* to judge the severity (mild, moderate, or severe) of a brain injury by objectively assessing improvement or deterioration. It consists of three subtests: best eye, *verbal*, and *motor* response.

Grandma Rule—*See* Premack Principle.

Gray Matter—The parts of the brain, including the outer surface of the *cerebral hemispheres*, made up of the bodies of the brain *cells*. *See also* Cortex.

Gross Motor—The use of the large muscles of the body, such as those of the back, legs, and arms. *See also* Fine Motor; Motor.

Growth Plate—The area near the end of a bone where the bone is still growing.

Guardian—A person appointed by law to manage the welfare, legal, and financial affairs of another person or his or her *estate*. *See also* Estate Planning.

Gyri—Ridges on the surface of the *right* and *left hemispheres* of the *cerebrum*.

Habilitation—The process of assisting someone with the acquisition of new skills and abilities.

Hallucination—The sensation of hearing or seeing something that is not real.

Handicap—An outdated term referring to some form of *disability*, including physical disability, *mental retardation*, *sensory* impairment, *behavioral* disorder, *learning disability*, or combination of the above. *See also* Multihandicapped.

Handicapped Children's Protection Act of 1986—A federal law that states that parents or *guardians* may be able to recover attorneys' fees when they prevail in any dispute concerning *special educational* services provided for their child under *IDEA*.

Head Injury—Trauma to the head that can result in a bone fracture in the skull or face, or bruises or cuts to the head and face. Does not necessarily result in a brain injury.

Hematoma—A blood clot situated outside a blood vessel.

Hemiparesis—A condition characterized by weakness on one side of the body.

Hemisphere—*See* Cerebral Hemisphere.

Hemorrhage—Bleeding where blood vessels have been torn or disrupted. *See also* Delayed Injury; Intracerebral Hemorrhage; Intraventricular Hemorrhage; Subarachnoid Hemorrhage.

Herniation Syndrome—A condition in which the brain's shape is deformed due to the pressure produced by a localized mass or area of swelling squeezing it into the remaining space within the *intracranial space*. *See also* Delayed Injury.

Heterotopic Ossification (HO)—When new bone forms in *abnormal* places, such as in the muscles of the body.

High Tone—Describes an increased tightness in muscles; the two types are *spasticity* and *rigidity*. *See also* Baclofen; Botulinum Toxin; Dantrolene; Tizanidine.

Hindbrain—The furthest back of the three major divisions of the brain, it contains the *cerebellum*. The hindbrain (not including the cerebellum) and *midbrain* make up the *brainstem*.

Hippocampus—Part of the *limbic system*, it is the seahorse-shaped structure in the *temporal lobe* that is essential in the formation of new *declarative memories*.

HO—*See* Heterotopic Ossification.

Homonymous Hemianopia—Loss of vision for the same half of the *visual* world in each eye that is caused by a lesion on the optic tract in the opposite side of the brain from the side of blindness. Moving the eyes can *compensate* for this condition.

Hormone—A chemical substance secreted by the glands of the *endocrine system* that regulates or controls certain important body functions.

Hydrocephalus—A condition in which there is too much *cerebrospinal fluid* under too much pressure in the brain, usually within enlarged *ventricles*. Also known as "*water on the brain*." *See also* Ventriculoperitoneal Shunt.

Hyperactivity—*Behavior* that includes frequent movement, flitting from one activity to another, or having difficulty remaining seated. *See also* ADHD.

Hyperextension—Injury caused by a joint bending beyond its normal range of extension.

Hyperphagia—Excessive eating. If this results from a *TBI*, it is referred to as *posttraumatic hyperphagia*.

Hypothalamus—The part of the *diencephalon* that is responsible for certain basic bodily functions such as the *autonomic* control over heart rate, body temperature, and fluid balance. It also plays a role in emotional control.

Hypoxic Ischemic Injury—*Delayed injury* to the brain that results from insufficient blood flow and *oxygenation*.

ICP—*See* Intracranial Pressure.

ICU—*See* Intensive Care Unit.

IDEA—*See* Individuals with Disabilities Education Act.

IEP—*See* Individualized Education Program.

IFSP—*See* Individualized Family Service Plan.

Immediate Injury—An injury that occurs immediately at the time of trauma and is due to the physical forces injuring or disrupting parts of the brain. The two main types of immediate injuries are *contusions* and *diffuse axonal injury*. *See also* Delayed Injury.

Immune System—The system that produces special proteins called *antibodies*, which protect the body from disease.

Impairment-Related Work Expenses (IRWE)—An *SSI* incentive program for individuals with *disabilities* that deducts the cost of special items and services the individual needs in order to work, when determining financial eligibility for SSI. *See also* Plans for Achieving Self Support.

Impulse Control—The ability to control automatic response to *stimuli*—to think before acting or speaking.

Impulsivity—Driven by impulse; acting without premeditation or thought to potential *consequences*.

Inclusion—Placing children with *disabilities* in the same schools and classrooms with children who are developing typically. The environment includes the special supports and services necessary for educational success. *See also* Least Restrictive Environment; Special Education.

Incontinence—The inability to control the release of urine from the bladder.

Individualized Education Program (IEP)—The written plan that specifies the education and *related services* the local education agency has agreed to provide a child with *disabilities* who is eligible under *IDEA*; for children ages three to twenty-one.

Individualized Family Service Plan (IFSP)—The written plan that specifies the education and *related services* the local education agency has agreed to provide a child with *disabilities* who is eligible under *IDEA*; for children birth to age three.

Individuals with Disabilities Education Act (IDEA)—A federal law originally passed in 1975 and subsequently amended that requires states to provide a *free appropriate public education* in the *least restrictive environment* to children with *disabilities*. *See also* Public Law 94-142, Education for All Handicapped Children Act of 1975.

Inhibition—An *executive function* controlled by the *frontal lobes* that allows us to not respond impulsively or automatically to a *stimulus*, but pause to consider the probable consequences of our actions. *See also* Disinhibition; Impulse Control.

Initial Course—The plan of care provided to a patient upon admission to an *acute care hospital*.

Inner Table—The rough inner surface of the skull.

Inpatient Rehabilitation Hospital—A medical facility that focuses on improving patients' *functional abilities* by means of intense therapy provided by a team of professionals.

Instructional Assistant—A person who assists a classroom teacher in providing supports for children with *disabilities* in educational settings. Also known as classroom aide. *See also* Inclusion; Least Restrictive Environment; One-to-One Assistant.

Intelligence Quotient (IQ)—A numerical measurement of intellectual capacity that compares a person's chronological age to his "mental age," as shown on *standardized* tests.

Intensive Care Unit (ICU)—The specialized unit within an *acute care hospital* in which critically ill patients receive aggressive medical treatment for life-threatening conditions.

Intracerebral Hemorrhage—Bleeding within the brain. Also known as *intraparenchymal hemorrhage*.

Intracranial Pressure (ICP)—Pressure within the space inside the head occupied by the brain, blood, and *cerebrospinal fluid*, due to swelling of the brain, bleeding, or accumulation of fluid.

Intracranial Pressure Monitor—A device surgically implanted inside the head that sends information about internal pressures to a monitor. This helps medical staff to recognize problems early so they can use appropriate medications and interventions to control *intracranial pressure*, and to recognize when there may be a problem that might be improved with surgery.

Intracranial Space—The space within the inner surface of the skull.

Intraparenchymal Hemorrhage—*See* Intracerebral Hemorrhage.

Intraventricular Hemorrhage—Bleeding into the *ventricles* of the brain.

Intrinsic Motivation—The desire to perform a particular action without promise of external reward or *reinforcement*.

Intrusive Thoughts—Unwanted yet persistent thoughts; can be *symptomatic* of depression.

Intubate—The process of inserting a tube, usually through the *larynx*, which allows the passage of air.

IQ—*See* Intelligence Quotient.

Irrelevant Conversational Speech—Information that is not relevant to a conversation. *See also* Confabulation; Expressive Language; Tangential Conversational Speech.

IRWE—*See* Impairment-Related Work Expenses.

IV Tube—A tube inserted directly into a vein for the purpose of injecting fluids.

Lability—*See* Emotional Lability.

Language—Any set of arbitrary symbols, in the form of spoken words, written symbols, or physical gestures, that people use to communicate with one another. *See also* Expressive Language; Receptive Language.

Larynx—The organ of voice production; contains the vocal cords, which vibrate to produce *speech,* and also constrict to close off and protect the airway during swallowing. *See also* Pharyngeal Phase.

Last Will and Testament—A written directive of how one wants their *estate* to be handled after their death; includes disposing of remains, naming of *beneficiaries* and *guardians* of minor dependents, and handling general affairs. *See also* Estate Planning.

LD—*See* Learning Disability.

Learning Disability (LD)—A condition that makes learning in one or more areas, such as math, reading, *language,* and writing, more difficult than would be expected based on child's overall level of intelligence. Students with a learning disability have a discrepancy between their intellectual ability and their academic achievement.

Least Restrictive Environment (LRE)—The requirement under *IDEA* that children receiving *special education* must be educated to the fullest extent possible with children who do not have *disabilities. See also* Inclusion.

Left Cerebral Hemisphere—One of the two *cerebral hemispheres,* separated anatomically and functionally, responsible for *verbal* functions, including producing and understanding spoken *language,* reading, writing, and verbal memory. *See also* Cerebrum; Right Cerebral Hemisphere.

Left Hemisphere—*See* Left Cerebral Hemisphere.

Lesion—An area of injury or damage.

Lethargy—*Abnormal* sluggishness or drowsiness.

Life Care Plan—A document that creates a global view of a child's future by summarizing the medical, psychosocial, educational, vocational, and daily living needs of the child who has sustained a catastrophic injury, such as *TBI*. *See also* Life Care Planner.

Life Care Planner—A qualified individual who assists in the development of your child's *life care plan*.

Limb Length Discrepancy—When one arm or leg is shorter than the other. *See also* Shoe Lift.

Limbic System—A group of brain structures that form the inner ring or core of the *cerebral hemispheres* and that are associated with emotional experience, emotional expression, memory, and the satisfaction of needs necessary for survival. *See also* Hippocampus.

Lioresal™—A trade name for *baclofen*.

Living Will—*See* Advance Medical Directive.

Lobe—Any of the main divisions of the brain, separated by *fissures*. *See also* Frontal Lobe; Occipital Lobe; Parietal Lobe; Temporal Lobe.

Long-Term Goal—In reference to an *IEP* or *IFSP*, a long-term goal is a statement of the skills or abilities that your child is expected to achieve over a period of time, generally one or two years or more. *See also* Short-Term Benchmarks.

Long-Term Memory—Information stored in the brain that can be recognized or recalled at a later time. *See also* Short-Term Memory.

LRE—*See* Least Restrictive Environment.

Magnetic Resonance Imagery (MRI)—A noninvasive technique that uses harmless magnetic energy to provide a detailed image of the brain or body. *See also* Neuroimaging.

Mediation—A voluntary process in which parents and school staff meet with an unbiased moderator in an attempt to resolve a dispute regarding a child's *special education* program.

Medicaid—A joint state and federal program that provides payments for medical care to people who are financially needy and therefore entitled to receive *SSI*.

Medicare—A federal health insurance program, not based on financial need, that provides payments for medical care to people who are over age 65, as well as some individuals who are covered by *SSDI* benefits.

Medulla Oblongata—Located at the point where the brain and *spinal cord* meet, the medulla oblongata controls breathing and circulation.

Membrane—Layer of tissue covering a *cell* or organ.

Memory Journal—A book that compiles important dates, times, events, photographs, and commentary relating to a child's brain injury and recovery process. Functions as a tool to help the child put his injury into perspective and resume *activities of daily living*.

Meninges—The three *membranes*, including the *arachnoid*, *dura mater*, and *pia mater*, that envelope the brain inside the skull.

Mental Retardation—A developmental disability associated with intellectual functioning significantly below average, as well as difficulties with adaptive functioning (acquiring the skills needed to function on an age-appropriate level in the real world). People diagnosed with mental retardation typically score below 70 on IQ tests.

Mental Status—Thinking abilities and processes.

Methylphenidate—A drug that stimulates the *central nervous system*. It is sometimes prescribed to treat *AD/HD*. Also known as *Ritalin*.

Midbrain—The midsection of the brain sandwiched between the *forebrain* and *hindbrain*. The midbrain and *hindbrain* (not including the *cerebellum*) make up the *brainstem*.

Migraine Headache—The experience of severe pounding or throbbing, usually localized to one side of the head, associated with strange *visual symptoms*, hypersensitivity to light and noise, and often nausea, with or without vomiting; often triggered or worsened by *TBI*.

Mild TBI—*Traumatic brain injury* characterized by less than one hour of *coma* (usually momentary loss of *consciousness* or none at all), as defined by the International Classification of Diseases. *See also* Moderate TBI; Severe TBI.

Moderate TBI—*Traumatic brain injury* characterized by one to twenty-four hours of *coma*, as defined by the International Classification of Diseases. *See also* Mild TBI; Severe TBI.

Modification—An alteration of the classroom environment, format, or situation, made to suit the needs of a student, that changes what that student is expected to learn or demonstrate. *See also* Accommodation.

Modified Barium Swallow—A test used to examine a child's swallowing ability after *TBI*. Different food types containing barium, which can be seen on an X-ray machine, are swallowed; how safely they pass through the *pharyngeal phase* is assessed and modifications are recommended.

Motor—Relating to the ability to use muscles to move oneself. *See* Fine Motor; Gross Motor; Oral Motor.

Motor Speech Disorders—Disorders that cause difficulties planning movements of the articulators (tongue, lips, and jaw) for *speech* production.

Motor Teacher—*See* Adaptive Physical Education Teacher.

MRI—*See* Magnetic Resonance Imagery.

Multidisciplinary Assessment—An evaluation conducted by a *multidisciplinary team* to determine a child's eligibility for *special education* services.

Multidisciplinary Team (MDT)—A group of professionals from a variety of disciplines (such as a speech-language pathologist, educator, psychologist, physical therapist) responsible for observing and evaluating your child's strengths and needs, making placement decisions, planning an educational program, monitoring progress, and revising the educational plan, as needed. *See also* Multidisciplinary Assessment.

Multihandicapped—Having more than one *handicap*, or *disability*.

Muscle Tone—The amount of tension, or resistance to movement, in a muscle.

Musculoskeletal—The system of the body consisting of bones, joints, and striated muscles.

Myelin—An insulating substance that coats *axons*, allowing them to send messages rapidly. *See also* White Matter.

Narrative Assessment—An *informal assessment* used by speech-language pathologists to evaluate a child's ability to tell or retell a story.

Nasogastric Tube (NG Tube)—A tube that is used to provide fluids and nourishment to an individual who is unable to adequately eat and drink on his own. The tube is inserted through the nose and down the throat into the stomach. It is the type of tube used most frequently during the *acute management stage* following *TBI*. *See also* Gastrostomy Tube; Percutaneous Endoscopic Gastrostomy Tube.

Neurochemical—Relating to the chemistry of the *central nervous system*. Brain *cells* communicate with each other primarily through the actions of neurochemicals.

Neuroimaging—Any process, such as *magnetic resonance imagery* or *computerized tomography scans*, used to create a picture or image of the *central nervous system*.

Neurolawyer—A lawyer who, through interest, education, and training, has developed a special expertise in representing clients with *TBI* or *spinal cord* injury.

Neurologic Status—Related to the integrity and functioning of the *central nervous system*.

Neuron—Nerve *cell*.

Neuropsychological Deficits—*Cognitive*, emotional, or mental disorders related to injury sustained by the *central nervous system*. Neuropsychological deficits that result from *TBI* typically occur in memory, *attention*, and organization, all of which are extremely important in learning new things.

Neuropsychological Evaluation—An evaluation of mental functions, particularly the extent to which they have been affected by brain damage or disorder; for the purpose of understanding brain-behavior relationships and treating brain-related dysfunction.

Neuropsychologist—A *psychologist* who has completed specialized training beyond the Ph.D. level in the *cognitive* and *behavioral* problems that result from changes in normal brain function. *See also* Pediatric Neuropsychologist.

Neurosurgeon—A doctor who specializes in surgical treatments for problems of the brain and *central nervous system*; sometimes referred to as a "brain surgeon."

Neurotoxic Cascade—A chain of events in the metabolism of a *neuron* that is set in motion by trauma and results in further injury and possible death of the neuron. *See also* Delayed Injury.

NG Tube   *See* Nasogastric Tube.

Nondominant Hemisphere—Either the right or left section of the *cerebrum*, depending on the individual, which usually controls the *visual* functions: copying, drawing, understanding things we see, visual memory, and rhythm. *See also* Cerebral Hemispheres; Dominant Hemisphere.

Nonnutritive Stimulation—Stimulating the mouth and other oral structures responsible for swallowing without using food in order to maintain the ability to tolerate things in the mouth and prepare an individual to begin eating by mouth again.

Normative Comparison—A means by which to compare your child's assessment scores to that of a "normative group," or large number of test-takers, whose scores represent an average.

Occipital Cortex—*See* Occipital Lobe.

Occipital Lobe—The farthest back (most posterior) of the four *lobes* in each *cerebral hemisphere*, which are devoted exclusively to vision. Where light, in the form of electrical signals from the *retinas* of the eyes, is received and interpreted. It is made up of three zones: *primary*, *secondary*, and *tertiary*. Also known as *visual cortex*, *visual zone*, *occipital cortex*, or *occipital zone*. *See also* Optic Chiasm; Optic Nerves; Optic Tracts.

Occipital Zone—*See* Occipital Lobe.

Occupational Therapist (OT)—A professional who provides *occupational therapy*.

Occupational Therapy (OT)—Treatment designed to develop and improve *fine motor* and self-help skills, and, sometimes, sensory integration.

Oculomotor—One of the three *cranial nerves* involved in movement of the eyeball and pupil. *See also* Abducens; Trochlear.

OHI—*See* Other Health Impaired.

One-to-One Assistant—A person who aids a classroom teacher and/or *instructional assistant* in providing support for a child with *disabilities* through direct and ongoing supervision and assistance in educational settings.

Open Head Injury—Injury to the head in which both the skull and *dura mater* have been penetrated.

Optic Chiasm—The area near the center of the brain where the *optic nerves* from each *retina* cross over and join. *See also* Optic Tracts.

Optic Nerves—Considered *cranial nerves*, these are bundles of fibers that originate from the *retina* of the eyeball that carry *visual* information to the brain. *See also* Occipital Lobe; Optic Chiasm, Optic Tracts.

Optic Tracts—Bundles of fibers formed when the *optic nerves* from the inside and outside halves of each *retina* join at the *optic chiasm*, on their way to the *occipital lobe*.

Oral—Relating to the mouth and *speech*.

Oral Motor—Relating to the muscles in and around the mouth. *See also* Motor; Oral Motor Therapy.

Oral Motor Therapy—Therapy administered by a *Speech-Language Pathologist* in which a child participates in exercises that strengthen the tongue, lips, and jaw to facilitate *speech* sound production. *See also* Motor Speech Disorders; Oral Motor.

Oral Phase—The phase of swallowing involving moving food around in the mouth, chewing it, and preparing it for passage through the *esophagus* by gathering it into a clump, or *bolus*.

Organized Behavior—Purposeful *behavior* that is governed by internalized language ("self-talk") and recognition of future plans and goals, rather than impulse.

Orthopedic—Relating to the bones, joints, ligaments, or muscles.

Orthopedic Surgeon—A doctor who specializes in diagnosing and treating *orthopedic* problems

Orthopedics—A branch of surgery related to problems of the *musculoskeletal* system.

OT—*See* Occupational Therapist; Occupational Therapy.

Other Health Impaired (OHI)—An eligibility category under IDEA used to describe a student with a chronic or *acute* condition that causes reduced vitality, strength, or alertness and affects the child's educational performance. This "catch-all" category is often used to grant eligibility for services to students with *TBI*.

Overactivation—*See* Overarousal.

Overarousal—A state of *disinhibition*, inattentiveness, irritability, agitation, *hyperactivity*, impulsiveness, inappropriate social *behavior*, and aggressiveness. Also known as *overactivation*. *See also* Underarousal.

Overcorrection—A strategy, used to discourage a *target behavior*, in which a child is expected to perform a physical act that, in some way, is related to or corrects the damage done by the misbehavior.

Oxygenation—The process by which something receives oxygen. *Cells* in the brain require oxygen to function properly.

P&A—*See* Protection and Advocacy System.

PADD—*See* Protection and Advocacy System for Individuals with Developmental Disabilities.

PAIMI—*See* Protection and Advocacy System for Individuals with Mental Illness.

PAIR—*See* Protection and Advocacy Program for Individual Rights.

Parietal Lobe—One of the four *lobes* in each *cerebral hemisphere*, which is important in the interpretation of *sensory* information (including high level skills such as reading and understanding *spatial* relationships) and *attention*.

Partial Complex Seizure—A *seizure* that begins in a localized area of the brain, then spreads throughout the entire brain. Also known as *partial seizure with secondary generalization*.

Partial Seizure—A *seizure* that remains *focal*, or localized to a part of the brain. Also known as *focal seizure*.

Partial Seizure with Secondary Generalization—*See* Partial Complex Seizure.

PASS—*See* Plans for Achieving Self Support.

Pediatric Neuropsychologist—A *neuropsychologist* who specializes in the problems of children with brain disorders, and how those problems will affect development.

Pediatric TBI—*Traumatic brain injury* that occurs in a child.

PEG Tube—*See* Percutaneous Endoscopic Gastrostomy Tube.

Percentile Rank—In formal testing, percentile rank is a converted score that expresses a child's score, relative to other test-takers, in percentile points. A score of 50 percent would mean that the child's performance was exactly average, or that he scored as well as, or better than, 50 percent of the children taking the test. *See also* Age Equivalent Score; Formal Assessment; Standard Score.

Percutaneous Endoscopic Gastrostomy Tube (PEG Tube)—A tube used to provide fluids and nourishment to an individual who is unable to adequately eat and drink on his own. The tube is inserted down the throat along with an *endoscope* and poked outward from inside the stomach. *See also* Gastrostomy Tube; Nasogastric Tube.

Performance IQ (PIQ)—Results from the seven Performance Scale subtests of the *Wechsler Intelligence Scale for Children-Third Edition* that require perceptual analysis and manual manipulation of *visually* presented materials. *See also* Full Scale IQ; Verbal IQ.

Persistent Vegetative State (PVS)—The term used to describe an individual who is able to open his eyes and has normal wake-sleep cycles, but does not engage in meaningful interactions with the environment.

Pharyngeal Phase—The phase of swallowing, following the *oral phase*, in which the *bolus* is transported from the mouth through the *pharynx* (the back of the throat), past the *larynx* (the opening into the airway), and into the *esophagus* (the tube leading from the throat to the stomach).

Pharynx—The throat; located below the back of the nose and mouth and above the *larynx* and *esophagus*. *See also* Pharyngeal Phase.

Phenobarbital—One of the less commonly prescribed *antiepileptic drugs* used to control *post-traumatic seizures*; may contribute to *cognitive* and *behavioral* problems.

Phonation—Voice production. *See also* Speech.

Phonation Exercises—Breath control techniques performed for the purpose of gaining control over the loudness or intensity level of *speech*. *See also* Motor Speech Disorders.

Phonemic Cue—A *verbal cue* that uses a "letter" sound to prompt a listener's response (e.g., saying "buh" to prompt the child to say "ball").

Physical Therapist (PT)—A professional who provides *physical therapy*.

Physical Therapy (PT)—Treatment designed to develop and improve *gross motor* skills. *See also* Physical Therapist.

Pia—Abbreviation of *pia mater*.

Pia Mater—The *membrane* inside the skull between the *arachnoid* and *dura mater* that helps protect the brain. *See also* Meninges.

PIQ—*See* Performance IQ.

Pituitary Gland—The "master" gland of the *endocrine system*, which secretes *hormones* influencing metabolism, growth, and the activity of other endocrine glands. Situated at the base of the brain, it is controlled by the *hypothalamus*.

Planned Ignoring—*See* Active Ignoring.

Plans for Achieving Self Support (PASS)—An *SSI* incentive program for individuals with *disabilities* that allows an individual to have more income or *assets* than usual when determining financial eligibility for SSI. *See also* Impairment-Related Work Expenses.

Plasticity—Flexibility; the ability of the brain to learn new things and adjust to change, despite injury.

Pons—*White matter* at the base of the brain that connects the *cerebellum, medulla oblongata,* and *cerebrum*.

Positive Practice—Socially acceptable or appropriate *behavior*.

Positive Reinforcement—Providing a pleasant *consequence* after a *behavior* in order to encourage the child to continue or repeat that behavior. *See also* Contingency Contract; Differential Reinforcement; Premack Principle; Reinforcement.

Postconcussion Syndrome—*Symptoms* that develop after a *concussion* such as: headache, dizziness, memory loss, *emotional lability,* increased sensitivity to sound, impaired concentration, *disinhibition,* depression, and tiredness.

Postictal Stage—The period following a *seizure* when the affected person experiences drowsiness and grogginess.

Post-traumatic—Occurring after the accident.

Post-traumatic Amnesia (PTA)—An episode of *amnesia* or memory disturbance, occurring after head trauma, leading to an inability to remember things, disorientation, confusion, and sometimes agitation. The length of PTA is a good indicator of the severity of the *TBI.*

Post-traumatic Epilepsy—*Epilepsy* caused by a *TBI. See also* Post-traumatic Seizure.

Post-traumatic Hyperphagia—*See* Hyperphagia.

Post-traumatic Seizure (PTS)—A *seizure* that occurs after *TBI.* Early PTS (those occurring within the first week after injury) are relatively common and do not correlate with severity of injury or predict whether *epilepsy* will develop. Late seizures (occurring after the first week) are more predictive of the chance of developing *post-traumatic epilepsy.*

Postural Skills—The ability to hold one's head up, to sit, and to stand.

Posturing—Assuming *abnormal* positions.

Pragmatic Language—Refers to social, conversational use of *language.*

Premack Principle—A form of *positive reinforcement* in which you insist a child complete a less preferred activity before allowing him to engage in a preferred activity. Also known as *grandma's rule.*

Premorbid History—Information regarding a child's performance prior to *TBI.*

Primary Zone—Located at the back of the brain, this is the area of the *occipital lobe* where electrical signals traveling from the *retina,* by way of the *optic nerve,* terminate. *See also* Secondary Zone; Tertiary Zone.

Procedural Memory—*Motor* skills, conditioning, and other types of memory that can be stored and retrieved without apparent *conscious* awareness or effort.

Progressive—Describes a condition that worsens over time.

Prompt—*See* Cue.

Prosthetic Organizer—An organizational device such as a calendar, list of rules, daily schedule, or alarm clock used to *compensate* for memory, *attention*, and organization problems.

Protection and Advocacy Program for Individual Rights (PAIR)—A national agency established to help enforce the *ADA* and the 1988 Fair Housing Act Amendments. Through PAIR, *P&A systems* nationwide protect and *advocate* for services for people with *disabilities* who are ineligible for *PADD, PAIMI,* or *CAP* programs.

Protection and Advocacy System (P&A)—A nationwide program of state and national offices that *advocates* for the civil and legal rights of people with *developmental disabilities.*

Protection and Advocacy System for Individuals with Developmental Disabilities (PADD)—State agencies established to provide information and referral for sources of assistance for *advocacy* training; representation in administrative and judicial proceedings; investigation of abuse and neglect; and legislative advocacy to people with *developmental disabilities.*

Protection and Advocacy System for Individuals with Mental Illness (PAIMI)—An agency established to protect the rights of persons with mental illness under federal and state statutes, and to investigate allegations of abuse and neglect of individuals residing in facilities.

Psychiatrist—A medical doctor who diagnoses and treats mental illness; he or she may utilize prescription medications in treatment.

Psychologist—A nonmedical professional who specializes in the study of human *behavior* and the treatment of behavioral disorders.

PT—*See* Physical Therapist; Physical Therapy.

PTA—*See* Post-traumatic Amnesia.

Ptosis—Drooping of the eyelid caused by damage to the nerves that help control the movements of the eyeball and pupil.

PTS—*See* Post-traumatic Seizures.

Public Law 94-142, Education for All Handicapped Children Act (EHA) of 1975—The predecessor of *IDEA*, this law established grants to states for the education of school-aged children with *disabilities* and entitled them to a *free appropriate public education.*

Punctate—Marked by spots the size of a pinpoint.

Punishment—A *consequence* that is applied following a *behavior* to reduce the probability of that behavior occurring again. Punishment can be very mild (a frown or scolding), more moderate (a brief time-out), or very severe (electric shock). *See also* ABC Method; Aversive; Behavioral Contingency.

PVS—*See* Persistent Vegetative State.

Rancho Los Amigos (RLA)—An assessment tool that functions as a "short hand" way for *rehabilitation* specialists to monitor daily changes in a *TBI* patient's *cognitive* and *behavioral* status and communicate that information to other medical professionals; useful in predicting the course of recovery. (See Appendix.)

Reasonable Accommodation—A requirement of the *ADA* that employers adapt the working environment to remove obstacles that may impede an otherwise qualified inividual's ability to work, despite his *disabilities*.

Receptive Language—The ability to understand spoken and written communication, as well as gestures. *See also* Expressive Language; Language.

Receptor Cells—Specialized *cells* in the *central nervous system* that convert various kinds of energy in the environment (e.g., light, sound waves) to chemical and electrical signals that the brain can interpret.

Redirection—Intentionally changing a child's focus of *attention* from one *stimulus* to another in an effort to avoid or curtail an unwanted *behavior*; a nonpunitive approach to shaping behavior.

Rehab—Abbreviation of *rehabilitation*.

Rehabilitation—The process of restoring abilities that someone used to have, but lost, due to injury or illness.

Rehabilitation Act of 1973, Title V—*Section 504* of this federal law prohibits *discrimination* against individuals with *disabilities* in federally funded programs. *See also* Client Assistance Programs.

Rehearsal—Repeatedly practicing something in order to transfer that information from *short-term memory* to *long-term memory*.

Reinforcement—Any *consequence* that increases the likelihood of the future occurrence of a *behavior*. A consequence is either presented or withheld in an effort to prompt the desired response. *See* Differential Reinforcement; Positive Reinforcement; Reinforcer.

Reinforcer—A reward, either edible, material, or in the form of attention, that effectively reinforces a desired *behavior*. *See also* Reinforcement.

Related Services—Developmental, corrective, and other supportive services that enable a child to benefit from *special education*. Related services may include *speech-language*, *occupational*, and *physical therapies*, as well as transportation.

Residual Functional Impairments— Physical, emotional, or mental problems that remain even after the child has worked with a *rehabilitation* team to improve them.

Resonance—The intensity and duration of sound created by air vibrations within the throat and head.

Respiration—Breathing. *See also* Speech.

Response Cost—A fine or penalty, usually in the form of a loss of privilege, for engaging in an undesirable *behavior*.

Response Output Unit—One of the three functional units of the brain, comprised mainly of the *frontal lobes*, that causes us to do something. Before a response is executed, the frontal lobes must select and put in correct order all the individual movements required by the response. *See also* Brainstem Arousal Unit; Sensory, Reception, Processing, and Storage Unit.

Resuscitate—To revive by artificial *respiration*.

Retina—The light-sensitive layer of tissue that lines the back of the eyeball; *cells* in the retina convert light to electrical signals, which are sent through the *optic nerves* to the brain for processing.

Retrieval—Accessing information from storage in *long-term memory*.

Right Cerebral Hemisphere—One of the two *cerebral hemispheres*, separated anatomically and functionally, responsible for the perception and memory of shape, texture, pattern, and three-dimensional *spatial* relationships, construction, such as copying, drawing and putting things together, and the understanding and expression of emotion. *See also* Cerebrum; Left Cerebral Hemisphere.

Right Hemisphere—*See* Right Cerebral Hemisphere.

Rigidity—A type of *high tone*, or stiff *muscle tone*, which produces the resistance you would feel when bending a lead pipe—constant resistance that does not change when you try to bend it more rapidly. This type of tone often decreases with sleep, and has a lower risk for *contracture* than *spasticity*.

Ritalinä—A trade name for *methylphenidate*.

RLA—*See* Rancho Los Amigos.

S-ADHD—*See* Secondary Attention Deficit/Hyperactivity Disorder.

Scoliosis—Curvature of the spine.

Scotoma—*See* Blind Spot.

Secondary Attention-Deficit/Hyperactivity Disorder (S-ADHD)—Symptoms of attention-deficit/hyperactivity disorder that are acquired later in life as a result of damage or changes to the brain. (This is in contrast to AD/HD, which is not diagnosed unless symptoms are present before the age of seven.)

Secondary Zone—The area of the *occipital lobe* where isolated sensations of lines or flashes of color received in the *primary zone* are built up into unified images of whole objects or scenes corresponding to something in the external world. *See also* Tertiary Zone.

Section 504—*See* Rehabilitation Act of 1973, Title V.

Sectioned—Severed completely.

SED—*See* Seriously Emotionally Disturbed.

Sedation—The administration of a chemical sedative designed to reduce anxiety and induce a state of calmness.

Seizure—*Abnormal* electrical discharges in nerve *cells* in the brain. This leads to abrupt changes in *neurologic* function, such as: shifts in level of alertness, abnormal sensations, or abnormal movements. *See also* Aura.

Selective Attention—The ability to stay focused on relevant *stimuli* in the presence of internal or external distractions. Also known as *freedom from distractibility*. *See also* Alternating Attention; Attention; Divided Attention; Sustained Attention.

Sensory—Relating to the senses.

Sensory Integration—The ability to receive *input* from the senses, to organize it into a meaningful message, and to act on it.

Sensory, Reception, Processing, and Storage Unit—One of the three functional units of the brain, comprised primarily of the *occipital*, *parietal*, and *temporal lobes*, responsible for the five senses and memory. *See also* Brainstem Arousal Unit; Response Output Unit.

Seriously Emotionally Disturbed (SED)—*See* Emotionally Disturbed.

Service Coordinator—*See* Case Manager.

Severe TBI—*Traumatic brain injury* characterized by twenty-four or more hours of *coma*, as defined by the International Classification of Diseases. *See also* Mild TBI; Moderate TBI.

Shaping—Promptly and generously *reinforcing*, through rewards and praise, each step a child takes toward acquiring a new skill. Eventually, reinforcement is offered only when the child's actions approximate the actual *behavior* you wish to create, or shape. *See also* Chaining; Task Analysis.

Shearing Injury—*See* Diffuse Axonal Injury.

Shoe Lift—A modification to a shoe that results in a thicker sole (either a removable insert inside the shoe or a modification of the sole itself), used on a shorter leg to *compensate* for *limb length discrepancy*.

Short-Term Benchmark—In reference to an *IEP* or *IFSP*, short-term benchmarks, which your child is expected to master within two months or a semester, are objectives that your child needs to meet in order to achieve her *long-term goals*.

Short-Term Memory—Believed to occur as patterns of electrical signals among *neurons*, this type of memory is not permanent. It lasts just a few seconds, though it can be extended indefinitely with *rehearsal*. *See also* Chunking; Long-Term Memory.

SIADH—*See* Syndrome of Inappropriate ADH.

"Silent" Aspiration—*See* "Silent" Penetration.

"Silent" Penetration—Refers to a situation in which an individual is unaware that food or fluid has gone "down the wrong way" and does not cough to regurgitate it. This can occur after *TBI*, when muscles involved in swallowing can be weak and uncoordinated. Also known as *"silent" aspiration*.

Sinusitis—Infection of the sinuses.

SLP—*See* Speech-Language Pathologist.

SNT—*See* Special Needs Trust.

Social Security Disability Insurance (SSDI)—Money that has been funneled into the Social Security system through payroll deductions on earnings. Workers who become disabled are entitled to these benefits. People who are born or become disabled before the age of twenty-two may collect SSDI under a parent's account if the parent is retired, disabled, or deceased.

Social Worker—A professional who assists families acquire the special services and funding they require for their child with a *disability* or mental disorder. They may also engage in family therapy with the goal of increasing positive communication and interaction within the family.

Spasticity—A type of *high tone*, or stiff *muscle tone*, that is "rate dependent," meaning the faster you stretch a muscle by moving it, the higher (tighter) the tone becomes. *See also* Rigidity.

Spatial—Existing or happening in space.

Special Education—Specialized instruction to address a student's educational *disabilities*, determined by a *multidisciplinary assessment*. Instruction must be precisely matched to the child's educational needs and adapted to his learning style.

Special Needs—Needs generated by a person's *disabilities*.

Special Needs Trust (SNT)—A *trust* that allows a parent to leave funds for a child with *disabilities* without disqualifying him from federal, state, and local benefit and assistance programs. Also known as *supplemental trust*.

Speech—The process of producing sounds and combining those sounds into words and sentences for the purpose of communication. *Articulation*, *phonation*, and *respiration* are necessary for effective speech.

Speech-Language Pathologist (SLP)—A professional who provides *speech-language therapy*. Also known as Speech/Language Pathologist or Speech and Language Pathologist.

Speech-Language Therapy—Treatment designed to improve *speech* and *language* development, as well as *oral motor* abilities.

Spinal Cord—The thick band of nerve tissue of the *central nervous system* that originates at the *medulla oblongata* and extends the length of the back; carries all of the messages, including *motor* and *sensory* impulses, between the body and the brain.

Spinal Tap—The process of using a needle, inserted into the back below the level of the *spinal cord*, to extract *cerebrospinal fluid*.

SSDI—*See* Social Security Disability Insurance.

SSI—*See* Supplemental Security Income.

Standard Score—A numerical score that is evaluated as being below average, low average, average, high average, or above average, depending upon the degree to which the score differs from the mean (average) score. Formal *standardized* tests are constructed so that a score of 100 is exactly average. *See also* Age Equivalent Score; Formal Assessment; Percentile Rank.

Standardized—relating to tests that are mathematically adjusted according to the *standard score*.

Standing Board—A device that provides a person who is unable to stand on his own with enough postural support to stand upright.

State Insurance Department—A designated state agency that acts as a go-between for consumers and insurance providers and is responsible for making sure all policies and contracts issued by private insurers fall within state insurance law guidelines.

Stimuli—Plural form of *stimulus*.

Stimulus—A physical object or environmental event that may trigger a response or have an effect upon the *behavior* of a person. Some *stimuli* are internal (earache pain), while others are external (a smile from a loved one).

Stoma—A hole or opening.

Strabismus—A condition in which both eyes cannot focus on the same point because one eye is deviated outward, inward, and/or upward. This results in double vision.

Stuttering—*See* Dysfluency.

Subarachnoid—The space occupied by *cerebrospinal fluid*, located between the *meninges, arachnoid*, and *pia mater*.

Subarachnoid Hemorrhage—Bleeding under the *arachnoid* layer of the *meninges* into the *cerebrospinal fluid*.

Subdural Hematoma—Bleeding under the *dura mater*.

Subluxation—A partial *dislocation* of a joint.

Subpoena—Official summons to appear in court.

Sulci—Grooves on the surface of the *right* and *left hemispheres* of the *cerebrum*.

Supplemental Security Income (SSI)—A program of payments available for eligible people who have disabilities, or are blind or elderly. SSI is based on financial need, not on past earnings. *See also* Disability Determination Service; Impairment-Related Work Expenses; Plan for Achieving Self Support.

Supplemental Trust—*See* Special Needs Trust.

Sustained Attention—The ability to keep responding consistently for the amount of time necessary to complete an age-appropriate task. *See also* Alternating Attention; Attention; Divided Attention; Selective Attention.

Symptom—An indication of a disease or disorder that is noticed by a patient and serves to help make a diagnosis.

Symptomatic Treatment—Treating and hopefully relieving the *symptoms* of illness or injury without necessarily treating or curing the cause of the problem.

Syndrome of Inappropriate ADH (SIADH)—Refers to the period following *severe TBI*, when too much *antidiuretic hormone* is often released by the *pituitary gland*, causing the body to become overloaded with fluid, threatening *edema*.

Tactile—Relating to touch.

Tangential Conversational Speech—Talking around a subject and switching topics frequently, leaving *tangents* or fragments of unfinished conversation. *See also* Confabulation; Expressive Language; Irrelevant Conversational Speech.

Target Behavior—A particular *behavior*, which is observable, measurable, and described in specific terms, that you want your child to modify or replace. *See also* ABC Method.

Task Analysis—A process in which an assignment is broken down into small, essential steps. Instructions and *cues* are delivered in order to make the task easier to accomplish. *See also* Chaining.

TBI—*See* Traumatic Brain Injury.

Tegretol™—A trade name for *carbamazepine*.

Temporal Lobe—One of the four *lobes* in each *cerebral hemisphere* that is important for memory, hearing, *receptive language*, and musical awareness. *See also* Hippocampus.

Tension Headache—The experience of pain in the head, which is less severe than a *migraine headache*, and often described as producing a dull, band-like ache; often triggered by stress related to *TBI*.

Tertiary Association Cortex—*See* Tertiary Zone.

Tertiary Cortex—*See* Tertiary Zone.

Tertiary Zone—The area of the *occipital lobe* where *visual* information is linked to many different types of input, including *auditory*, touch, and body-sense (position of joints and muscles). Also known as *tertiary association cortex* and *tertiary cortex*. *See also* Primary Zone; Secondary Zone.

Thalamus—The part of the *diencephalon* that functions as the "relay station" and distribution center for sensations traveling from the body to the *cortex*.

Thrush—A yeast infection in the mouth.

Time-Out—A strategy for influencing *behavior* based on "time-out" from *positive reinforcement*. In order to stop a *target behavior* in progress, the child is taken to a chair or other designated area to sit quietly for a designated amount of time.

Tizanidine—*Oral* medication used to reduce *high tone* in muscles throughout the body. Also known as *Zanaflex™*.

Transependymal Edema—A condition in which the fluid in the *ventricular system* is under so much pressure that it begins to flow out of the *ventricles* directly into the brain tissue. *See also* Edema.

Transportation Specialist—A representative of the school system's transportation department with knowledge regarding accessibility of, and modifications to, transportation vehicles.

Traumatic Brain Injury (TBI)—Damage to the brain, caused by an external force, that can result in functional *disability* or social impairment. *See also* Mild TBI; Moderate TBI; Pediatric TBI; Severe TBI.

Trochlear—One of the three *cranial nerves* involved in movements of the eyeball and pupil. *See also* Abducens; Oculomotor.

Trust—A legal arrangement in which a person or institution (*trustee*) maintains responsibility for money or property for another's benefit (*beneficiary*).

Trustee—A person or institution responsible for governing a *trust*. *See also* Beneficiary.

Underactivation—*See* Underarousal.

Underarousal—A state of apathy, poor motivation, and social withdrawal; experiencing anxious, depressive *symptoms* and physical complaints may also be present. Also known as *underactivation*. *See also* Overarousal.

Unilateral Visual Neglect—The tendency to ignore *visual* stimulation on the side of the body opposite the side of a brain lesion. This behavior cannot be explained by damage to the visual system; the individual seems unaware of the presence of something in that half of space and may behave as if his whole world "left or right of center" is missing.

Valproic Acid—One of the most commonly prescribed *antiepileptic drugs* used to control *post-traumatic seizures*. Also known as *Depakene™*.

Vegetative State—A rare, irreversible condition resulting from massive destruction of the *cerebral hemispheres.* The individual shows no awareness of internal or external events, but sleep/wake cycles may continue.

Ventilator—A mechanical support device that delivers oxygen necessary to sustain *respiratory* function.

Ventricle—Space in the brain where *cerebrospinal fluid* is produced. *See also* Ventricular System.

Ventricular System—The system of *ventricles* or spaces within the brain that produces *cerebrospinal fluid.*

Ventriculoperitoneal (VP) Shunt—A *catheter* that drains fluid from the *ventricles* and empties into the abdominal space around the stomach and intestines, reducing the pressure on the brain; frequently used to combat *hydrocephalus.*

Verbal—Relating to words and *speech.*

Verbal IQ (VIQ)—Results from the six Verbal Scale subtests of the *Wechsler Intelligence Scale for Children-Third Edition* that require the understanding and use of *oral language* for various types of thinking and reasoning. *See also* Full Scale IQ; Performance IQ.

VIQ—*See* Verbal IQ.

Vision Specialist—A professional who assesses and treats *visual* difficulties as they affect a child's school and educational activities.

Visual—Relating to the ability to see.

Visual Cortex—*See* Occipital Lobe.

Visual Field—The total area that can be seen without moving the eyes or head.

Visual Zone—*See* Occipital Lobe.

Voluntary Muscle Activity—Movement of skeletal muscles in response to *conscious*, volitional processes.

VP—*See* Ventriculoperitoneal Shunt.

Water on the Brain—*See* Hydrocephalus.

Wechsler Intelligence Scale for Children-Third Edition (WISC-III)—The most frequently used individual test of intelligence for children, consisting of ten to thirteen (three are optional) subtests, which in turn cluster into two broad domains of ability: *Verbal IQ* and *Performance IQ. See also* Full Scale IQ.

"What" System—The system of vision that combines *visual* and *auditory* information and allows us to label and describe what we see, using words.

"Where" System—The system of vision that combines *visual*, touch, and position information and allows us to understand *spatial* relationships and to perform movements guided by our vision.

White Matter—The parts of the brain made up of *axons*, which are coated with *myelin*. *See also* Pons.

Will—*See* Last Will and Testament.

WISC-III—*See* Wechsler Intelligence Scale for Children-Third Edition.

Working Memory—A mental "scratch-pad" where all stored and incoming information relevant to a particular situation can be called up into *consciousness*, represented, combined, and manipulated. Working memory, along with *impulse control*, helps us organize our *behavior*.

Zanaflex™—A trade name for *tizanidine*.

READING LIST

■ Chapter 1

Acorn, Sonia, ed. **Living with Brain Injury: A Guide for Families and Caregivers.** Toronto: University of Toronto Press, 1998.

A reference book put together by health-care and legal experts from Canada and the United States that guides the reader through the process of brain injury rehabilitation, discussing physical abilities and psychological make-up, relationships and family roles, school and employment, recreation and leisure, and more.

Bellenir, Karen, ed. **Head Trauma Sourcebook: Basic Information for the Layperson about Open-Head and Closed-Head Injuries, Treatment Advances, Recovery, and Rehabilitation, along with Reports on Current Research Initiatives.** Detroit, MI: Omnigraphics, Inc., 1997.

Written for the patient, family, and friends, this very comprehensive book covers explanations about common causes and prevention of TBI, different types of head trauma and their consequences, rehabilitation and research, special information for families, and source listings for further help and information.

Burke, William, ed. **HDI Professional Series.** Houston, TX: HDI Publishers, 1996.

A series written primarily for professionals in the fields of health care and education, which includes books on the topics of Managing Anger and Aggression, Managing Attention Deficits, Management of Memory Disorders, Developing Social Skills, Head Injury Rehab with Children and Adolescents, The Role of the Family in TBI Rehab, and Management of Communication and Language Deficits, among others.

Coleman, Jeanine G. **The Early Intervention Dictionary.** 2nd ed. Bethesda, MD: Woodbine House, 1999.

Words and abbreviations from the fields of medicine, child development, early intervention, special education, and various therapies are defined in parent-friendly terms. A useful companion when deciphering medical reports, evaluations, or textbooks.

John, Delores. **Head Injury Guide for Survivors, Families, & Caregivers.** Collingdale, PA: DIANE Publishing Co., 1990.

This book discusses what happens to the brain as a result of trauma, brain injury rehabilitation, levels of recovery, financial and legal resources, and survivor and family support resources, and includes a directory of organizations and glossary of terms.

Ryan, Cathy E., and Richard C. Senelick. **Living with Brain Injury: A Guide for Families.** Birmingham, AL: Healthsouth Corp., 1998.

This resource is excellent for describing head trauma and how different functions can be affected. It also explains how a person actually comes out of a coma in gradual stages.

Sellars, Carole Wedel, Candace Hill Vegter, Susan Sivertsen Ellerbusch, and Annette Angland Flaig. **Pediatric Brain Injury: The Special Case of the Very Young Child.** Houston, TX: HDI Publishers, 1997.

This book, written primarily for professionals, presents a clinical definition of pediatric brain injury, case studies along with MRI and CT scans, and information on normal pediatric development, specific therapeutic activities, injury prevention, and transitional programs from hospital to school. The focus is on infants, toddlers, and preschoolers with traumatic brain injuries.

Sturm, Christopher, Thomas R. Forget, and Janet L. Sturm. **Head Injury: Information and Answers to Commonly Asked Questions: A Family's Guide to Coping.** St. Louis, MO: Quality Medical Publishing, Inc., 1998.

This book provides general information and answers to commonly asked questions regarding important aspects of severe head injury. Topics include: the accident, types of head injury, symptoms and behavior, intensive care setting, prognosis and outcomes, emotional reactions, aspects of therapy, prevention, and a glossary of terms.

Sweeney, Wilma. **The Special Needs Reading List: An Annotated Guide to the Best Publications for Parents and Professionals.** Bethesda, MD: Woodbine House, 1998.

A helpful guide to publications, organizations, and websites for parents seeking information on a wide variety of disability issues, including hydrocephalus, seizures, physical disabilities, daily care, family life, special education, technology, and more.

■■ Chapter 2

Batshaw, Mark L. **Children with Disabilities.** 4th ed. Baltimore: Paul H. Brookes, 1997.

This parent-friendly reference book contains information on a variety of childhood disabilities. It includes a chapter on traumatic brain injury, as well as information relating to hydrocephalus, learning disabilities, seizures, attention deficit disorders, and more.

Brain Injury Association. **National Directory of Brain Injury Rehabilitation Services.** Distributed by HDI Publishers.

HDI Publishers disseminates copies of the Brain Injury Association's "National Directory of Brain Injury Rehabilitation Services," with relevant listings by state, for $16.00/copy. Can be ordered by calling (800) 321-7037.

CNS Familyworks! LLC. **Transfer Techniques: A Step-By-Step Procedure.** Bakersfield, CA: CNS Familyworks! LLC, 1999.

This manual gives detailed descriptions and illustrations of ways to transfer an injured or recovering person from one location to another in the safest, most efficient manner. Minimum, moderate, and maximum assistance transfers are detailed; two-person transfers, floor lifts, and transfers for special environments, such as bathtubs, toilets, recliners, and cars, are covered in a step-by-step, fully illustrated format.

Davies, Patricia M. **Starting Again: Early Rehabilitation after Traumatic Brain Injury or Other Severe Brain Lesion.** New York: Springer-Verlag, 1994.

Written primarily for physical therapists, this book may be useful to highly motivated parents and caregivers as well. Filled with numerous photographs of patients, this book illustrates a broad spectrum of treatment, ranging from the intensive care unit to the reeducation of walking. Chapters cover perceptual disturbances; positioning, moving, and standing the unconscious patient; teaching the patient to eat, drink, and speak again; and ways in which contractures and deformities can be overcome.

Freeman, John M., Eileen P. Vining, and Diana J. Pillas. **Seizures and Epilepsy in Childhood: A Guide for Parents.** 2nd ed. Baltimore: Johns Hopkins University Press, 1997.

An optimistic guide to raising a child with epilepsy, this book covers causes, diagnosis, treatment, and coping strategies.

Guilmette, Thomas J. **Pocket Guide to Brain Injury, Cognitive, and Neurobehavioral Rehabilitation.** San Diego, CA: Singular Publishing Group, 1997.

Designed for psychology, neuropsychology, and rehabilitation practitioners, this book is technical but may be useful to parents during the rehabilitation phase of their child's recovery.

Mindell, Amy, and Robert King. **Coma: A Healing Journey.** Portland, OR: Lao Tse Press, 1999.

The authors of this book consider coma to be a meaningful altered state of consciousness, rather than a helpless vegetative condition, and suggest ways to communicate with patients who are considered unresponsive.

Toporek, Chuck, and Kellie Robinson. **Hydrocephalus: A Guide for Parents, Families, and Friends.** Sebastopol, CA: O'Reilly & Associates, 1998.

Topics covered in this practical guide include selecting a neurosurgeon, understanding treatment options, keeping records to aid in home monitoring, and living with hydrocephalus.

Ylvisaker, Mark, ed. **Traumatic Brain Injury Rehabilitation: Children and Adolescents.** Woburn, MA: Butterworth-Heinemann Publishers, Ltd., 1998.

Functioning as a broad reference for health care providers, patients, and family, this is a collaborative work between a group of clinicians and young people and their parents, recounting their experiences with survivors of TBI. Topics include: rehabilitative medical management, a nursing perspective on the recovery continuum, intervention for motor disorders, assistive technologies, cognitive rehabilitation, school reentry, career development, and support networks.

∷ Chapter 3

Abrahamson, Patt, and Jeffery Abrahamson. **Brain Injury: A Family Tragedy.** Houston, TX: HDI Publishers, 1997.

In this personal account, a mom describes her son's life before he was injured, the injury itself, and the rehabilitation process.

Brandt, Avrene L. **Caregivers Reprieve: A Guide to Emotional Survival When You're Caring for Someone You Love.** Atascadero, CA: Impact Publishers, 1998.

This book is an excellent resource for anyone facing the challenges of caring for a loved one who needs long-term support. It highlights the fact that care-giving is a difficult task and that the emotions caregivers feel are common and normal.

Capossela, Cappy. **Share the Care: How to Organize a Group to Care for Someone Who Is Seriously Ill.** New York: Simon & Schuster Books, 1995.
This book is a step-by-step guide to creating a care-giving network for the survivor of TBI, including how to meet the people who care, organize the first group meeting, use all the hidden skills in the group, and more. Offers valuable guidelines, compassionate suggestions, and a workbook that details how to help free the patient from worry and the caregiver from burnout.

Deboskey, Dana S., ed. **Coming Home: A Discharge Manual for Families of Persons with a Brain Injury.** Houston, TX: HDI Publishers, 1996.
An informative guide to dealing with the practical and emotional issues surrounding your child's discharge from the hospital following a traumatic brain injury.

Dell Orto, Arthur E., and Paul W. Power. **Head Injury and the Family: A Life and Living Perspective.** Delray Beach, Florida: GR/St. Lucie Press, 1997.
Critical topics covered in this book include the impact of head injury on the family and individual members, adjustment considerations, assessment, families in crisis, group counseling, respite care, alcohol abuse, loss, grief, hope, and optimism.

Gronwall, Dorothy, Philip Wrightson, and Peter Waddel. **Head Injury: The Facts: A Guide for Families and Care-Givers.** New York: Oxford University Press, 1998.
This book explains the effects of injury in nontechnical terms and suggests practical ways of overcoming these effects. The authors walk you through the stages of patient recovery and explain the procedures and techniques used to chart progress. This book also examines how head trauma affects families and friends, the return to work or school, and discusses the head injury rehabilitation system, and long-term adjustments.

Klein, Stanley, and Maxwell Schleifer. **It Isn't Fair: Siblings of Children with Disabilities.** Westport, CT: Bergin & Garvey, 1993.
Written from the perspective of parents, young adult siblings, younger siblings, and professionals, this book tackles the complex issues regarding family and disability, including expectations, rewards, punishments, fairness, care-taking responsibilities, guilt, and worry.

Kushner, Harold S. **When Bad Things Happen to Good People.** New York: Avon Books, 1994.
Written by a rabbi whose son died of a rare disorder (progeria) in his early teens, this book can be helpful in working through all the "why's" that parents feel when facing unexpected news.

Lash, Marilyn. **When Your Child is Seriously Injured: The Emotional Impact on Families.** Houston, TX: HDI Publishers, 1991.
This publication chronicles a child's admission to the hospital following injury and ends after discharge. Chapters include: The Hospital Stay, Helping Brothers and Sisters of the Child with an Injury, Getting Help and Coping, and Planning for Discharge from the Hospital.

Marsh, Jayne D.B., ed. **From the Heart: On Being the Mother of a Child with Special Needs.** Bethesda, MD: Woodbine House, 1995.

Included in this book are many short reflections and anecdotes contributed by mothers of children with a variety of disabilities. Among the topics covered are coping, education, family life, and relationships with professionals.

Meyer, Donald J. **Living with a Brother or Sister with Special Needs: A Book for Sibs.** 2nd ed. Seattle, WA: University of Washington Press, 1996.

An introduction to a variety of disabilities written for siblings in upper elementary school or middle school grades. Chapters cover neurological problems, mental retardation, hearing and visual impairments, and laws and services for people with disabilities. Common feelings of siblings are acknowledged and discussed throughout.

Meyer, Donald J. **Views from Our Shoes: Growing Up with a Brother or Sister with Special Needs.** Bethesda, MD: Woodbine House, 1997.

For siblings who are in third to seventh grade, this book is an excellent source of information and support. Included are short essays by nearly fifty children, aged four to nineteen, about what it's like to have a brother or sister with special needs.

Meyer, Donald J., ed. **Uncommon Fathers.** Bethesda, MD: Woodbine House, 1995.

A variety of fathers whose children have a variety of diagnoses reflect—sometimes humorously, sometimes ruefully—on how having a child with a disability has shaped their life.

Osborn, Claudia L. **Over My Head: A Doctor's Own Story of Head Injury from the Inside Looking Out.** Kansas City, MO: Andrews McMeel Publishing, 1998.

An inspiring personal account of a woman, who used to be a doctor and clinical professor of medicine, coming to terms with the loss of her identity as a result of brain injury and learning to rebuild her life.

▪▪ Chapter 4

Baker, Bruce L., et al. **Steps to Independence: Teaching Everyday Skills to Children with Special Needs.** 3rd ed. Baltimore: Paul H. Brookes, 1997.

In step-by-step fashion, this useful guide explains how to teach children with disabilities daily living skills such as dressing, using the toilet, playing, and more. The book includes sections on managing behavior problems at home and using technology to enhance children's learning.

CNS Familyworks! LLC. **Basic Self-Care: Dressing, Eating, Toileting, Hygiene, and Grooming Skills.** Bakersfield, CA: CNS Familyworks! LLC, 1999.

This book offers step-by-step teaching procedures and illustrated instructions to simplify basic self-care tasks. Included are check sheets for evaluating and charting the person's progress and a list of useful adaptive equipment.

Monahon, Cynthia. **Children and Trauma: A Guide for Parents and Professionals.** San Francisco, CA: Jossey-Bass, 1997.

This book teaches parents and professionals about the effects of psychological trauma on children, including fearfulness, nightmares, and dramatic behavioral or personality changes, and offers a blueprint for restoring a child's sense of safety and balance.

Schleien, Stuart J., M. Tipton Ray, and Frederick P. Green. **Community Recreation and People with Disabilities: Strategies for Inclusion.** 2nd ed. Baltimore: Paul H. Brookes, 1996.

Designed for professionals and advocates, this book offers creative ideas and new techniques for including people with disabilities in community recreation programs. Includes information on friendship and recreation, collaboration, intervention strategies, and how to foster social inclusion in recreation settings and build bridges between families and recreation professionals.

Snyder, Heather. **Elvin: The Elephant Who Forgets.** Wake Forest, NC: Lash Publishing Associates/Training, 1998.

This picture book is designed to help children, friends, and classmates understand what it's like to have a brain injury. Written for kindergarten through elementary school age children. To order online, visit: http://www.lapublishing.com/books.htm.

▪▪ Chapter 5

CNS Familyworks! LLC. **Brain Injury Rehabilitation: Basic Principles and Techniques.** Bakersfield, CA: CNS Familyworks! LLC, 1998.

This manual teaches families how to maximize the rehabilitation of a family member recovering from brain injury. It includes: detailed instructions on creating the best possible learning environment, optimal teaching techniques and methods, and responses to behavioral, emotional, cognitive, and physical problems that interfere with the learning process. Written in a clear, easy-to-read format.

Healy, Jane M. **Your Child's Growing Mind: A Practical Guide to Brain Development and Learning from Birth to Adolescence.** New York: Doubleday, 1994.

This very readable guide for parents covers research about how children develop memory, language, and other cognitive skills, and also explores differences in academic abilities and learning styles.

Hodgdon, Linda. **Visual Strategies for Improving Communication: Practical Supports for Home and School.** Troy, MI: Quirk Roberts Publishing, 1995.

This "how-to" book is designed to assist teachers, SLP's, and parents in devising solutions to the communication and self-management challenges that are common to children with learning, sensory, and processing difficulties. It explains in detail the importance of visual communication and recommends techniques and strategies that will help these students participate more effectively in social interactions and life routines.

Sattler, Jerome M. **Assessment of Children.** 3rd edition. La Mesa, CA: Jerome M. Sattler Publisher, 1992.

This is the book that psychologists and other professionals involved in assessing children's cognitive skills turn to for information on administering specific IQ, achievement, and other tests. For parents, it is a good source of information about what the different tests measure, and what scores on the various subsections might indicate. Pricey, so look for this in your library.

Wodrich, David L. **Children's Psychological Testing: A Guide for Nonpsychologists.** 3rd edition. Baltimore: Paul H. Brookes, 1997.

In nontechnical language, this book discusses many of the tests used to assess intelligence, academic achievement, emotional, and behavioral status in children—

how they are administered, what they measure, how results are interpreted, draw-backs. A separate section describes tests often used to evaluate children who have had brain injuries.

■■ Chapter 6

Cera, Roselyn M., Nova N. Vulanich, and William A. Brady. **Patients with Brain Injury: A Family Guide to Assisting in Speech, Language, and Cognitive Rehabilitation.** 2nd ed. Austin, TX: Pro-Ed, 1995.

This booklet serves as a general guide to help families and the patient with brain injury understand the process of recovery and rehabilitation. It identifies eight levels of recovery using the Rancho Los Amigos Cognitive Scale. In addition, this publication provides families with simple cognitive, speech, and language activities and therapy goals for the patient. Includes a progress chart.

Hamaguchi, Patricia, M. **Childhood Speech, Language & Listening Problems: What Every Parent Should Know.** New York: John Wiley & Sons, 1995.

A thorough overview of many different types of speech, language, and listen-ing problems is provided in this reader-friendly book, with information on reading evaluation reports, diagnosis, legal issues, and treatment.

McKrell, Judith L. **Communication Problems after Brain Injury or Stroke.** Atlanta, GA: Pritchett and Hull Associates, 1996.

Speech-language pathologists, family, and caregivers will find this a valuable tool in working together for the benefit of a child who has had a TBI. For each problem identified, including aphasia, speaking, writing, reading, dysarthria, apraxia, and cog-nitive problems, a list of easy-to-follow tips to help improve communication is given.

Murdoch, Bruce, and Deborah G. Theodoros. **Traumatic Brain Injury: Associ-ated Speech, Language, and Swallowing Disorders.** San Diego, CA: Singular Publishing Group, 2000.

This book provides holistic and synthesized coverage of communicative and swallowing disorders associated with TBI. Includes coverage of the latest thinking regarding the relationship between cognitive and linguistic impairments, and de-tailed information regarding the assessment and treatment of communication and swallowing disorders following TBI. Targeted at professionals, but may be of interest to some parents.

Schoenbrodt, Lisa, and Romayne A. Smith. **Communication Disorders and In-terventions in Low Incidence Pediatric Populations.** San Diego, CA: Singu-lar Publishing Group, 1995.

This book, coauthored by the editor of **Children with Traumatic Brain Injury,** includes a chapter on how TBI affects communication skills in children. It includes a thorough discussion of how a child with TBI differs from a child with learning disabilities. Written primarily for SLPs, but not overly technical.

Schwartz, Sue, and Joan E. Heller Miller. **The New Language of Toys: Teaching Communication Skills to Children with Special Needs.** 2nd edition. Bethesda, MD: Woodbine House, 1996.

The authors of this book explain how to use commonly available toys and games to teach communication skills to children who are at the developmental age of about birth to age six.

■■ Chapter 7 and 8

Barkley, Russell A. **Taking Charge of ADHD: The Complete, Authoritative Guide for Parents.** Revised ed. New York: Guilford Press, 2000.

A guide to the nature and treatment of ADHD, with useful strategies for managing behavior at home and at school.

Clark, Lynn. **SOS! Help for Parents: A Practical Guide for Handling Common Everyday Behavior Problems.** Bowling Green, KY: Parents Press, 1996.

Practical strategies for dealing with challenging behavior in young children, including time out, reward systems, and behavior contracts.

Dendy, Chris A. Zeigler. **Teaching Teens with ADD and ADHD: A Quick Reference Guide for Teachers and Parents.** Bethesda, MD: Woodbine House, 2000.

This book contains concise summaries of over seventy-five key issues related to AD/HD and school success such as: intervention strategies, IEP troubleshooting tips, maximizing medication effectiveness, strategies for behavior management, and common learning problems. Particularly helpful for the home-school partnership are the many blank forms and checklists, suitable for photocopying.

Duke, Marshall P., Elisabeth A. Martin, and Stephen Nowicki. **Teaching Your Child the Language of Social Success.** Atlanta: Peachtree Publishers, 1996.

An excellent book for children with TBI who are having trouble with nonverbal social skills. This book teaches basic and critical emotional intelligence skills and offers good explanations and exercises that any patient parent or teacher can use to help the child who is often misunderstood.

Gruen, Andrew K., and Lynn S. Gruen. **Functional Communication Series.** Eau Claire, WI: Thinking Publishers, 1994.

This series uses natural storylines to make intervention more effective for survivors of TBI with cognitive, learning, or language disabilities. The hands-on activities in Traumatic Brain Injury Activities: Back into Life rebuild reasoning, memory, judgment, organization, and self-confidence. Daily Problem Solving Activities: Transitioning to Independence helps students with their efforts to resolve problems as they transition toward independence in various social contexts. These books are written at a fourth-grade level for survivors of TBI in grades ten to twelve. Can be used by educators and motivated parents and caregivers.

Mannix, Darlene. **Social Skills Activities for Special Children.** New York: Center for Applied Research in Education, 1993.

Designed with teachers in mind, but also helpful for parents, this book is a collection of lessons, activities, and ideas designed to help elementary children with special needs become aware of acceptable social behavior and to help them develop proficiency in acquiring basic social skills. A social skills book for secondary students is also available. In addition, a book including life skills activities, by the same author, is available for elementary and secondary students.

Nowicki, Stephen, and Marshall P. Duke. **Helping the Child Who Doesn't Fit In.** Atlanta, GA: Peachtree Publishers, 1992.

This book is targeted at the parents of children who are having trouble with nonverbal social skills, particularly kids who have difficulty making friends because they are unaware of nonverbal social "rules." This book offers suggested activities and practical advice.

Osborn, Claudia L. **Over My Head: A Doctor's Own Story of Head Injury From the Inside Looking Out.** Kansas City, MO: Andrews McMeel Publishing, 1998.
The author offers very personal insights into how a TBI can change one's personality, behavior, and thought processes, and the effects those changes have on the individual herself, as well as friends and family.

Staub, Debbie. **Delicate Threads: Friendships between Children with and without Special Needs in Inclusive Settings.** Bethesda, MD: Woodbine House, 1998.
The author of this book followed seven pairs of friends, with and without developmental disabilities, at an inclusive elementary school over the course of several years. The children's stories provide clues as to why some such friendships fail and some succeed.

Voss, Judith, Elizabeth Cooley, Bonnie Todis, Ann Glang, and Marilyn Lash. **Building Friendships When Students have Special Needs.** Wake Forest, NC: Lash & Associates Publishing/Training Inc., 1999.
This manual and video present an innovative program for building peer support, decreasing social isolation, and developing friendships. Using a friendship facilitator, it takes the reader through how to recruit participants, involve families and peers, run effective meetings, and troubleshoot potential problems. To order online, visit: http://www.lapublishing.com/books.htm.

■■ Chapter 9

Anderson, Winifred, Stephen Chitwood, and Deidre Hayden. **Negotiating the Special Education Maze: A Guide for Parents and Teachers.** 3rd ed. Bethesda, MD: Woodbine House, 1997.
This practical, step-by-step guide explains how to obtain an appropriate education for children who are eligible for early intervention or special education services. The authors offer helpful information about special education laws, meeting with school officials, planning IEPs, choosing a program, and resolving conflicts.

Bigler, Erin D., Elaine Clark, and Janet Farmer. **Childhood Traumatic Brain Injury: Diagnosis, Assessment, and Intervention.** Austin, TX: Pro-Ed, 1997.
This book outlines basic mechanisms of traumatic brain injury, how to assess deficits, implementing school and social programs, providing community support for children with TBI, and includes a clinical guide to managing resulting behavior problems.

Block, Martin E. **A Teacher's Guide to Including Students with Disabilities in Regular Physical Education.** Baltimore, MD: Paul H. Brookes, 2000.
Offers general strategies for inclusion, suggestions for adapting specific sports activities, and examples of goals and objectives for IEPs. Emphasizes collaborative teaming, including families and their goals in the physical education curriculum, and raising the expectations for children with disabilities. Also included is information on behavior management, classroom safety, adapted aquatics, and the social aspects of inclusion.

Des Jardins, Charlotte. **How to Get Services by Being Assertive.** 2ⁿᵈ ed. Chicago, IL: Family Resource Center on Disabilities, 1993.

This is must read before attending an IEP or IFSP meeting. The author also explains how to prepare for a due process hearing and includes the stories of many parents who were able to get appropriate services for their children by being assertive. The book can be ordered form Family Resource Center on Disabilities, 200 S. Michigan Ave., Ste. 1520, Chicago, IL 60604.

Gerring, Joan P. and Joan M. Carney. **Head Trauma: Strategies for Educational Reintegration.** 2ⁿᵈ ed. San Diego: Singular Publishing Group, 1992.

Written primarily for SLPs and other professionals, but accessible to parents, this book offers an overview of how returning to school fits into the recovery process. Includes case studies.

Glang, Ann, George H.S. Singer, and Bonnie Todis, eds. **Students With Acquired Brain Injury: The School's Response.** Baltimore, MD: Paul Brookes, 1997.

Written mostly for educators but informed and involved parents also, this publication covers assessment, transition issues, challenging behaviors, building friendships, and preparing school staff.

Goldberg, Alan L., ed. **Acquired Brain Injury in Childhood and Adolescence: A Team and Family Guide to Educational Program Development and Implementation.** Springfield, IL: Charles C. Thomas Publishing, 1997.

This book includes approaches, techniques, and procedures that are useful for students with TBI. Topics include options for educational service delivery, practical discussions of educational program development, school reentry and staff training, transitions from school to adult life, and the critical role of parents.

Lash, Marilyn, and Bob Cluett. **A Manual for Managing Special Education for Students with Brain Injury.** Wake Forest, NC: Lash & Associates Publishing/Training Inc., 1998.

This publication details skills used by professional case managers that are adapted for parents and applied to special education. They include: assessment, information gathering, referral, service coordination, advocacy, and evaluation. Includes many worksheets. To order online, visit: http://www.lapublishing.com/books.htm.

Leff, Patricia Turner, and Elaine H. Walizer. **Building the Healing Partnership.** Cambridge, MA: Brookline, 1992.

The focus of this book is on helping parents and professionals learn to respect each other's values and perspectives in working together for the good of a child with disabilities.

Ray, John, and M. Kathleen Warden. **Technology, Computers and the Special Needs Learner.** Stamford, CT: Wadsworth Publishing Co., 1994.

This book, written mainly for teachers, includes information on multidisciplinary teams, learning and instruction, computer hardware and software, assistive devices, vision, hearing, speech and language, and mobility.

Savage, Ronald C., and Gary F. Wolcott. **Educational Dimensions of Acquired Brain Injury.** Austin, TX: Pro-Ed, 1994.

This book provides teachers and parents with specific models and strategies to help respond to the educational and lifelong needs of students with brain injury.

Includes information on cognitive assessment and intervention, speech and language, behavior, sense of self, physical interventions, classroom environment, school administration involvement, and transitions to work.

Todis, Bonnie, McKay Moore Sohlberg, and Ann Glang. **Making the IEP Process Work for Students with Brain Injuries.** Wake Forest, NC: Lash & Associates Publishing/Training Inc., 1998.

This manual provides practical suggestions for gathering information and developing effective educational plans for students with brain injuries in middle, junior high, and high school. To order online, visit: http://www.lapublishing.com/books.htm.

Tyler, Janet S., and Mary P. Mira. **Traumatic Brain Injury in Children and Adolescents: A Sourcebook for Teachers and Other School Personnel.** Austin, TX: Pro-Ed, 1992.

This book offers an overview of the entire spectrum of issues related to TBI. In addition to describing the causes and short-term and long-term consequences of TBI, this sourcebook presents techniques and procedures to successfully return the child to school following an injury.

Wolcott, Gary, Marilyn Lash, and Sue Pearson. **Signs and Strategies for Educating Students with Brain Injuries: A Practical Guide for Teachers and Schools.** Houston, TX: HDI Publishers, 1995.

Not just for educators, this book gives a basic overview of the consequences that brain injuries can have on a child's learning, behavior, and adjustment in school and home. It explains common changes that can occur and gives strategies for dealing with these differences and challenges. A special section on transition strategies helps prepare the student for moving from teacher to teacher, grade to grade, and school to school. Includes many worksheets for families and educators.

▪▪ Chapter 10

Baldwin, Ben. **The Complete Book of Insurance: The Consumer's Guide to Insuring Your Life, Health, Property, and Income.** Chicago: Irwin Professional Publishing, 1996.

Designed to help consumers make intelligent insurance-buying decisions, this book covers: determining how much coverage you need; disability, medical, liability, life, and other types of insurance; selecting an insurance agent and company.

Bateman, Barbara, and Mary Anne Linden. **Better IEPs: How to Develop Legally Correct and Educationally Useful Programs.** 3rd ed. Longmont, CO: Sopris West, Inc., 1998.

A useful and practical guide to the IEP process, written for parents. Contains information on the 1997 IDEA amendments.

Goldberg, Daniel, and Marge Goldberg. **The Americans with Disabilities Act: A Guide for People with Disabilities, Their Families, and Advocates.** Minneapolis: Pacer Center, 1993.

Provides explanations of how the ADA applies to employment, public services, public accommodations, and telecommunications.

Knowlen, Barbara Bradford. **How to Kick Ass and Win: A Consumer's Guide to Getting Services and Equipment from the State Vocational Rehabilitation Agency by Using the Appeals Process.** Oriskany Falls, NY: Barrier Breakers, 1998.

   Order from: Barrier Breakers, 4239 Camp Rd., Oriskany Falls, NY 13425; 315-821-2460.

Rose, F. David, and D.A. Johnson, eds. **Brain Injury and After: Towards Improved Outcome.** New York: John Wiley & Son, Ltd., 1996.

   An informative discussion on brain damage and the factors that can affect outcome following a TBI. Topics include assessment, long-term management, therapy, legal considerations, and legislative and policy factors.

Russell, L. Mark, Arnold E. Grant, Suzanne M. Joseph. **Planning for the Future: Providing a Meaningful Life for a Child with a Disability after Your Death.** Evanston, IL: American Publishing Co., 1995.

   Developing a comprehensive estate plan for a child with disabilities is the focus of this practical guide. Topics covered include: writing a Letter of Intent, deciding whether to appoint a guardian, writing a will, establishing trust funds, and getting the most out of government benefits.

Sbordone, Robert J. **Neuropsychology for the Attorney.** Delray Beach, FL: St. Lucie Press, 1991.

   Written specifically for attorneys, this book provides an insider's guide to what one may anticipate during essential testimony in any head injury case. Includes information on cases involving mild head injury, traumatic brain injury, toxic exposure, post-traumatic stress disorder, hypoxia, memory or intellectual loss, postconcussion syndrome, and more. Very technical.

Schlachter, Gail. **Financial Aid for the Disabled and Their Families.** San Carlos, CA: Reference Service Press, 1998.

   A guide to a wide range of financial aid programs offered to people with disabilities and their families.

Stengle, Linda. **Laying Community Foundations for Your Child with a Disability.** Bethesda, MD: Woodbine House, 1996.

   This guide looks at the human side of estate planning—ensuring that your child will have a network of caring friends to look after his best interests after your death. The book also looks at planning for living arrangements, jobs, and activities that will give your child a secure place in the community.

■■ Online Publications *(Guides, Booklets, Downloadable Forms)*

Coma Guide for Caregivers

Delaware Health and Social Services, Division of Services for Aging and Adults with Physical Disabilities
Email: DSAAPDinfo@state.de.us
Web: http://www.dsaapd.com/COMAGUIDE.pdf

   Visit website to download a free copy of this very informative book on coma and TBI. Includes an extensive and useful resource guide.

Emergency Information Forms (EIF) for Children with Special Health Care Needs
American Academy of Pediatrics & American College of Emergency Physicians (1999)
The American Academy of Pediatrics
141 Northwest Point Boulevard
Elk Grove Village, IL 60007-1098
(847) 434-4000; (847) 434-8000 (Fax)
Email: kidsdocs@aap.org
Web: http://www.aap.org/advocacy/emergprep.htm
   Visit website to download a free copy of an EIF form which provides parents and medical professionals immediate and easy access to your child's pertinent medical information. Website also offers a Q&A section regarding the EIF, as well as other information on its history and intended use.

Facts about Concussion and Brain Injury: Where to Get Help
National Center for Injury Prevention and Control at the Centers for Disease Control and Prevention (1999)
Mailstop K65
4770 Buford Highway NE
Atlanta, GA 30341-3724
(770) 488-1506, (770) 488-1667 (Fax)
Email: OHCINFO@cdc.gov
Web: http://www.cdc.gov/ncipc/tbi; http://www.cdc.gov/safeusa/siteindex.htm
   Visit website to download a free copy of this booklet, which contains common symptoms following mild to moderate brain injury, describes danger signs, provides tips for recovery and resources for help.

A Guide to the Individualized Education Program
Office of Special Education and Rehabilitative Services, U.S. Department of Education (2000)
U.S. Department of Education
330 C Street, SW
Washington, DC 20202
(202) 205-5465; (202) 205-9252 (Fax)
Web: http://www.ed.gov/offices/OSERS/OSEP/IEP_Guide
   Visit website to download a free copy of this guide, which assists parents and educators design and implement an IEP, based on what is required by IDEA.

Helping Parents and Professionals Communicate after a Child Has Been Injured
Research and Training Center in Rehabilitation and Childhood Trauma of the New England Medical Center (1997)
750 Washington Street, #75K-R
Boston, MA 02111
(617) 636-5031; (617) 636-5513 (Fax)
Email: bhastings@hrsa.gov
Web: http://www.tbigrants.com/tip_card.htm
   Visit website to download a free copy of this set of five tip cards, which provide parents and health care professionals with suggestions for positive communication within the ICU, hospital, rehabilitation center, and community.

IDEA Practices Home Page
Educational Development Center (EDC)
Superintendent of Documents
U.S. Government Printing Office
Washington, DC 20402
(617) 332-5321 (Fax)
Email: ideapractices@ideapractices.org
Web: http://www.ideapractices.org
This website's goal is to offer service providers, local administrators, and other interested parties information and support for IDEA-related concerns, issues, and strategies. Visit website to download a free copy of IDEA Public Law and its associated regulations, answers to frequently asked questions about IDEA, a "User's Guide to the 1999 IDEA Regulations," a publication entitled "To Assure the Free Appropriate Public Education of All Children with Disabilities," and much more.

Key Transition Issues for Youth with Disabilities and Chronic Health Conditions
Maternal and Child Health Bureau's Institute for Child Health Policy's Healthy and Ready to Work
National HRTW Initiative
HHS/HRSA/MCHB/DSCSHN
Parklawn Building, Room 18A-18
5600 Fishers Lane
Rockville, MD 20857
(301) 443-2370;(301) 443-0832 (Fax)
Web: http://www.mchbhrtw.org/materials/default.htm; http://www.mchb.hrsa.gov
Visit website to download a free copy of this policy paper regarding SSI programs that affect adolescents. This paper assists families and service providers ensure successful transitions to work and independence for youth with disabilities and chronic illness.

A Parent's Guide: Accessing Programs for Infants, Toddlers, and Preschoolers with Disabilities
National Information Center for Children and Youth with Disabilities (NICHCY) (1994)
P.O. Box 1492
Washington, DC 20013-1492
(202) 884-8200 (V/TTY); (800) 695-0285 (V/TTY); (202) 884-8441 (Fax)
Email: nichcy@aed.org
Web: http://www.nichcy.org/pubs/parent/pa2.htm
Visit website to download a free copy of this guide, which provides information about IDEA, early intervention services for children ages birth to two, special education and related services for children ages three to five years, and services for underserved populations. Available in English and Spanish.

A Parent's Guide: Special Education and Related Services: Communicating Through Letter Writing
National Information Center for Children and Youth with Disabilities (NICHCY) (1991)
P.O. Box 1492
Washington, DC 20013-1492
(202) 884-8200 (V/TTY); (800) 695-0285 (V/TTY);
(202) 884-8441 (Fax)
Email: nichcy@aed.org
Web: http://www.nichcy.org/pubs/parent/pa9.htm

Visit website to download a free copy of this publication, which identifies when it is useful for parents to write letters to key players in the special education process. Available in English and Spanish.

Paying the Bills: Tips for Families on Financing Health Care for Children with Special Needs, 2nd Edition
Maternal and Child Health Clearing House
(888) 434-4624
Web: http://www.nmchc.org/html/order.htm
Offers information regarding getting started, medical bills, alternative sources of funding, influencing decision-makers, and connecting with other families. Also other publications from the Maternal and Child Health Clearing House available online.

Pediatric Brain Injury Reading List
Research & Training Center in Rehabilitation and Childhood Trauma
Department of Physical Medicine & Rehabilitation at the New England Medical Center
750 Washington Street, #75 K-R
Boston, MA 02111-1901
(617) 636-5031
Web: http://www.neuro.pmr.vcu.edu/reflists/PEDREF.html
Offers a listing of easy to-read guides and booklets on brain injury, hospital care, and rehabilitation.

Traumatic Brain Injury in Children and Teens: A National Guide for Families
New Hampshire EMS for Children Grant Project (1999)
Web: http://www.ems-c.org/family/framefamily.htm
Visit website to download a free copy of this guide, which walks parents of children with TBI through each step of their child's recovery, from the hospital to the home. Includes information on understanding and coping with the diagnosis, how to access appropriate health care services, and options for payment of short- and long-term care.

When Your Child's Head Has Been Hurt
Arizona Governor's Council on Spinal & Head Injuries (1999)
Web: http://www.tbigrants.com/arizonaproduct.htm
Visit website to download a free copy of this fact sheet, which identifies symptoms of postconcussive disorders. It addresses common physical, behavioral, and cognitive signs that may indicate a more serious problem.

RESOURCE GUIDE

The organizations and web sites listed below offer support, information, and services that can be of help to you and your child with TBI. For further information about any of these organizations, call, write, or visit their web page and request a copy of their newsletter or other publications.

■ National Organizations

ABLEDATA
Macro International
8630 Fenton Street, Suite 930
Silver Spring, MD 20910
(800) 227-0216; (301) 608-8958 (Fax)
Email: adaigle@macroint.com
Web: http://www.abledata.com
ABLEDATA is a database containing information on assistive technology and rehabilitation equipment. Parents can search the database free of charge from the website, or can pay a small fee to have a search performed for them. ABLEDATA offers low-cost information packets on selected subjects.

American Occupational Therapy Association (AOTA)
4720 Montgomery Lane
P.O. Box 31220
Bethesda, MD 20824-1220
(301) 652-2682 (V); (800) 377-8555 (TDD)
Email: humanres@aota.org
Web: http://www.aota.org
The AOTA is a professional organization for occupational therapists. It can refer you to a qualified Occupational Therapist in your area.

American Physical Therapy Association (APTA)
1111 N. Fairfax Street
Alexandria, VA 22314-1488
(703) 684-2782 (V); (800) 999-APTA (V); (703) 683-6748 (TDD); (703) 684-7343 (Fax)
Email: humanresources@apta.org
Web: http://www.apta.org
The APTA has a free list of patient education publications. They can also direct you to the APTA chapter in your area. Call and ask for Information Central.

American Speech-Language-Hearing Association (ASHA)
10801 Rockville Pike
Rockville, MD 20852
(800) 498-2071 (V); (301) 571-0457 (TTY); (877) 541-5035 (Fax)
Email: actioncenter@asha.org
Web: http://www.ASHA.org
ASHA researches communication disorders. It has fifty state affiliates that can provide information about speech-language pathology services available locally. The organization offers brochures on speech/hearing disorders and information on computer software and augmentative communication.

Bicycle Helmet Safety Institute (BHSI)
4611 Seventh Street South
Arlington, VA 22204-1419
(703) 486-0100; (703) 486-0576 (Fax)
Email: info@helmets.org
Web: http://www.bhsi.org
This organization provides information about bicycle helmet safety, including laws, standards, recalls, statistics and research, information from *Consumer Reports*, plus a number of publications and documents.

Brain Injury Association (BIA)
105 North Alfred Street
Alexandria, VA 22314
(703) 236-6000; (703) 236-6001 (Fax)
Email: FamilyHelpline@biausa.org; PublicRelations@biausa.org
Web: http://www.biausa.org
The association strives to create a better future through brain injury prevention, research, education, and advocacy. It produces a Catalog of Educational Resources, available online and in a print version. It also publishes a bimonthly newsletter as well as the *National Directory of Brain Injury Rehabilitation Services*, which lists over 350 facilities and programs. It has affiliates in most states; see list under State Resources below.

Brain Injury Society (BIS)
1901 Avenue N, Suite 5E
Brooklyn, NY 11230
(718) 645-4401
Email: BISociety@aol.com
Web: http://www.bisociety.org
The Brain Injury Society is a not-for-profit organization that works with clients, families, and caregivers to identify strategies and techniques to maximize newfound potential for a stronger recovery from brain injury. This organization sponsors events, as well as provides general information on TBI, a quarterly newsletter, links to other relevant sites, and important contact information for government officials in a position to affect legislation.

Centers for Disease Control and Prevention (CDC)
1600 Clifton Road
Atlanta, GA 30333
(404) 639-3311; (404) 639-3534; (800) 311-3435
Web: http://www.cdc.gov/health/injuries.htm

The CDC's primary goal is to promote health and quality of life by preventing and controlling disease, injury, and disability. Specifically, the CDC can provide information on and prevention, and vital statistics on incidence, causes, and cost of care of TBI.

Children and Adults with Attention-Deficit/Hyperactive Disorder (CHADD)
8181 Professional Place, Suite 201
Landover, MD 20785
(301) 306-7070; (800) 233-4050; (301) 306-7090 (Fax)
Web: http://www.chadd.org
CHADD is a membership organization for families and individuals with attention deficit disorders which provides support and education for families, advocates for the rights of individuals with AD/HD, supports research, and offers a variety of publications.

Children's Defense Fund (CDF)
25 E Street, NW
Washington, DC 20001
(202) 628-8787; (800) CDF-1200
Email: cdfinfo@childrensdefense.org
Web: http://www.childrensdefense.org/
CDF is a far-reaching, nonprofit legal organization that works to expand the rights of children, including children with disabilities. It can provide information on topics such as insurance and childcare.

Coma Recovery Association, Inc. (CRA)
807 Carman Avenue
Westbury, NY 11590
(516) 997-1826; (516) 997-1613 (Fax)
Web: http://www.comarecovery.org
This nonprofit organization's main mission is to help people out of coma, resolve their postcomatose problems, and help them to achieve the best lives possible through rehabilitation, new technologies, medicines, and methods. This group provides referrals and general information regarding coma, networking with coma/brain injury professionals and other families, advocacy, and support.

Consortium for Appropriate Dispute Resolution in Special Education (CADRE)
P.O. Box 51360
Eugene, OR 97405-0906
(541) 686-5060; (541) 686-5063 (Fax)
Email: cadre@directionservice.org
Web: http://www.directionservice.org/cadre
CADRE provides technical assistance to state departments of education on the implementation of mediation requirements under IDEA. CADRE also supports parents, educators, and administrators by proposing options that will facilitate resolution for issues of conflict in special education programs. Offers pertinent articles and lists state contacts for CADRE projects.

Council for Exceptional Children (CEC)
1920 Association Drive
Reston, VA 22091-1589
(703) 620-3660 (V); (888) CEC SPED (V); (703) 264-9446 (TDD); (703) 264-9494 (Fax)
Email: service@cec.sped.org
Web: http://www.cec.sped.org

This international membership organization for educators focuses on the educational needs of children who are gifted or have disabilities. Their publications catalog includes a variety of materials on education-related topics such as Inclusion, AD/HD, At Risk Students, Early Childhood, Social Skills, Behavior Management, and Assessment.

Educational Resources Information Center—Clearinghouse on Disabilities and Gifted Education (ERIC EC)

US Department of Education/National Library of Education
The Council for Exceptional Children (CEC)
1920 Association Drive
Reston, VA 20191
(800) 328-0272 (V/TTY)
Email: ericec@cec.sped.org
Web: http://www.accesseric.org; http://ericec.org

ERIC EC gathers and disseminates professional literature, information, and resources on the education and development of individuals of all ages who have disabilities and/or who are gifted.

Epilepsy Foundation of America (EFA)

4351 Garden City Drive
Landover, MD 20785
(301) 459-3700 (V); (800) EFA-1000 (V-Out of state only); (800) 332-2070 (TDD)
Email: postmaster@efa.org
Web: http://www.efa.org

The EFA answers questions and provides information on seizure disorders and medications. The professionals on staff can also refer you to other organizations and agencies depending on your needs. A catalog of publications is available.

Families USA—The Voice for Health Care Consumers

1334 G Street, NW
Washington, DC 20005
(202) 628-3030; (202) 347-2417 (Fax)
Email: info@familiesusa.org
Web: http://www.familiesusa.org/index.html

This national nonprofit, nonpartisan organization provides information and resources related to healthcare public policy and tracks the progress of legislation affecting managed care and Medicaid. Lists links to pertinent web sites and has publications, which can be mailed or downloaded on computer, regarding health insurance, especially Medicaid, and prescription medications. Lists relevant information state by state.

Family Voices

National Office
P.O. Box 769
Algodones, NM 87001
(505) 867-2368; (888) 835-5669; (505) 867-6517 (Fax)
Email: kidshealth@familyvoices.org
Web: http://www.familyvoices.org

A grassroots clearinghouse for information and education concerning the health care of children with special health needs. They monitor public and private sector healthcare changes, and serve on boards and task forces, bringing the family perspective to policy discussions and decisions. Offers a newsletter, fact sheet, list of publications, and an advocacy handbook.

Hydrocephalus Association
870 Market St., Suite 705
San Francisco, CA 94102
(415) 732-7040; (888) 598-3789; (415) 732-7044 (Fax)
Email: hydroassoc@aol.com
Web: http://www.hydroassoc.org
This membership organization educates, advocates for, and provides support for families. They have a booklet in English and Spanish discussing all facets of hydrocephalus, publish a quarterly newsletter, and offer many other services and resources.

International Brain Injury Association (IBIA)
700 Harris Street, Suite 205
Charlottesville, VA 22903
(804) 296-IBIA; (804) 296-4546 (Fax)
Email: info@internationalbrain.org
Web: http://www.internationalbrain.org
The IBIA works with medical and clinical professionals, advocates, policy makers, and consumers, striving to provide international leadership for creative solutions to the issues associated with brain injury. The IBIA publishes the *International NeuroTrauma Letter*, a quarterly newsletter, and *Brain Injury*, a professional journal, and sponsors many international programs and conferences related to TBI.

National Association for Parents of Children with Visual Impairments (NAPVI)
P.O. Box 317
Watertown, MA 02471
(617) 972-7441; (800) 562-6265; (617) 972-7444 (Fax)
Email: napvi@perkins.pvt.k12.ma.us
Web: http://www.spedex.com/napvi
This national organization of parents promotes the development of parent groups, provides information and publications about visual impairments, maintains a national support and information network, and sponsors workshops and conferences.

National Association of Private Schools for Exceptional Children
1522 K Street, NW, Suite 1032
Washington, DC 20005
(202) 408-3338; (202) 408-3340 (Fax)
Email: napsec@aol.com
Web: http://www.napsec.com
This professional association publishes a newsletter and a directory of private schools for children with special needs.

National Association of Protection & Advocacy Systems (NAPAS)
900 Second Street, NE, Suite 211
Washington, DC 20002
(202) 408-9514 (V); (202) 408-9521 (TDD); 202-408-9520 (Fax)
Email: napas@earthlink.net
Web: http://www.protectionandadvocacy.com/;
   http://www.protectionandadvocacy.com/pa12.htm
NAPAS can refer you to your local protection and advocacy office for help with IDEA disputes, discrimination complaints, etc.

National Association of State Head Injury Administrators (NASHIA)
98 Corporate Lake Drive
Columbia, MO 65203
(573) 882-3807; (801) 912-4168 (Fax)
Web: http://www.nashia.org
    The goal of this association is to establish sound national head injury policy and assist government programs in the development of state and local prevention, rehabilitation and community support services programs and policies for people with traumatic head injury and their families. Their web site recommends many relevant web sites, lists state government services and federal agencies, and provides explanations for pertinent federal laws.

National Attention Deficit Disorder Association (ADDA)
1788 Second Street, Suite 200
Highland Park, IL 60035
(847) 432-ADDA; (847) 432-5874 (Fax)
Email: mail@add.org
Web: http://www.add.org/index.html
    ADDA is an organization focused on the needs of adults and young adults with AD/HD and their families. This organization offers relevant articles, answers to frequently asked questions, means to contact AD/HD professionals, and information regarding support groups, conferences, books, and other resources.

National Center of Medical Home Initiatives for Children with Special Needs
The American Academy of Pediatrics (AAP)
141 Northwest Point Boulevard
Elk Grove Village, IL 60007-1098
(847) 434-4000; (847) 434-8000 (Fax)
Email: medical_home@aap.org
Web: http://www.aap.org/advocacy/medhome/aap.htm
    The mission of the National Center is to work in cooperation with federal agencies, particularly the Maternal and Child Health Bureau (MCHB), to ensure that children with special needs have access to a medical home where health care services are accessible, family-centered, continuous, comprehensive, coordinated, compassionate, and culturally competent.

National Council on Disability
1331 F Street, NW, Suite 1050
Washington, DC 20004-1107
(202) 272-2004 (V); (202) 272-2074 (TTY); (202) 272-2022 (Fax)
Email: mquigley@ncd.gov
Web: http://www.ncd.gov
    The NCD is an independent federal policy agency that makes recommendations to the president and congress on disability policy and represents all people with disabilities, regardless of severity, age, or cultural background. Lists links to other major federal agencies concerned with disabilities, lists resources including means to contact your state senators and representatives, a guide to disability rights laws, information regarding IEPs and IFSPs, etc.

National Council on Independent Living
1916 Wilson Boulevard, Suite 209
Arlington, VA 22201

(703) 525-3406; (703) 525-4153; (703) 525-3409 (Fax)
Email: ncil@ncil.org
Web: http://www.ncil.org
A source of information on affordable and accessible housing for people with disabilities.

National Easter Seal Society
230 West Monroe, Suite 1800
Chicago, IL 60606
(312) 726-6200 (V); (800) 221-6827 (V); (312) 726-4258 (TTY); (312) 726-1494 (Fax)
Email: info@easter-seals.org
Web: http://www.easter-seals.org
The National Easter Seal Society is dedicated to helping people with disabilities and their families by offering screening, advocacy, public education, and other services. Local chapters offer rehab services, childcare, and recreational programs. The society publishes many valuable booklets and pamphlets.

National Headache Foundation (NHF)
428 West St. James Place, 2nd Floor
Chicago, IL 60614-2750
(888) NHF-5552; (773) 525-7357 (Fax)
Web: http://www.headaches.org
Email: info@headaches.org
This organization's goal is to serve as an information resource to individuals with headaches, their families, and the healthcare providers who treat them; to promote research into potential headache causes and treatments; and to educate the public about the causes and consequences of headaches. They offer educational resources, information about upcoming events, programs, and clinical trials, and pharmaceutical links.

National Information Center for Children and Youth with Disabilities (NICHCY)
P.O. Box 1492
Washington, DC 20013-1492
(202) 884-8200 (V/TTY); (800) 695-0285 (V/TTY); (202) 884-8441 (Fax)
Email: nichcy@aed.org
Web: http://www.nichcy.org
This clearinghouse provides information on educational programs and other special services to parents of children with disabilities. You may call or send in questions. For a nominal charge, NICHCY also produces fact sheets, information packets, and "State Sheets," which list each state's resources for people with disabilities. Publications can be downloaded for free from the web site and some are available in Spanish.

National Organization on Disability (NOD)
910 Sixteenth Street, NW, Suite 600
Washington, DC 20006
(202) 293-5960 (V); (202) 293-5968 (TDD); (202) 293-7999 (Fax)
Email: ability@nod.org
Web: http://www.nod.org
NOD is a national disability network organization concerned with all disabilities, all age groups, and all disability issues. Provides a fact sheet on ADA, as well as answers to frequently asked questions regarding disability and accessibility.

National Parent Network on Disabilities (NPND)
1130 17th Street, NW, Suite 400
Washington, DC 20036
(202) 463-2299; (202) 463-9403 (Fax)
Email: shepard_linda@hotmail.com
Web: http://www.npnd.org
This organization serves as a national voice for parents of children and adults with disabilities. A major goal is to empower parents to obtain inclusive educations for their children. Offers publications.

National Rehabilitation Information Center (NARIC)
1010 Wayne Avenue, Suite 800
Silver Spring, MD 20910
(301) 562-2400 (V); (800) 346-2742 (V); (301) 495-5626 (TT); (301) 562-2401 (Fax)
Email: dwendling@kra.com
Web: http://www.naric.com
Funded by the National Institute on Disability and Rehabilitation Research (NIDRR), this organization provides quick reference and referral to nearby rehabilitation facilities and relevant newsletters and support groups, rehabilitation database searches, document delivery, and access to commercially published books, journal articles, and audiovisuals.

National Resource Center for Traumatic Brain Injury (NRC for TBI)
Medical College of Virginia Campus of Virginia Commonwealth University
P.O. Box 980542
Richmond, VA 23298-0542
(804) 828-9055; (804) 828-2378 (Fax)
Email: mbking@hsc.vcu.edu
Web: http://www.neuro.pmr.vcu.edu
Provides a catalog of books and videos on TBI. Titles include: *The Brain Injury Source Book, Getting Better and Better After Brain Injury* (separate editions for Survivors and Family), *For Kids Only: A Guide to Brain Injury, Guidelines for Educational Services for Students with TBI*. Website offers an opportunity for families to write in with questions about coping with TBI.

New Visions
1124 Roberts Mountain Road
Faber, VA 22938
(804) 361-2285; (800) 606-3665; (804) 361-1807 (Fax)
Email: sem@new-vis.com
Web: http://www.new-vis.com
New Visions provides continuing education and therapy services to professionals and parents working with infants and children with feeding, swallowing, oral-motor, and prespeech problems. This organization provides workshops, clinical services, a Mealtimes Catalogue, information papers, and links to related websites.

Office of Americans with Disabilities Act (ADA)
Civil Rights Division
U.S. Department of Justice
P.O. Box 66118
Washington, DC 20035-6118
(202) 514-0301 (V); (202) 514-0383 (TDD)

Web: http://www.usdoj.gov/crt/ada/adahom1.htm
This is the federal agency charged with distributing information and answering questions about the Americans with Disabilities Act. Information can be obtained on the web site or sent by fax or U.S. mail. Spanish language service is also available.

Office of Special Education and Rehabilitative Services (OSERS)
U.S. Department of Education
330 C Street, SW
Washington, DC 20202
(202) 205-5465; (202) 205-9252 (Fax)
Web: http://www.ed.gov/offices/OSERS
This federal organization offers information on civil rights, federal benefits, medical services, education, and support organizations. It publishes *OSERS News in Print*, a newsletter regarding federal activities affecting people with disabilities, and *Pocket Guide to Federal Help for Individuals with Disabilities*, a summary of services and benefits available to individuals who qualify.

Parent Advocacy Coalition for Educational Rights (PACER)
8161 Normandale Boulevard
Minneapolis, MN 55437-1044
(952) 838-9000 (V); (800) 537-2237 (V); (952) 838 0190 (TTY); (952) 838-0199 (Fax)
Email: pacer@pacer.org; fape@pacer.org
Web: http://www.pacer.org; http://www.fape.org
This organization offers twenty-one programs to expand opportunities that enhance the quality of life for children and young adults with all types of disabilities. Offers a catalog of publications, a computer resource center, relevant articles, and workshops. Sponsors a new project called Family & Advocates Partnership for Education (FAPE), which aims to inform and educate families and advocates about IDEA.

Rehabilitation Engineering and Assistive Technology Society of North America (RESNA)
1700 N Moore Street, Suite 1540
Arlington, VA 22209-1903
(703) 524-6686 (V); (703) 524-6639 (TTY); (703) 524-6630 (Fax)
Email: info@resna.org
Web: http://www.resna.org
RESNA promotes research, development, education, advocacy, and the provision of technology, and supports the people engaged in these activities. It disseminates a number of publications, including an assistive technology journal. In addition, its web site includes downloadable legislative documents, and lists states funded under the Assistive Technology Act of 1998 along with addresses and contacts.

Research and Training Center in Rehabilitation and Childhood Trauma
Department of Physical Medicine and Rehabilitation
New England Medical Center
750 Washington Street, #75K-R
Boston, MA 02111-1901
(617) 636-5031; (617) 636-5513 (Fax)
Web: http://www.nemc.org/rehab/homepg.htm
The purpose of this organization is to conduct research to increase knowledge about the causes, treatment, and outcomes of injuries to children, increase access to available services, and disseminate this information to involved parties.

Senate Document Room
Hart Building
2nd and C Street, NE
Washington, DC 20515
(202) 224-7860; (202) 225-1772 (Legislative information regarding bill numbers);
(202) 228-2815 (Fax)
Web: http://www.senate.gov
    You can obtain a copy of any federal bill or law, including IDEA or ADA, by contacting this office. Requests must be submitted by fax, by mail, or in person (not by phone).

Social Security Administration
Office of Public Inquiries
6401 Security Boulevard
Room 4-C-5 Annex
Baltimore, MD 21235-6401
(800) 777-1213 (V); (800) 325-0778 (TTY)
Web: http://www.ssa.gov
    A government program offering economic protection to retired and disabled persons, as well as their survivors. Web site offers online application for SSI and Medicare, downloadable forms and many pertinent publications, and an explanation of Social Security statements.

Starbright World
The Starbright Foundation
11835 West Olympic Boulevard, Suite 500
Los Angeles, CA 90064
(310) 479-1212; (310) 479-1235 (Fax)
Web: http://www.starbright.org
    Starbright World is dedicated to the creation of projects that empower seriously ill children and teens to address the medical and emotional challenges that accompany prolonged illness and injury. This organization produces a number of videos and interactive programs for kids, teens, and healthcare professionals that discuss hospital life, medical procedures, communicating with doctors, and going back to school.

TASH—Disability Advocacy Worldwide
29 W. Susquehanna Avenue, Suite 210
Baltimore, MD 21204
(410) 828-8274 (V); (410) 828-1306 (TDD); (410) 828-6706 (Fax)
Email: nweiss@tash.org
Web: http://www.tash.org
    TASH is an international advocacy organization that works for the inclusion of people with disabilities in every aspect of life. The organization promotes inclusive education, advocates for opportunities and rights, and publishes a journal and a newsletter.

Think First
5550 Meadowbrook Drive, Suite 110
Rolling Meadows, IL 60008
(847) 290-8600; (800) THINK56; (847) 290-9005 (Fax)
Email: thinkfirst@thinkfirst.org
Web: http://www.thinkfirst.org/

This foundation's mission is to prevent brain, spinal cord, and other traumatic injuries through the education of individuals, community leaders, and the creators of public policy. They provide public education in the form of video programs for kids and teens.

U.S. Department of Education
Clearinghouse on Disability Information
330 C Street, SW
Washington, DC 20202
(800) USA-LEARN; (202) 205-8245 (Clearinghouse); (800) 437-0833 (TTY); (202) 401-0689 (Fax)
Email: National_Library_of_Education@ed.gov
Web: http://www.ed.gov/index.html; http://cricec.org
The mission of the U.S. Department of Education is to ensure equal access to education and to promote educational excellence for all Americans. Its website provides information regarding initiatives, grant opportunities, research, statistics, and publications. ERIC, the clearinghouse on disability information, gathers and disseminates professional literature, information, and resources on the education and development of individuals of all ages who have disabilities and/or who are gifted.

U.S. Department of Justice
Civil Rights Division
Coordination and Review Section
P.O. Box 66560
Washington, DC 20035-6560
(202) 307-2222 (V); (202) 307-2678 (TDD); (888) TITLE-06 (V/TDD)
Web: http://www.usdoj.gov/crt/cor/index.htm
This is the agency to contact if you believe you or your child has been discriminated under Title II or III of the ADA. From the web site, you can download a complaint form, in English or Spanish. You can also send a letter of complaint to the address above.

U.S. Equal Employment Opportunity Commission (EEOC)
1801 L Street, NW
Washington, DC 20507
(202) 663-4900 (V); (202) 663-4494 (TTY)
Web: http://www.eeoc.gov
The mission of this organization is to promote equal opportunity in employment through administrative and judicial enforcement of the federal civil rights laws and through education and technical assistance. You can send a letter of complaint regarding discrimination under Title I of the ADA to the address above.

University of Kansas
Department of Special Education—Traumatic Brain Injury Project
521 J.R. Pearson
1122 W Campus Road
Lawrence, KS 66045
(913) 588-5943
Project Director: Janet Tyler
Email: jtyler@kumc.edu
Web: http://www.sped.ukans.edu

The Kansas State Department of Education's Student Support Services addresses the training needs of professionals working with students with TBI through the services provided by the Traumatic Brain Injury Project.

:: International Organizations

CANADA

Brain Injury Association of Alberta (BIAA)
136 17th Avenue, NE
Calgary, AB
T2E-1L6
(403) 207-5606; (888) 533-5355 (In AB); (403) 207-3444 (Fax)
Email: biaa@cadvision.com
Web: http://www.biaa.net
The BIAA is a nonprofit charitable organization and provincial advocacy group dedicated to improving the quality of life for individuals with the effects of acquired brain injury. This group promotes research, public awareness, and the creation of new services, represents the needs of affected families, and advocates for brain injury survivors.

Brain Injury Association of Toronto
#500-1 St. Clair Avenue E.
Toronto, ON
M4T 2V7
(416) 513-1903; (416) 964-2492 (Fax)
Email: biatinfo@volnetmmp.net

Epilepsy Canada
1470 Peel Street, Suite 745
Montreal, Quebec
H3A 1T1
(514) 845-7855
A nonprofit organization dedicated to improving the quality of life for people with epilepsy, this organization publishes a newsletter and several informational brochures.

Northern Alberta Brain Injury Society (NABIS)
Alberta Brain Injury Help Line
Suite 301
10106 – 111 Avenue
Edmonton, AB
T5G 0B4
(870) 474-5678; (877) 474-5678; (870) 474-4415 (Fax)
Email: nabis@abihelp.org
Web: http://www.abihelp.org
This helpline provides information and referrals to community services for brain injury survivors, families, and professionals.

Ontario Brain Injury Association (OBIA)
P.O. Box 2338
St. Catharines, ON
Canada

L2R 7R9
(905) 641-8877; (905) 641-0323 (Fax)
Email: obia@obia.on.ca
Web: http://www.obia.on.ca/default.html
    This organization is dedicated to preventing traumatic brain injuries and to improving the quality of life for survivors of acquired brain injury, their families, and the community with which they interact. They provide encouragement, direction, resources, advocacy, and access to the Caregiver Information Support Link (1-800-263-5404).

UNITED KINGDOM

Brain Injury Association of London and Region
(London, Middlesex, Huron, Perth, Oxford, and Elgin)
111 Waterloo Street, Suite 307
London Ontario
N6B 2M4
(519) 642-4539; (519) 642-4124 (Fax)
Email: braininj@skynet.ca
Web: http://www.braininjurylondon.on.ca/
    This charitable organization and support group offers information regarding available services, resources, and programs, an Internet chat room, a monthly newsletter, and a resource center with books, articles, tapes, and videos about brain injury and recovery.

Headway—The Brain Injury Association of the UK
+44 (0)115-924-0800;+44 (0)115-947-1903
Email: information@headway.org.uk; gen.administration@headway.org.uk
Web: http://www.headway.org.uk/
    Headway is a charitable organization and support group, the aim of which is to promote understanding of all aspects of head injury and to provide information, support, and services, especially rehabilitation and resettlement, to people with head injury, their family and caregivers. Headway National produces a large selection of publications on many issues related to head injury and its aftermath.

■■ State and Local Resources

    Listed below are some national organizations and agencies that can give you contact information for state and local organizations. You may also contact the National Information Center for Children and Youth with Disabilities (NICHCY) listed under National Organizations, for a "state sheet" listing disability resources in your state.

State Departments of Education/Offices of Special Education Systems:
    These are the state agencies responsible for ensuring that the requirements of the Individuals with Disabilities Education Act (IDEA) are followed. These agencies oversee how local school districts implement IDEA. For contact information for your state agency, write or call:
U.S. Department of Education/National Library of Education
400 Maryland Avenue, SW
Washington, DC 20202-5523
(202) 205-5015; (800) 424-1616; (202) 205-7561 (TTY); (202) 401-0547 (Fax)
Email: library@inet.ed.gov
Web: http://www.ed.gov/NLE/; http://www.ed.gov

State Vocational Rehabilitation Agencies:

These agencies provide education, training, and counseling, as well as medical, therapeutic, and other services, to prepare people with disabilities to work. Locate your state agency by contacting:
Office of Special Education and Rehabilitative Services
Rehabilitative Services Administration (RSA)
U.S. Department of Education
330 C Street, SW
Room 3026
Washington, DC 20202
(202) 205-5482; (202) 205-9874 (Fax)
Web: http://www.ed.gov/offices/OSERS/RSA/; http://www.resna.org/taproject/at/statecontacts.html

Protection & Advocacy Agencies:

P&A offices are legal organizations established to protect the rights of people with disabilities. They can supply information about the educational, health care, residential, social, and legal services available for children with head injuries in your state. In some cases, attorneys from these offices can provide representation on behalf of your child. For information regarding your state P&A agencies for CAP, PADD, PAIMI, PAIR (see Chapter 11) contact:
National Association of Protection & Advocacy Systems (NAPAS)
900 Second Street, NE, Suite 211
Washington, DC 20002
(202) 408-9514 (V); (202) 408-9521 (TDD); 202-408-9520 (Fax)
Email: napas@earthlink.net
Web: http://www.protectionandadvocacy.com

State Chapters of the National Brain Injury Association, Inc. (BIA):

These organizations serve as centralized advocacy, educational, and information sources for persons with TBI and their families. Parent Programs include privately and publicly funded groups that offer support, information, and referral services to parents of children with disabilities. If your home state does not have an active BIA chapter, information necessary to contact local representative(s) for the National Brain Injury Association is listed.

Alabama
Alabama Head Injury Foundation (AHIF)
3600 8th Avenue South
Birmingham, AL 35222
(205) 328-3505; (800) 433-8002; (205) 328-2479 (Fax)
Email: info@ahif.org
Web: http://www.ahif.org

Alaska
Brain Injury Association of Alaska
1251 Muldoon Road, Suite 103
Anchorage, AK 99504
(907) 338-9800 (V); (907) 338-9801 (TTY/Fax); (888) 945-HEAD;
(907) 283-5711 (Kenai Chapter)
Web: http://www.alaska.net/~drussell/bia-ak/

Arizona
Brain Injury Association of Arizona
3320 E. Roeser Road
Phoenix, AZ 85040
(602) 323-9165; (888) 305-0073; (602) 323-9378 (Fax)
Web: http://www.biausa.org/Arizona/index.htm

Arkansas
Brain Injury Association of Arkansas
P.O. Box 26236
Little Rock, AR 72221-6236
(501) 771-5011; (501) 227-8632 (Fax)
Email: BIAofAR@aol.com
Web: http://www.biausa.org/Arkansas/index.htm

California
Brain Injury Association of California
P.O. Box 160786
Sacramento, CA 95816-0786
(916) 442-1710; (800) 457-2443; (916) 442-7305 (Fax)
Email: biac@juno.com
Web: http://www.biausa.org/California

Colorado
Brain Injury Association of Colorado
4200 West Conejos Place, Suite 524
Denver, CO 80224
(303) 355-9969; (800) 955-2443 (In state)
Email: BIACOLO@aol.com
Web: http://www.biacolorado.org

Connecticut
Brain Injury Association of Connecticut
1800 Silas Deane Highway, Suite 224
Rocky Hill, CT 06067
(860) 721-8111; (800) 278-8242; (860) 721-9008 (Fax)
Web: http://www.biact.org

Delaware
Brain Injury Association of Delaware
P.O. Box 95
Middletown, DE 19709-0095
(302) 537-5770; (800) 411-0505;
Web: http://www.biausa.org/Delaware/bia.htm

District of Columbia
BIA Representative of the District of Columbia: Karen Tyner
2100 Mayflower Drive
Lake Ridge, VA 22192
(202) 877-1464; (202) 291-5366 (Fax)

Florida

Brain Injury Association of Florida
North Broward Medical Center
201 East Sample Road
Pompano Beach, FL 33064
(954) 786-2400; (800) 992-3442; (954) 786-2437 (Fax)
Email: info@biaf.org
Web: http://www.biaf.org

Georgia

Brain Injury Association of Georgia
1447 Peachtree Street, NE, Suite 810
Atlanta, GA 30309
(404) 817-7577; (404) 817-7521 (Fax)
Email: biag@BrainInjuryGA.org
Web: http://www.braininjuryga.org

Hawaii

Brain Injury Association of Hawaii
1775 South Beretania Street, #203
Honolulu, HI 96826
(808) 941-0372
Web: http://www.geocities.com/biahawaii/

Idaho

Brain Injury Association of Idaho
P.O. Box 414
Boise, ID 83701-0414
UPS Packages: 1547 E. Holly Street, Boise, ID 83712
(208) 336-7708; (888) 374-3447 (In state); (208) 333-0026 (Fax)

Illinois

Brain Injury Association of Illinois
1127 S Mannheim, Suite 213
Westchester, IL 60154
(708) 344-4646; (800) 699-6443 (In state); (708) 344-4680 (Fax)
Email: info@biail.org; membership@biail.org
Web: http://www.biausa.org/Illinois/bia.htm

Indiana

Brain Injury Association of Indiana
Mickolon Building, First Floor
1525 N. Ritter Avenue
Indianapolis, IN 46219
(317) 356-7722; (800) 407-4246; (317) 356-4241 (Fax)
Email: BIAI@iquest.net
Web: http://www.biausa.org/Indiana/bia.htm

Iowa

Brain Injury Association of Iowa
2101 Kimball Avenue LL7
Waterloo, IA 50702

(319) 272-2312; (800) 475-4442; (319) 272-2109 (Fax)
Email: info@biaia.org
Web: http://www.biaia.org

Kansas
Brain Injury Association of Kansas and Greater Kansas City
1100 Pennsylvania, Suite 4061
Kansas City, MO 64105-1336
(816) 842-8607; (800) 783-1356; (816) 842-1531 (Fax)
Web: http://www.brain-injury-ks-gkc.org

Kentucky
Brain Injury Association of Kentucky
4229 Bardstown Road, #330
Louisville, KY 40218
(502) 493-0609; (800) 592-1117; (502) 499-8995 (Fax)
Email: info@braincenter.org
Web: http://www.braincenter.org; http://www.braincenter.org

Louisiana
Brain Injury Association of Louisiana
217 Buffwood Drive
Baker, LA 70714-3755
(225) 775-2780

Maine
Brain Injury Association of Maine
211 Maine Street, Suite 200
Farmingdale, ME 04344
(207) 582-4696; (800) 275-1233 (In state); (207) 582-4803 (Fax)
Email: biaofme@ctel.net
Web: http://www.biausa.org/Mainc/bia.htm

Maryland
Brain Injury Association of Maryland
2200 Kernan Drive
Baltimore, MD 21207
(410) 448-2924; (800) 221-6443 (In state); (410) 448-3541 (Fax)
Email: info@biamd.org
Web: http://www.biamd.org

Massachusetts
Massachusetts Brain Injury Association
484 Main Street, #325
Worcester, MA 01608
(508) 795-0244; (800) 242-0030; (508) 797-0101 (TTY/TDD); (508) 757-9109 (Fax)
Email: mbia@mbia.net
Web: http://www.mbia.net

Michigan
Brain Injury Association of Michigan
8619 W. Grand River, Suite I

Brighton, MI 48116-2334
(810) 229-5880; (800) 772-4323 (In state); (810) 229-8947 (Fax)
Email: biaofmi@cac.net
Web: http://www.biausa.org/Michigan

Minnesota
Brain Injury Association of Minnesota
43 Main Street SE, Suite 135
Minneapolis, MN 55414
(612) 378-2742; (800) 669-6442 (In state); (612) 378-2789 (Fax)
Email: info@braininjurymn.org
Web: http://www.braininjurymn.org

Mississippi
Brain Injury Association of Mississippi
P.O. Box 55912
2727 Old Canton Road
Jackson, MS 39296
(601) 981-1021; (800) 641-6442
Email: biaofms@aol.com
Web: http://members.aol.com/biaofms/index.htm

Missouri
Brain Injury Association of Missouri
10270 Page, Suite 100
St. Louis, MO 63132
(314) 426-4024; (800) 377-6442 (MO, IL, and KS only); (314) 426-3290 (Fax)
Email: braininjy@aol.com
Web: http://www.biausa.org/Missouri/bia.htm

Montana
Brain Injury Association of Montana
University of Montana
52 Corbin Hall, Room 333
Missoula, MT 59812
(406) 243-5973; (800) 241-6442 (In state); (406) 243-2349 (Fax)
Web: http://www.biausa.org/Montana

Nebraska
Brain Injury Association of Nebraska
1108 Avenue H
P.O. Box 124
Gothenburg, NE 69138
(308) 537-7875; (308) 537-7663; (888) 642-4137; (308) 537-7663 (Fax)
Web: http://www.biausa.org/Nebraska/bia.htm

Nevada
BIA Representative of Northern Nevada: Carol Swan
P.O. Box 2789
Gardenerville, NV 89410
(775) 782-8336

BIA Representative of Southern Nevada: Dr. Leif Leaf
NV Community Enrichment Program
2820 W. Charleston Boulevard, Suite D-37
Attn: Robert Hogan
Las Vegas, NV 89102
(702) 259-1903

New Hampshire
Brain Injury Association of New Hampshire
109 North State Street, Suite 2
Concord, NH 03301
(603) 225-8400; (800) 773-8400; (603) 228-6749 (Fax)
Email: mail@bianh.org
Web: http://www.bianh.org

New Jersey
Brain Injury Association of New Jersey
1090 King George Post Road, Suite 708
(732) 738-1002; (800) 669-4323 (In state); (732) 738-1132 (Fax)
Email: info@bianj.org
Web: http://www.bianj.org

New Mexico
Brain Injury Association of New Mexico
11000 Candelaria Boulevard NE, Suite 113-W
Albuquerque, NM 87112
(505)292-7414; (888) 292-7415 (In state)
Email: headway@aol.com

New York
Brain Injury Association of New York State
10 Colvin Avenue
Albany, NY 12206-1242
(518) 459-7911; (800) 228-8201; (518) 482-5285 (Fax)
Web: http://www.bianys.org

North Carolina
Brain Injury Association of North Carolina
State Resource and Administration Center
133 Fayetteville Street Mall
Raleigh, NC 27601
(919) 833-9634
Email: info@bianc.org
Web: http://www.bianc.org

North Dakota
Brain Injury Association of North Dakota
Open Door Center
209 2nd Avenue, SE
Valley City, ND 58072
(701) 845-1124; (701)-845-1175 (Fax)
Email: opendoorctr@hotmail.com

Ohio
Brain Injury Association of Ohio
1335 Dublin Road, Suite 217-D
Columbus, OH 43215-1000
(614) 481-7100; (800) 686-9563 (In state); (614) 481-7103 (Fax)
Email: help@biaoh.org
Web: http://www.biaoh.org

Oklahoma
Brain Injury Association of Oklahoma
P.O. Box 88
Hillsdale, OK 73743-0088
(580) 233-4363; (800) 765-6809; (580) 233-4546 (Fax)
Email: biaok@ionet.net
Web: http://www.biaok.org

Oregon
Brain Injury Association of Oregon
1118 Lancaster Drive NE, PMB 345
Salem, OR 97301
(503) 585-0855; (800) 544-5243 (In state); (503) 585-0888 (Fax)
Email: biaor@open.org
Web: http://www.open.org/~biaor

Pennsylvania
BIA Representative of Eastern Pennsylvania: Suedell Cirwithen
33 Rock Hill Road
Bala Cynwyd, PA 19004
(800) 383-8889
Email: suedell@brain-rehab.com

BIA Representative of Western Pennsylvania: Ed Crinnion
(412) 884-8937

Rhode Island
Brain Injury Association of Rhode Island
Independence Square
500 Prospect Street
Pawtucket, RI 02860
(401) 725-2360; (401) 727-2810 (Fax)
Email: BuckleUp1@aol.com
Web: http://www.oso.com/community/groups/brainin/index.html

South Carolina
Brain Injury Association of South Carolina
1030 St. Andrews Road
Columbia, SC 29210
(803) 731-0588; (800) 290-6461; (803) 731-0589 (Fax)
Email: scbraininjury@mindspring.com

South Dakota
South Dakota Brain Injury Association

RR 2, Box 449
Aberdeen, SD 57401-9702
(605) 229-2177

Tennessee
Brain Injury Association of Tennessee
699 W Main Street, Suite 112
Hendersonville, TN 37075
(615) 264-3052; (877) 885-7511 (In state); (615) 264-1693 (Fax)
Email: mail@tnbiat.org
Web: http://www.tnbiat.org

Texas
Brain Injury Association of Texas
1339 Lamar Square Drive, Suite C
Austin, TX 78704
(512) 326-1212; (800) 392-0040; (512) 326-8088 (Fax)
Email: info@biatx.org
Web: http://www.biatx.org

Utah
Brain Injury Association of Utah
1800 SW Temple, Suite 203, Box 22
Salt Lake City, UT 84115
(801) 484-2240; (800) 281-8442 (In state); (801) 484-5932 (Fax)
Email: biau@sisna.com
Web: http://www.biau.org

Vermont
Brain Injury Association of Vermont
P.O. Box 8388
Essex Junction, VT 05451
(802) 872-9999; (802) 879-3355 (Fax)
Email : BIAVT@aol.com
Web: http://www.biavt.org

Virginia
Brain Injury Association of Virginia
3212 Cutshaw Avenue, Suite 315
Richmond, VA 23230
(804) 355-5748; (800) 334-8443; (804) 355-6381 (Fax)
Web: http://www.bia.pmr.vcu.edu

Northern Virginia Brain Injury Association (NVBIA)
P.O. Box 2148
Springfield, VA 22152
(703) 569-1855; (703) 352-1656
Email: info-nvbia@nvbia.org
Web: http://www.nvbia.org

Washington
Brain Injury Association of Washington

16315 NE 87th, Suite B-4
Redmond, WA 98052
(425) 895-0047; (800) 523-LIFT (In state); (425) 895-0458 (Fax)
Email: biawa@biawa.org
Web: http://www.biawa.org

Washington, DC
See District of Columbia

West Virginia
Brain Injury Association of West Virginia
P.O. Box 574
Institute, WV 25112-0574
(304) 766-4892; (800) 356-6443 (In state); (304) 766-4940 (Fax)
Email: biawv@aol.com
Web: http://www.biausa.org/Wvirginia

Wisconsin
Brain Injury Association of Wisconsin
2900 North 117th Street, Suite 100
Wauwatosa, WI 53222
(414) 778-4144; (800) 882-9282 (In state); (414) 778-0276 (Fax)
Email: biaw@execpc.com
Web: http://www.biaw.org

Wyoming
Brain Injury Association of Wyoming
111 West 2nd Street, Suite 106
Casper, WY 82601
(307) 473-1767; (800) 643-6457; (307) 237-5222 (Fax)
Email: gloriad@trib.com
Web: http://www.biausa.org/Wyoming

■ Internet Resources

ADA Technical Assistance Project
Web: http://adata.org
 This website provides an overview of the Americans with Disabilities Act and offers links to dozens of online government publications about different aspects of the ADA.

Ask a Neurosurgeon—Questions and Answers on Head Injury
Department of Neurosurgery
University of Utah
50 North Medical Drive
Salt Lake City, UT 84132
(801) 581-6908
Web: http://www.neurosurgery.org/pubpages/patres/askaneuro/jan98.html
 This website answers hard-hitting questions about head injury and includes a list of neurosurgeons in your area.

Balance Check's ADD/ADHD Page
Web: http://user.cybrzn.com/~kenyonck/add/Links
This website includes an extensive links page and book guide on AD/HD.

Bandaides and Blackboards
Web: http://funrsc.fairfield.edu/~jfleitas/contents.html
This site, designed for kids and teens with disabilities and chronic illness and their families, includes stories, poems, and other expressions of what it's like to be different. Also includes information on disease, disability, and available supports.

Bikes 'n' Blades: The Safety Scene
Web: http://pages.prodigy.net/sosberg/index.htm
This website includes statistics and articles about biking, skating, and skateboarding safety and links to related sites.

The Brain Injury Information NETwork
Web: http://tbinet.org/index.html
An international network of information, support groups, and listserv regarding brain injury.

Brain Injury Information Page
Web: http://www.tbilaw.com
This is the home page of Attorney Gordon S. Johnson, Jr. and the Brain Injury Law Office. More than just an advertisement, this site provides information about brain injury, concussion, and coma for TBI survivors, spouses, and caregivers. Also sponsors the site *Waiting While Someone is in Coma*.

Centre for Neuro Skills
2658 Mt. Vernon Avenue
Bakersfield, CA 93306
(661) 872-3408; (800) 922-4994;
(661) 872-5150 (Fax)
Email: bakersfield@neuroskills.com
Web: http://www.neuroskills.com

Disability Resource Library
Web: http://www.disabilityresource.com
This online shopping resource offers books about various disabilities and links to related web rings.

Dr. Diane Roberts Stoler on Mild Brain Injury
Web: http://www.drdiane.com; http://www.health-helper.com
This website features a reference book on brain trauma, *Coping with Mild Traumatic Brain Injury: A Guide to Living with Problems Associated with Brain Trauma*, which includes an extensive resource section. The site also includes answers to frequently asked questions about brain injury, articles, resources, and links to chat rooms and other related sites.

Family Village—A Global Community of Disability-Related Resources
Waisman Center
University of Wisconsin-Madison
1500 Highland Avenue
Madison, WI 53705-2280
Web: http://www.familyvillage.wisc.edu/index.htmlx
This site provides information, resources, and communication opportunities on the Internet for persons with cognitive and other disabilities, for their families, and for those that provide them services and support.

Half the Planet—The Disability Resource Network
350 Fifth Avenue
New York, NY 10118
(212) 643-0650; (212) 643-6704 (Fax)
Web: http://www.halftheplanet.com
An authoritative online source of tools for independent living for the entire disability community. This web site provides access to reliable services and products, allows people to connect with peer support, and keep up with disability-related news and information.

Head Injury Hotline
212 Pioneer Building
Seattle, WA 98104-2221
(206) 621-8558
Email: brain@headinjury.com
Web: http://www.headinjury.com
This website, geared toward persons with head injury, survivors, and families, provides information, education, and support while promoting self-advocacy, and self-care, centered around collaborative partnerships with family, loved ones, and professional service providers.

Lash and Associates Publishing/Training
708 Young Forest Drive
Wake Forest, NC 27587-9040
(919) 562-0015 (Phone/Fax)
Email: lapublishing@earthlink.net
Web: http://www.lapublishing.com
This site offers manuals, books, newsletter articles, answers to frequently asked questions, and resources for educators, clinicians, parents, and survivors of TBI.

LD Online
Web: http://www.ldonline.org
This very user-friendly site, designed for families and teachers of students with learning disabilities and/or AD/HD, offers hundreds of online articles on assessment, treatment, coping, and other issues, as well as links to other pertinent websites. The lists and explanations of accommodations and modifications are helpful for students with a variety of learning differences, not just LD.

Neuropsychology Central
Web: http://www.neuropsychologycentral.com
The goal of this website is to increase public awareness of the relatively new field of neuropsychology, which investigates the role of individual brain systems in

complex forms of mental activity. Discusses how and why a neuropsychological evaluation is important for TBI patients and when one should be considered.

The Neurotrauma Law Nexus
Web: http://www.neurolaw.com
This website provides information about the incidence, causes, and consequences of TBI and spinal cord injury (SCI), new developments in diagnosis and treatment, a glossary of TBI and SCI terms, medico-legal issues affecting survivors and their families, the role of a neurolawyer, and information about resources available to TBI/SCI survivors and family members.

New Beginnings
Web: http://www.geocitics.com/nbsobl
This website is dedicated to survivors of TBI and their caregivers, family, and friends. It chronicles personal stories of survival, daily challenges, and coping strategies. It also connects visitors to TBI web rings.

Parents and Special Education
Ameri-Corp Speech and Hearing
1442 E Lincoln Avenue, #363
Orange, CA 92865
Email: superpal@parentpals.com
Web: http://www.parentpals.com
Offers some basic information about brain injury, explanations of special education terminology, recommends books on the subject of TBI, and provides links to related web sites.

The Perspectives Network (TPN)
Web: http://www.tbi.org
This organization's primary focus is positive communication between persons with brain injury and those who care for, support, and treat them. In addition, their goal is to increase public awareness and knowledge of TBI. The website features a message board, articles of interest, reference materials, survivor tools, an on-line book and video store and lending library, and artwork and poetry by survivors and family members.

SafetyTips.com
Web: http://www.safetytips.com
This website provides up-to-date information on sports and recreation safety, auto and travel safety, and personal and family safety.

School Psychology Resources Online
Office of Psychological Services
Baltimore County Public Schools
Towson, MD 21204
Web: http://www.schoolpsychology.net
This website functions as a vehicle for researching learning disabilities, mental retardation, functional behavioral assessment, mental health, special education, and much more.

The TBI Chat Room & Homepage
Email: sagasha@tbichat.org; wecare@tbichat.org
Web: http://www.tbichat.org

This website features links to chat rooms, message boards, email lists, member stories, poems and writings, and related websites.

This website provides information on current neurological news and research, rehabilitation, assessment scales, grants, support groups, and access to articles and newsletters. The Centre for Neuro Skills has rehabilitation facilities in California and Texas.

Waiting While Someone Is in Coma

(800) 992-9447

Email: rm@berlinwi.com

Web: http://www.waiting.com

This website provides information on brain injury: intracranial pressure, coma, the Rancho Los Amigos Scale, neurosurgery, the ICU, legal issues, brain anatomy, brain functions and pathology, and a complete glossary of terms you may encounter. Also includes a message board, sources of support, other resources, and links to related sites.

The Whole Brain Atlas

Web: http://www.med.harvard.edu/AANLIB/home.html

This site provides high quality brain images and clinical information. Can be viewed on the website or ordered in CD-ROM form.

CONTRIBUTOR'S NOTES

CYNTHIA HEDEMAN BONNER, LCSW-C, graduated from Gettysburg College and the University of Maryland School of Social Work. Her social work practice of five years has focused on a range of areas including developmental disabilities, inpatient and outpatient neurorehabilitation, and therapeutic foster care and adoptions for children with special needs. Currently, she provides child and family mental health services at the Kennedy Krieger Institute in Baltimore, MD, with a special interest in serving children experiencing issues of grief and loss.

KATHLEEN BRADY is a psychologist at the Kennedy Krieger Institute Specialized Transition Program and Kennedy Krieger School in Baltimore, MD. She provides neuropsychological evaluations, treatment planning, rehabilitation therapy, and staff and parent consultation for children with traumatic brain injury and other acquired and developmental neurological disorders. Dr. Brady received a Ph.D. in Developmental Psychology at the George Washington University, and completed postdoctoral work in neuropsychology at the Kennedy Krieger Institute. Her primary area of research activity and interest is pediatric traumatic brain injury rehabilitation. Beyond formal training, Dr. Brady has learned about TBI firsthand through family experience.

JOAN CARNEY is a special educator who taught eight years in the Prince George's County public school system in Maryland before taking a position in brain injury rehabilitation at the Kennedy Krieger Institute in Baltimore, MD. In her fifteen years with the Kennedy Krieger Institute, the focus of Joan's various positions has always been to assist families and schools in providing appropriate services to students with specialized health needs, including TBI. Ms. Carney is the director of several outpatient programs in the Kennedy Krieger Institute's rehabilitation continuum of care.

JAMES R. CHRISTENSEN obtained his medical degree from the University of Nebraska in 1975. He completed his Pediatric residency and Developmental Pediatrics fellowship at Johns Hopkins, and his Physical Medicine and Rehabilitation residency in the Johns Hopkins/ Sinai program. He is Director of Rehabilitation at the Kennedy Krieger Institute (KKI) and an Assistant Professor at the Johns Hopkins University School of Medicine. He is responsible for the rehabilitation care provided to children at KKI and Johns Hopkins Hospital, including the KKI Pediatric Brain Injury Program for children with Traumatic Brain Injuries and other acquired brain injuries. His areas of interest and research include brain injury outcome and models of care.

JEAN SHULTZ CHRISTIANSON graduated from Pennsylvania State University and the University of Maryland School of Social Work. Her social work practice of twenty-seven years has focused on developmental disabilities and pediatric neurorehabilitation. She provides clinical social work services, graduate social work training, staff supervision, and interdisciplinary education at Kennedy Krieger Institute in Baltimore, MD.

NATHANIEL FICK is a Civil Trial Specialist certified by the National Board of Trial Advocacy. He is a frequent lecturer to health care providers, case managers, and rehabilitation professionals regarding the medicolegal issues of catastrophic injury. He is currently President of Brain Injury Association of Maryland, a member of the American College of Legal Medicine, the International Brain Injury Association, Brain Injury Association (USA), National Spinal Cord Injury Association, and the American Trauma Society. He practices in Towson, MD. His web site is the Neurotrauma Law Nexus: www.neurolaw.com [800-757-7699, nfick@neurolaw.com].

PATRICIA PORTER has taught special education classes for fourteen years in a public school system in Baltimore, MD. She is currently an educational specialist at the Kennedy Krieger Institute, where she has worked for nine years on the inpatient rehabilitation unit with children with traumatic brain injuries. Her current position involves evaluation, school placement, and advocacy for children with TBI.

LISA SCHOENBRODT is an associate professor and chair of the Department of Speech Pathology and Audiology at Loyola College in Maryland. She teaches courses in communication disorders with children and adolescents, technical writing courses, and those which involve service-learning in the community. She has practiced as a speech-language pathologist in the public school system, private practice, and rehabilitation centers for over fifteen years. Her research interests include communication disorders in children with TBI, narrative language intervention in children with TBI, children with language learning disabilities, and children who use English as a second language. She has written several articles and a resource book related to the above topics.

CINDY L. TUCKER is an Instructor in the Department of Psychiatry and Behavioral Science at the Johns Hopkins University School of Medicine and a psychologist in the Department of Behavioral Psychology at The Kennedy Krieger Institute in Baltimore. From 1992 to 1997, Dr. Tucker provided services, assessment, training, and consultation for the Pediatric Comprehensive Neurorehabilitation Unit at Kennedy Krieger, working extensively with TBI survivors and their families. Presently, she is Project Coordinator on a NICHD Grant studying Behavioral Medicine Approaches to Pediatric Acute Pain. She holds a Ph.D. in Counseling Psychology from The State University of New York at Buffalo, as well as an M.S. in Nursing from the same university.

INDEX